"This book could not have come at a better time. *Succeeding in Your Psychotherapy Practicum and Internship* is a must read for graduate students in mental health and related fields, supervisors, and practicum/internship instructors. Packed with practical tips, useful exercises, and real-world examples, it will be the go-to text for graduate students navigating their transition into the mental-health field. I can't wait to use this book in my future practicum and internship courses!"

Jon Sperry, PhD, *Lynn University, co-editor of the* Journal of Individual Psychology

"Better than having a friend a few years ahead of you in the program! This book answers all the questions—and then some—about the nuts and bolts of what to expect in your practicum and internship training experience. A truly useful guidebook for students in any mental-health professions who are required to have external clinical training."

Christopher Burnett, PsyD, Associate Professor of human relationship systems, Nova Southeastern University

Succeeding in Your Psychotherapy Practicum and Internship

Succeeding in Your Psychotherapy Practicum and Internship is a book about what students can often expect from their psychotherapy internship and how they can make the most of their experience.

The book is written from two perspectives—one, that of a seasoned therapist, professor, and supervisor of therapy, and two, the perspective of a registered intern therapist who just went through the internship process. *Succeeding in Your Psychotherapy Practicum and Internship* covers the basics of psychotherapy internships, from the beginning stages of finding and starting at an internship site, to navigating the common experiences at an internship, to reflecting on therapeutic growth and the ending of an internship, and much more. Students will come away from this book with a deep understanding of each perspective, one that will enhance their appreciation of the practicalities and possibilities of their practicum and internship experiences.

Michael D. Reiter, PhD, LMFT, is an AAMFT-approved supervisor with more than 30 years of experience as a therapist and more than 20 years as a full-time faculty member. He currently teaches and supervises at Capella University.

Kayleigh Sabo is an LMFT in the State of Florida. She has a master's degree in family therapy and is a doctoral candidate in couple and family therapy at Nova Southeastern University.

Succeeding in Your Psychotherapy Practicum and Internship

Tips, Tools, and Tales From Supervisors and Interns

Michael D. Reiter and Kayleigh Sabo

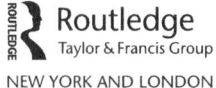

Routledge
Taylor & Francis Group

NEW YORK AND LONDON

Designed cover image: Benjavisa © Getty Images

First published 2025
by Routledge
605 Third Avenue, New York, NY 10158

and by Routledge
4 Park Square, Milton Park, Abingdon, Oxon, OX14 4RN

Routledge is an imprint of the Taylor & Francis Group, an informa business

ISBN: 978-1-032-55992-6 (hbk)
ISBN: 978-1-032-55990-2 (pbk)
ISBN: 978-1-003-43348-4 (ebk)

DOI: 10.4324/9781003433484

Typeset in Optima
by Apex CoVantage, LLC

Michael dedicates this book to all of the supervisees he has worked with who have helped him learn how to be a supervisor.

Kayleigh dedicates this book to her parents, Jennifer and Nathan, who have supported her endeavors throughout her entire life.

Contents

Preface

We (Michael and Kayleigh) met in August of 2015. Kayleigh was entering Nova South-eastern University as a freshman undergraduate student, and Michael was an established faculty member there. They were introduced through a mutual acquaintance (a high school friend of Kayleigh's who was already at the university in the Honors program and had taken Michael as an instructor). Originally, Kayleigh was intending to pursue a career in environmental science and planned her program around this major. She took one Honors course per year with Michael, a couple of which focused on families and relationships and one which focused on the therapeutic relationship. During her junior year, she requested a meeting with Michael and revealed she wanted to switch her career path and become a therapist. During her senior year, Kayleigh shadowed in the university's therapy clinic, where Michael was the supervisor for a team of doctoral students who engaged in live supervision (one of the therapists would be in the room working with the client while the supervisor and rest of the team watched behind the mirror and provided immediate feedback).

Through these experiences, Kayleigh decided, upon graduation, to enter into the master's family therapy program. Here, she did practicum experiences both in the clinic and outside at a community agency. She and Michael had a supervisory relationship in both contexts. After graduating, Kayleigh entered the PhD program in couple and family therapy and worked with Michael for more internal practica in the university clinic. We then wrote several articles and book chapters together as well as presented on our work at international conferences.

Michael has written many textbooks (see Reiter, 2014, 2018, 2019a, 2019b, 2022, 2023a, 2023b). These were mainly to introduce therapy students to the skills and theories of conducting therapy. He had supervised hundreds of students in a variety of therapy programs (family therapy, mental health counseling, and psychology) and contexts (e.g., university clinic, private practice, substance abuse clinics, inpatient hospital programs) and wanted to write a book helping students to succeed in their placements. However, he realized that there was a bit of a disconnect between the day-to-day experience of being a practicum/internship student today and his own experience in his practicum and internship experiences from 30 years ago. He wanted the book to portray the reality of the practicum/internship experience rather than just one point of view (from a supervisor). So the impetus for this book was born. Given that Michael and Kayleigh had worked together for so long, kismet was in place. We decided to try to provide practicum and internship students (you!) with some of the tips that we believe are useful. We also wanted to expose you to some of the common dilemmas and situations that you might find yourself in during your field placement. Thus, we recruited a variety of interns and supervisors from a variety of fields (clinical social work, mental health counseling, clinical and counseling psychology, and family therapy) to provide tales from their experiences that will hopefully resonate for you and provide you fodder when thinking about your own field placement.

We want to thank Desiree Barrionuevo, Lauren Jordan, and Bailey Rich for suggestions of what might be useful to include in the book. To all of the student interns who provided a tale or two, we express our utmost appreciation. These individuals included Grazia Acosta, Goldie Barajas, Sonia Burgos, Chris Cantergiani, Aubrey Glover, Lauren Jordan, Amanda Mohammad, Victoria Nichols, Alexandra Pestano, Shauna Putzy, Bailey Rich, and Erin Zubia. And to the supervisors who contributed a tale or two, we give our heartfelt thanks to continuing to give to the next generation of therapists. These supervisors were Limor Ast, Kristi Mueller, Janice Nuss, Lori Pantaleao, Jessica Popham, Kelsey Railsback, Carlos Ramos, Natalie Rothman, Annalynn Schooley, Yukari Tomozawa, Chris Valls, Dale Wayman, and Ben Wilson. We also want to thank Heather Evans and Julia Giordano at Routledge for their editorial role in the development and completion of this work.

While we are both marriage and family therapists, this book is intended for anyone going into the psychotherapy field. We hope we've made the book general enough that just about everything presented within will be pertinent for you on your clinical journey. This is an amazing field. You will be helping people who are desperate to get on a positive path. For both of us, we believe that the most important tool in therapy to help this happen is you. This book is your opportunity to really explore yourself and learn who you are as a therapist. The more you do that, the more you will succeed in your practicum/internship.

References

Reiter, M. D. (2014). *Case conceptualization in family therapy*. Pearson.

Reiter, M. D. (2018). *Family therapy: An introduction to process, practice, and theory*. Routledge.

Reiter, M. D. (2019a). *Substance abuse and the family* (2nd ed.). Routledge.

Reiter, M. D. (2019b). *Systems theories for psychotherapists*. Routledge.

Reiter, M. D. (2022). *Therapeutic interviewing: Essential skills and contexts of counseling* (2nd ed.). Routledge.

Reiter, M. D. (2023a). *A therapist's guide to writing in psychotherapy*. Routledge.

Reiter, M. D. (2023b). *Family therapy: The basics*. Routledge.

About the Authors

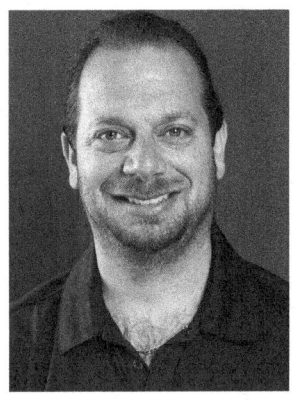

Michael D. Reiter, PhD, LMFT, has been a practicing family therapist for the past 30 years. He earned his MS and EdS in counselor education from the University of Florida with specializations in marriage and family therapy and mental health counseling. He then earned his PhD in family therapy from Nova Southeastern University. Michael is a licensed marriage and family therapist in the state of Florida, an approved supervisor through the American Association of Marriage and Family Therapy, and a state of Florida approved supervisor for both marriage and family therapy and mental health counseling. For 25 years he has been a full-time faculty member, first at Nova Southeastern University and currently at Capella University, where he has supervised hundreds of undergraduate, master's, and doctoral students working in a wide range of mental health settings. Michael has written 12 books, over 20 articles, and was the editor for three books, all on various aspects of psychotherapy.

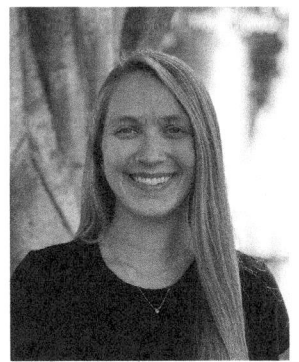

Kayleigh Sabo is a Licensed Marriage and Family Therapist in the state of Florida and is also a certified yoga instructor (RYT-200). She has her MS in family therapy and is currently a PhD candidate in couple and family therapy. Kayleigh has worked in various therapy settings, including private practice, school-based programs, a nonprofit facility, and a university clinic. She is writing her dissertation on therapists' incorporation of yoga into therapy.

Chapter 1

The Importance of Practicums and Internships

This is it! You are about to start the part of your graduate program that will make it all worthwhile. When you first thought about applying to your psychotherapy program, this was most likely what you were thinking about: going into a therapy room, sitting across from a client, and somehow being helpful to them. Depending on your program, you've taken several or many classes to give you enough information to think about what you will do with your client and why. Now, it is time for the *doing* part.

This is what your practicum/internship is all about: applying what you have learned and starting to develop your stance and style as a therapist. And that is what this book is all about: walking with you as you navigate the wide variety of situations, complications, and possibilities that occur during your field placement. In this book, we will talk about all the ins and outs of what we—and other student therapists and supervisors—find most important to know before going into and during your practicum/internship. The first step in this process is to talk about the various fields of psychotherapy, how and why they utilize practicums and internships, and what all the fuss is about.

Myth About the Field

"I will learn everything I need to know about therapy in my school courses."

This is probably one of the mythiest myths that there can be about this field because it implies that practicums/internships are not going to teach you anything new. You will certainly learn a lot during your academic courses in your psychotherapy program, and they will give you the foundation to start providing therapy. However, actually giving therapy and being in a real therapy clinic is a completely different ball game. You will come across situations with your clients, situations with your site, and situations within yourself (all of which we will detail throughout the book) that classroom learning simply cannot fully prepare you for. That is why the practicum/internship experience is so important: You will not only be able to apply what you have learned in the classroom but also learn how to adapt to new circumstances that only a practice-based experience can provide.

The Fields of Psychotherapy

We have intentionally written this book in a general manner so that it will be useful for you regardless of which specific field of psychotherapy you are in (we will use the terms

DOI: 10.4324/9781003433484-1

"therapy" or "psychotherapy" to refer to working clinically with people, but the word "counseling" could also be used). Michael received his master's degrees in counselor education with specializations in mental health counseling and family therapy. He then received a doctorate in family therapy. Over his 25 years as a faculty member, he has taught in the following programs: marriage and family therapy, mental health counseling, school counseling, and clinical psychology. Kayleigh earned her master's degree in family therapy and is completing her doctoral degree in couple and family therapy. We want to take just a minute to talk about each field and what makes them unique (see Figure 1.1). However, our view is that, at their core, there are more similarities than differences between the fields. We are all in the helping professions.

Clinical and counseling psychology degrees lead to someone being able to call themselves a psychologist (the other fields cannot; however, that is how most people will think of you). They usually work with people dealing with mental, emotional, and behavioral disorders. Clinical psychologists, more than professionals from other fields, are able to engage in psychological testing, such as neuropsych, personality, and IQ testing. The mean annual wage for clinical and counseling psychologists in the United States for 2022 was $102,740. This is probably the highest salary for any of the therapy professions (besides psychiatrists).

Couple and family therapy attempts to understand people's behaviors within their relevant contexts, primarily their interpersonal relationships. You can practice and get licensed with a master's degree. While, for most states in the United States, the license is LMFT (Licensed Marriage and Family Therapist), many programs are moving toward changing their program titles to Couple and Family Therapy instead of Marriage and Family Therapy to be more

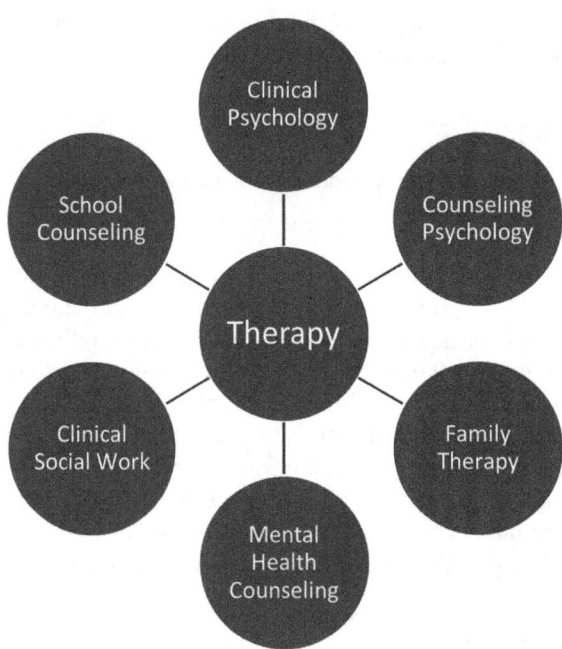

Figure 1.1 There are a variety of fields wherein you will be able to provide therapy services for clients.

inclusive in the language. Many people go on for a doctoral degree either to teach or take on greater administrative roles. All fields have at least one course in their curriculum focusing on couple and family therapy. Those who specialize in this area can work with multiple people at the same time, but they can also work with individuals and groups. In 2022, the mean annual wage for a marriage and family therapist was $63,000.

Mental health counseling trains people to be able to work with a range of issues including mental disorders, addictions, anxiety, depression, and more. To be licensed, you need a master's degree along with the pertinent clinical hours. In 2021, the median pay for a mental health counselor was $48,520.

School counseling is a field that trains individuals to work with students to enhance their academic and social skills. They help students develop skills to improve their academic, career, and social and emotional development. A master's degree is needed for licensure. In 2021, the median salary for a school counselor was $60,510.

Clinical social work is a subbranch of social work designed to understand the individual within the various contexts in which they are located. The social worker appreciates how the person's environment impacts their current situation. Clinical social workers need to attain a master's degree, obtain supervised clinical experience, and become licensed in their state. In 2021, the median pay for a social worker was $50,390.

Depending on your state and/or country, there might be another field in which you can earn a certificate or degree and provide psychotherapy services. Whichever field you are going into, you will need to learn how to be with clients and how you can navigate the process of becoming a therapist. Our hope is that this book will be a trusted companion for you on that journey.

What Is a Practicum/Internship?

Whichever of these fields that you are going into, you need to be trained clinically. That is, there needs to be oversight to ensure that you are properly utilizing the skills and theories you are learning in the classroom while you work with actual clients. To do so, most every psychotherapy program will have at least one practicum and/or internship that you will need to take. This course is designed to provide you with the training you need to become competent in the field.

You might have noticed that we have used both the words "practicum" and "internship" in these first few paragraphs. This is intentional because some programs have practicums, some have internships, and some have both. And what each university defines as a practicum and internship may differ as well.

For example, in the master's and doctoral programs in which we were a supervisor (MR) and student (KS) together, we had both practicums and internships. That university has an on-site clinic that provides psychotherapy services to the community—this was our practicum. The student therapists provide therapy at this clinic, which has a therapy room on one side and a consultation/observation room on the other connected by a one-way mirror. With the mirror, the supervisor and other students in the practicum are able to watch sessions unfold and provide live supervision and feedback. The students in these programs also had to participate in two semesters of "internship" outside of the university (i.e., in the field). These internships were at sites such as hospitals, agencies, private practices, and schools in the community.

Having a practicum or internship at your university is not the case for everyone as many programs do not have an on-site clinic. A practicum may be on-site or off-site; the same holds for internships. According to the *Merriam-Webster* dictionary, a **practicum** is "a course of study designed especially for the preparation of teachers and clinicians that involves the supervised practical application of previously studied theory" (Merriam-Webster, n.d.). During your practicum, you will be supervised as you attempt to take your book learning and put it in practice while working with actual clients (and not having to solely rely on role-plays). While similarly defined, the *Cambridge* dictionary states that an **internship** is "a period of time spent receiving or completing training at a job as a part of becoming qualified to do it" (Cambridge, n.d., Intermediate English Definition). Usually, people do a practicum before they do an internship, as internships tend to be viewed as more advanced. Depending on the program, you may do a practicum or an internship or both.

Because of the differences in the usages/examples of these two experiential learning settings, we will generally address both practicum/internship at the same time and/or use them interchangeably (unless we are intentionally making a distinction). Again, overall, both practicums and internships "are supervised discipline- and career-related work experiences that involve active learning (i.e., learn by doing), critical reflection, and professional development" (Simons et al., 2012, p. 325).

The practicums and internships we described previously are just examples from one university. The setup of a practicum/internship is likely to differ between each psychotherapy program. Therefore, it is impossible for us to say exactly what your practicum/internship will look like. For instance, some may have you engage in therapy sessions on your own (with a supervisor present on site), or they may require you to shadow other therapists in their sessions. Each state and accrediting institution have differing laws and guidelines stipulating what student therapists are allowed to do at a practicum/internship, so that will probably lead to some differences as well. Your specific program or specific site will give you the breakdown for the structure of your practicum/internship.

We also want to address that different therapy programs—for example, mental health counseling, clinical psychology, marriage and family therapy, clinical social work—obviously have some differences in their academic content and ways of approaching therapy. It is important to make clear that this book is not a manual on how to apply different therapy theories or talk about how to be a therapist at your practicum/internship. Rather, this book is a general guide to succeeding in your psychotherapy practicum/internship no matter the specific therapy field you are in.

Why Do We Have Practicums/Internships?

The academic/classroom learning is usually the first chunk of a psychotherapy graduate program. This is the "textbook" learning in which you are in the classroom being taught the theories, diagnoses, ethical/legal considerations, and more. This is clearly a very important element of your schooling because it provides the basis of your know-how for when you eventually enter a therapy room. The next step—entering the therapy room to implement this knowledge—is where internships/practicums come into your therapeutic journey.

The practicum/internship phase of your graduate program provides a space for the practical application of what you have learned so far. It also starts to get you in the groove of seeing clients for the first time and, slowly but surely, developing your sense of self as a therapist. Basically, you can't be a therapist without being a therapist! You have to give the knowledge that you have accumulated a test run and put it into practice.

The psychotherapy practicum/internship experience is a special one in which you aren't just thrown to the wolves and expected to go through this process alone. Part of what makes your practicum/internship so helpful in developing your skills as a therapist is the supervision that you receive along the way. As mentioned, some practicums/internships may have **live supervision** (i.e., another therapist/supervisor is in the room with you or watching the session from behind a one-way mirror). This creates an amazing opportunity for useful feedback from a supervisor who has seen you in action. Other practicums/internships may require you to have weekly supervision sessions with your supervisor during which you either present audio or video from a session or verbally detail what happened. This is also extremely beneficial, as you engage in your ability to describe a case and then conceptualize it. This supervision element of the practicum/internship is integral to your therapeutic development.

We can also talk about the networking advantages that often result from a practicum/internship (depending on the type of practicum/internship your program requires). Practicums/internships not only provide the experience of putting your skills into practice, but they also introduce you to what the field is like in "real life." Basically, you experience the field of psychotherapy outside of a classroom setting. Because you are now in a "real life" setting (again, depending on what your program's practicum/internship consists of), you are likely to be at an actual workplace—for example, an agency, a private practice, a nonprofit—that has graduated/licensed therapists being paid for their therapeutic services. If you do well at your internship and your internship site is hiring once you graduate (and you liked your experience at your site, of course), you may be an easy hire for them right after you get your degree. Even if this is not the case, you may meet professionals in the field at this site who have connections elsewhere.

Tips From an Intern

This is (most likely) the beginning of your journey through your psychotherapy practicum/internship. As we talk about the importance of the practicum/internship experience as a whole, I think it might be helpful to reflect on some general advice that I discovered (and wish I realized earlier) while I was engaging in my own practicums and internships. While we will give various tips and tales throughout the entirety of this book, this particular advice seems most appropriate to consider at the start of your practicum/internship: Be humble *and* intuitive.

The classroom information, the supervision discussions, and the relevant books (including this one, hopefully!) will impart the necessary knowledge and wisdom for you to successfully navigate your practicum/internship. It is absolutely imperative that you remain humble and open to all feedback and teachings throughout this process—the information and words of wisdom from your teachers/supervisors are there for a reason. You are a beginner, and learning from experienced clinicians is a privilege. At the same time, it is also necessary to listen to your own intuition. No therapist is exactly the same; you will likely have different ideas compared to some professors/supervisors on how therapy would be most effective for your clients. This is okay, as you will start developing your own philosophy of change and therapeutic style. Blindly following another's way of doing things prevents your own ideas/style from emerging, and thinking you know best and ignoring what mentors say is equally ineffective. The balance of both listening to/consulting with others and listening to your gut will, I think, be a huge component that allows you to make the most of your psychotherapy practicum/internship.

Who Does Practicums/Internships?

You guessed it: students! Yes, student therapists (whether they are in a bachelor's, master's, or doctoral program) are the ones who engage in a practicum/internship. Some undergraduate programs, such as social work, will have their students complete a practicum experience. For master's students, this is usually their first time dipping their toes in the therapeutic world, which means it is also usually the first time they will be working with clients.

Sometimes, there are students who already have a graduate degree in one therapy field (e.g., mental health counseling) and are working toward a second degree in another therapy field (e.g., marriage and family therapy); they may also be obtaining a higher degree (such as a doctoral degree). When this is the case, these students have already typically worked with clients before. They most likely have done so through whatever practicum/internship was a part of their original program, and they may have seen clients at a job after graduation as well. Perhaps we are referring to you right now.

Just because you have your graduate degree in a psychotherapy field, have likely engaged in a practicum/internship before, and/or have had a job working with clients, that doesn't mean this book can't be helpful. Some time is likely to have passed in between obtaining your first degree and beginning this new one, so it is expected that the field of therapy has changed in some ways. Additionally, different therapy fields have different ways of conceptualizing how to work with clients—engaging in a practicum/internship for a new therapy program is certainly going to be different than it was the first time. They will be applying different knowledge in different ways, so a refresher of the ins and outs of practicums/internships is probably going to be helpful.

You Are Not Alone

Not only are you excited about your field placement, but your supervisor is as well. They are going to have a unique experience by working with you as you navigate your journey. They will have wisdom to share with you, provide tips on how you can better succeed, and support and challenge you while you grow as a clinician. Your supervisor will have a very different perspective of your field placement than you. They likely have had many years of training, therapy, and supervision experience. However, they are not you. They know more about therapy than you, but they don't know more about you than you. This is why we have chosen to write this book: To bring together these different perspectives. Supervisors and interns tend to see what happens during field placement through different lenses. One tends to be more global. The other is more specific. And both of these lenses are useful. They bring a binocular vision to you (de Shazer, 1982). The combination of your viewpoint and your supervisor's viewpoint brings a new understanding to both of you.

At your university, you are probably registered for a practicum or internship course. This includes a faculty member at your university as well as fellow students who are also beginning to work with clients. This provides you with an opportunity to learn from many people. Likely, most of the students in your cohort are doing their field placement somewhere different than you. Hearing their experiences at their sites and with their clientele enables you to vicariously learn about a wider range of clinical practice than what you will get at just your site.

At your placement, you may be in contact with your site supervisor, the clientele, other interns, support staff (e.g., administration), and staff therapists. Larger sites such as agencies, schools, and medical settings are likely to have a more expansive network of employees with whom you may interact (as compared to a smaller private practice, for example). If your practicum/internship site happens to be one of these larger-staffed facilities, then you really won't feel alone. There will be an abundance of support through these individuals in addition to your school supervisor and colleagues.

Quick Tip: Reach out to someone in your program that is a year ahead of you. They are either in their practicum/internship or have completed it. See if you can talk with them about their experience. Ask them what they would have liked to have known before they started the process. They may even have some networking opportunities to connect you to sites. If not, they will have stories from their colleagues about which sites their classmates liked and which they did not.

Succeeding in Your Practicum/Internship

What does it mean to succeed in your practicum/internship? It means that you learn—learn about your clients, learn about therapy, and learn about who you are as a therapist. Therapy is a field in which the expectation is that you are continually enhancing your skills, theoretical understanding, and competencies. This requires you to be present in all of your therapeutic encounters in and outside the therapy room. You might do extra readings beyond what you are assigned in class, watch therapy videos on your own, or attend various therapeutic trainings.

However, not everyone is this engaged in their own learning. People come into the therapy field for a variety of reasons. Most do so for good reasons, a few not so much. They may not have the right mindset, aptitude, or attitude. One of the greatest comedians of all time, George Carlin, had a joke that went something like this:

Somewhere in the world, based upon how you measure it, is the world's worst doctor. And someone has an appointment with them tomorrow.

The same must be true in the therapy field. Our belief is that utilizing this book is one of the many ways that you can not only assure that that person won't be you but that you will become one of the better therapists out there.

This brings us to an important message: It is vital to put intention into your beginning experiences as a therapist. This intention can manifest in many ways, including utilizing supervision/asking for feedback, taking notes, or even reading this book. You will get what you put into this experience, so this is necessary to keep in mind if you want to succeed in your practicum/internship. If you approach this experience with lackluster energy or with a purposeless attitude, then you will likely not gain much from it or grow as much as you could as a therapist.

Exercise 1.1 Success in Your Practicum/Internship

You, your school, your supervisor, and your future clients all want you to succeed in your practicum/internship. But what does success here mean? Answer the following questions to explore your perceptions and expectations for yourself and your field experience.

1. What are you hoping to get out of this clinical experience?
2. Six months from when you finish your placement, how would you know that it was successful? What would you get from it?
3. What will be three signs for you that, within the first month, you are on track to succeed?
4. How have you prepared for your practicum/internship?
5. What are the various resources available for you to succeed in your field placement?
6. Whom can you ask questions of in your program?
7. Whom can you ask questions of at your university?
8. Whom can you ask questions of at your (potential) site?
9. How fluent are you in navigating your university's library so that you can access articles and books that relate to your placement?

Tips From a Supervisor

My tip comes from being a faculty member for 25 years and having supervised hundreds of student therapists in many different programs who worked in hundreds of different agencies. And the tip is this: Use this book! I have seen a lot of students just go to their sites to collect their hours and to learn something about doing therapy. This isn't a book about doing therapy. You've had a lot of classes, read a lot of books and articles, and watched a lot of videos for that purpose. You probably just want to do the therapy and not have to do any accompanied reading.

This book is designed to help frame your experience so that you can function better at your site and have a greater takeaway from it. We've written it so that it is not so "textbooky." Hopefully you find it interesting. Let it become your companion on your internship journey. If you're reading this chapter, then you already have the book. Don't let it collect dust (or at least not until your field placement is over)! As a reader of books, I know it is sometimes easy to skip over some of the sections, such as the exercises or the What Would You Do? scenarios. Don't. When you feel that urge, slow down and appreciate that they were developed to help expand your understanding of your practicum/internship experience. See how much you can get out of this book. If something doesn't seem to apply to you, pause and adapt it.

Before We Embark

Before we embark on this practicum/internship journey, we want to make a few notes about the structure of this guide. Throughout this book, you will see that we use the first-person perspective through the use of "we." That is because we are referring to the two of us (both Michael and Kayleigh). Michael has been a professor of family therapy and a supervisor of therapy students for many years. Kayleigh has completed her master's degree in family therapy, is currently a doctoral candidate, and has gone through the practicum/internship process quite recently. What we wanted to do with this book, unlike many other related books, is to include the ideas and tips from both an experienced therapist, teacher, and supervisor *and* a newly licensed therapist (who is still also a student at the time we are writing this book) who just went through this entire process.

So we say "we" throughout the book because we work as a team and are providing a collaborative, comprehensive guide based on both of our experiences and knowledge. At the same time, we also want to highlight the fact that we are two individuals at different stages in our therapeutic careers. That is why we have included a Tips From a Supervisor and a Tips From an Intern section in each chapter. These sections will provide an extra bit of guidance from us separately that reflect our journeys as a seasoned therapist who teaches student interns and a newly licensed therapist who was recently a student intern herself. In these sections, we will use "I" instead; the former section will be in Michael's perspective, and the latter section will be in Kayleigh's.

Additionally, each chapter has two Tales From the Field sections. We understand that we are not the only two people in this field with helpful tips, information, and stories to share about succeeding in your psychotherapy practicum/internship. To make this book as comprehensive as possible, we also added two of these sections in each chapter to provide further stories that relate to each chapter topic. Each Tales From the Field is written by a different therapist. These individuals are from varying therapy backgrounds to provide perspectives from each particular concentration within the mental health field as well. Additionally, one Tales is written by a student intern talking about their own experience, and the other Tales is written by a supervisor talking about one of their supervisees. This is the case for all chapters except the last one, Chapter 17, as we believe that an intern's story about the next steps after a practicum/internship is sufficient.

We also have at least two exercises per chapter which we believe, once you do them, will help you to better navigate your site. Each chapter also has a What Would You Do? section. Here, we present you with a situation that has happened either to one of us, a colleague, or a supervisee during their practicum/internship. These sections are designed to put you into the field and think about how you might navigate a situation that has a high likelihood of happening to you (to one degree or another). While your own contemplation of this scenario is useful, we encourage you to talk about them with your intern colleagues as well as your site and faculty supervisors. The more prepared you can be before a situation happens, the greater likelihood you will have of navigating that situation successfully. Lastly, we want to wish you well on this important therapeutic journey that you've just begun. We hope this book helps you to successfully navigate your practicum/internship experience.

References

Cambridge. (n.d.). Internship. In *Cambridge.org dictionary*. Retrieved May 12, 2023, from https://dictionary.cambridge.org/us/dictionary/english/internship

de Shazer, S. (1982). *Patterns of brief family therapy: An ecosystemic approach*. Guilford.

Merriam-Webster. (n.d.). Practicum. In *Merriam-Webster.com dictionary*. Retrieved May 12, 2023, from www.merriam-webster.com/dictionary/practicum

Simons, L., Fehr, L., Blank, N., Connell, H., Georganas, D., Fernandez, D., & Peterson, V. (2012). Lessons learned from experiential learning: What do students learn from a practicum/internship? *International Journal of Teaching and Learning in Higher Education, 24*(3), 325–334. www.isetl.org/ijtlhe/pdf/IJTLHE1315.pdf

Chapter 2

Attaining an Internship Site

In our discussion of the different definitions/types of practicums and internships, we noted that some are internal to your program (e.g., a school clinic). These are often fixed in your degree plan/program, so you will likely not need to interview at these places—it is expected that you will be a student intern at these sites. For the semesters in which the practicum/internship is not internal to/affiliated with the program, you will need to find your own site, which is a similar process to a job hunt.

Even if you have had an internship before (perhaps for your undergraduate degree) and have some knowledge of the internship application process, that does not mean that this chapter can't be helpful for you. While some of what we discuss in this chapter applies to internships as a whole, some of it is specific to the psychotherapy field and psychotherapy graduate programs. We encourage you to not skip over this chapter, even if you have applied for multiple jobs and/or internships before.

This chapter details the main considerations that you should make to obtain an internship site. We are using only the word "internship" in this chapter because, in our experience, most psychotherapy graduate programs call these external therapy experiences internships. Remember, this chapter still applies even if your school calls this external experience "practicum" or even "externship."

Myth About the Field

"Every site will want me since I am free labor."

While this would make your life easier, this is sadly not the case. First, there are often many students applying to the same sites around the same time (especially if you find your placement from a master list of approved sites from your program). This means that multiple people may be vying for the same internship. Second, your site will (hopefully) be taking this process seriously and want to find the best fit based both on your resume and personal engagement during the interview. Because the previous quote is a myth, the information in this chapter becomes all the more helpful because it will assist you in bolstering your chances in getting your preferred site.

Researching a Site

The first step in attaining an internship site involves finding sites that pique your interest. Your program will most likely help you with this endeavor, as they often offer some sort of internship fair where you can talk to representatives from some of the sites or provide a list

DOI: 10.4324/9781003433484-2

of internship sites with their information. This list includes the sites that are approved internship sites with your program.

If you come across and are interested in a facility that is not on the list, some programs allow sites to apply to become an approved internship site. If this is the route you take, talk with the facility first and make sure they are all right with becoming an approved site for your program. If so, start this approval process sooner rather than later as it can sometimes take a while (depending on how long your program takes to process the necessary paperwork or how long the site takes to fill out this paperwork). We've seen it take several months for the full approval process in some circumstances.

In addition to reviewing any information that your program provides about the approved sites, it is also a good idea to peruse the sites' websites to learn about them further. This is where you will really get more of a vibe about an internship site. You can see their general website presence, the type of information they choose to include, and the content of the information itself (e.g., staff, mission statements, About Us sections, services offered).

When looking at this information, consider what you are hoping to get from your practicum/internship experience. For example, if you are interested in going into private practice after graduation, looking into private practices is probably a good idea. The same goes for other settings (e.g., schools, medical settings, nonprofits). Researching an internship site involves purposefully reflecting on your hopes and goals for your therapy experience and then seeing what sites will help promote the achievement of those goals.

There will probably be a few sites that stand out to you once you have reviewed their information and compared this information to your hopes for your internship experience. From here, you have to obtain even more detail about these select sites to narrow them down further. A helpful way to do this is to consult with students who have interned at these sites already. They can give you the inside scoop on their experience, including what they liked about working there and what they didn't. We suggest that you even ask your professors about their knowledge of these sites. They can share what they know about the site or even provide recounts of past students' experiences if they know anyone who interned there.

As mentioned, your graduate program may also offer an internship fair of some sort. We highly recommend going to this fair, as it usually consists of representatives from the internships sites themselves coming to give their spiel about their site to potential interns (i.e., you!). This is a great way to meet someone who works at that site to ask further questions and to get your name out there. These representatives will then have already seen your face and experienced your interest in their site.

If you find that you are wanting two different therapy experiences (for example, perhaps you want to gain experience both at a hospital and a school), then you usually can have more than one internship site with your program. That means that you should keep multiple options open and interview at each of these places. If you are set on having two sites, then you will need to know the number of hours you can work at each site prior to your interview. We will talk about this in more detail when we discuss the interview process.

Exercise 2.1   Research a Site

While there are times that you do not have a choice of which placement you will go to, other times you do. For this exercise, think about the aspects of the site that are important for you when you consider whether to do a placement with them.

1. What type of clients are you hoping to work with?
2. How far from your home are you willing to travel to get to the site?
3. How able are you to engage in a variety of activities, such as intakes, case consultation, individual sessions, group sessions, and family sessions?
4. What type of supervisor would you like to have? What are their qualities?
5. What are the rules and regulations of the site?

Tips From a Supervisor

I am over 30 years into my therapy career. My first clinical work happened at the University of Florida in the Counselor Education Department, where we saw some cases in our actual classrooms. I then did two different practicum experiences, one being in a hospice setting and the other at an agency for children. My internship in this program was at an outpatient substance and sexual abuse program for adolescents.

These experiences gave me experience but did not define my future clinical pathway. In the years since, I have become a supervisor of hundreds of master's students who were going into their first placements. I saw the anxiety of the students in trying to figure out what was the "right" placement for them. I'm not quite sure there is a "right" placement. Each placement is an opportunity to learn. Now, I have had supervisees who had a bad experience at their sites. Even then, that was a learning opportunity for them to think about who they are as a therapist, the context they want to work in, and how they want to be treated.

My tip for you is to not take so long to struggle over a site, especially if you are thinking about what population you are wanting to work with. You are not getting married! You might think of this as "talking to" a client population or a site context (e.g., outpatient agency, inpatient facility, private practice). Now, if you know that there is a certain population you want to work with and there is a placement that will get you that experience, then sure, go for it. You will gain experience in that area as well as the ability to network with professionals in that specialty. This could set you up for a potential job once you graduate. However, for most of you, while you would like to work with a specific population in your placement, you have your whole career to do so. For now, see how many boxes a particular site checks off: location, times, supervisor, clientele, and variety of therapy experiences you will get. While your hope is that all boxes are checked, that is sometimes a rarity. Thus, my other tip is to not view this practicum/internship experience as one that will define your whole career.

Developing a Resume

At this point in your life, you may have some experience with creating a resume. If not, that is okay, too. That is what this section is all about—going over the basics of developing a resume whether it be as a refresher or a first-time learning experience.

First things first: What is a resume? This may seem like a silly question to pose to graduate students, but it can actually help to reorient yourself to the definition and parameters of a resume before writing one. **Resumes** are essentially documents that show your qualifications and experiences relevant to a particular position that you are attempting to attain. They are succinct ways to market yourself to potential employers—a representation of what you have to offer to the position to which you are applying.

Whether this is your first time writing a resume or your tenth, we recommend that you go to your school's writing and/or career office for help. These individuals are trained in the presentation/grammatical elements of the resume to make sure it looks and sounds professional, and they also know how to structure and present your content in the most effective way. In addition to these school resources, it would probably be helpful to have a trusted professor or two review your resume as well. While the writing/career centers know the basics of any resume, your professor may be able to help you specifically word certain things to best reflect your particular field.

Though we encourage you to go to the writing and/or career centers, we will still provide some general tips and tricks when it comes to developing a resume. First, keep it short, sweet, and to the point. Resumes are usually around one or two pages at the maximum; don't go over this range. Practicum/internship sites want to be able to see that you can give them the highlights of your accomplishments and experience.

Second, structure your resume so that it is easy to read. There isn't one universal resume template, so each person's resume is going to look a little different. However, you always want your resume to be noticeable yet clean. This might include boldening, capitalizing, and/or underlining certain sections (e.g., INTERNSHIPS) and then boldening certain titles within those sections (e.g., **Therapy Office Receptionist**). You can also look at examples online of resumes that you find are understandable and clear. Have someone else look at your resume to see if they can easily see the relevant information. Most resumes have bullet points under each major section instead of paragraphs because bullet points are easier to read.

Third, utilize action verbs that represent what you did/do at any past or present jobs, internships, or other relevant work. Make sure the tense is representative of whether you *did* the action or whether you are still currently *doing* the action. For example, if you are talking about an internship that you completed and are no longer interning at, use the past tense. If you are still currently working at that internship, use the present tense. Additionally, incorporate language that the site itself uses (which can be found on their website, any flyers they hand out at an internship fair, etc.). This creates a connection between what you have done/do and what the internship site does. This means that you may need to submit a slightly different version of your resume to each site.

Depending on what you are applying for, the major information that you include in your resume will change. Since you are applying for therapy-based internships, you will clearly want to include any and all therapy-related experience and education. This will include your current schooling (notating in some way that your degree is in progress) and any past schooling/degrees you received (at the college level, no need to include high school). Put your highest level of education first—you want to lead with your best foot forward. Even if you have never had any direct therapy-related jobs or internships in the past, you can still include jobs or internships at which you did tasks that relate to therapy skills. For example, Kayleigh was a resident assistant in the residence halls during her undergraduate program; this job included leading roommate conflict resolution meetings, helping students who were homesick, and providing resources for students at the university. These can all be connected to therapy skills (e.g., conflict resolution, rapport building, resource providing), so she put this job on her resume when applying for internship sites.

Cover Letter

In the twenty-first century, there has been a move away from the traditional ways of job searching (we are including practicums/internships here). It used to be that you would mail (snail mail) a cover letter with your resume. That doesn't really happen anymore. Most everything occurs electronically, usually through email. Some internships will directly tell you that you only need to submit a resume and do not need a cover letter. However, if they don't specify, a cover letter may be helpful if you have had no contact with the site yet (such as at an internship fair) and want them to hear your interest in the site instead of just seeing your credentials on your resume.

A **cover letter** briefly introduces you to the other person, highlighting your key strengths along with your goals/purpose for applying to that organization. In essence, the cover letter provides a written overview of who you are, your past training, and your future hopes.

For most places, you don't want your cover letter to be too long. It will probably be one page at the longest. If you are submitting to a clearinghouse through a matching program, your cover letter will probably be a bit longer than this. Let's talk about what you might put in your cover letter.

You should start the cover letter with your contact information including your name, degree, address, phone number, and email address. Please make sure that your email address is appropriate: littlefunkygirl27@hotmail.com or beerguzzlingguy@yahoo.com are not appropriate. Consider using your university email as this placement will be related to your school. Next, you will have a salutation. If you know the specific person who makes decisions about field placement, put them here. If not, you can use "To Whom It May Concern" or some other such address.

Next, you will write your opening paragraph. Try to get the person interested in you. Introduce yourself and explain the purpose of the inquiry—that you are seeking a practicum/internship (and perhaps for how long) with their organization. Your next paragraph should explain your qualifications and skills that will help you succeed in the placement. Either in this paragraph or the following, discuss your therapeutic interests and how they align with the organization's mission. Then you might have a closing paragraph where you summarize the position you are seeking, your qualifications, and how you think the field placement will be mutually beneficial. Provide a closing signature, such as "Sincerely" or "Yours Truly," followed by your name.

Before you send out your cover letter, put it through spell-check and grammar-check. You don't want to scare off the site by having them think you are not a good student or not conscientious. Any errors in your cover letter might do so. Have other people look it over and provide feedback. If you can, work with one or more people at your university, such as a faculty member, the internship coordinator, or the career center.

Interviewing for Success

If a site that you applied to likes the looks of your resume, the next step is usually the **interview**. This is basically an in-person (or virtual) version of your resume, as the interviewer asks a variety of questions related to the information on your resume and then expands this information to the specifics of the site as well. Whether you have interviewed for something before or not, we want to go over some helpful tips in preparing for any interviews you may have while applying to your internship sites.

One of the logistics of interviewing that you can get out of the way early on is your interview outfit. Even if it may seem obvious, we want to emphasize that you need to present professionally at an interview. Now, based on our experiences, some sites are going to be more casual than others in terms of clothing once you actually start working there. It may be more appropriate for a therapeutic relationship with a teenager, for example, to dress a bit more casually than to be in full suit and tie. However, you want to err on the side of dressing more professionally for the interview, as this is likely your first visual impression with the site.

Business casual and/or business professional are usually the way to go for an interview. Business casual allows for a bit more flexibility in terms of fashion and excludes formal items of dress such as ties. Button-down shirts and blouses are usually good for the top half, and regular pants (aside from jeans) or length-appropriate skirts are good for the bottom half. Loafers, dress shoes, heels, or flats can work. It's a bit more versatile in terms of color as well—you can add a pop of color in your blouse, for example, if you'd like. Business professional is a bit more classic in the color scheme (usually black and white). This dress code is stricter with suits and ties, pencil skirts, blazers, and the like. Run your potential outfit by a professor or colleague whom you trust to get their opinion.

Site coordinators/supervisors are looking for someone that they think is capable, personable, professional, and engaged. While you will not know exactly what they want to hear, you can prepare yourself for some common interview questions. Having been in plenty of interviews, both as the interviewer and interviewee, we will provide a few of them here for you in Exercise 2.2. We encourage you to slow down at this point, take time to think through your answers, write them down or video record them, and then have someone who has interviewing experience go over them and provide you with feedback.

Exercise 2.2   Interview Preparation

For the following potential interview questions, develop at least one answer. Try to provide depth without going too long and without being too brief.

1. What draws you to wanting to do your practicum/internship at our site?
2. What would you say are your three most useful attributes?
3. What are your main strengths and your main weaknesses?
4. Tell us about a time when you were involved in a conflict and how you handled it.
5. How would you describe your theoretical orientation?

In addition to preparing to answer the interviewer's questions, you should also prepare some questions to ask during the interview as well. This brings up an important point: You are also the interviewer. Read that again. *You are also the interviewer.* While you are a student looking for an internship, the internship site is also looking for an intern. You need to make sure that the internship site is a good fit for you as much as the internship site will make sure you are a good fit for them. It also shows initiative and genuine interest in the site to come prepared with your own questions.

The specifics of your questions will probably vary somewhat between each site. There are some general questions, however, that we can go over here. First, ask questions about the logistics of the site to make sure they fit with what you need your practicum/internship experience to be. For instance, you should probably ask about the number of hours that the site is able to offer. If they can't offer the hours you need, you need to either find a different site that can offer this number of hours or get two sites. On the flipside, you should also find out what hours they are expecting you to be able to work. As we talked about, if you are set on having two different sites for the different experiences, then you will obviously have to split your time at each site. This time split has to match up with each site's expectations of how many hours you will be contributing to them.

Unless they go over this during the interview (as sites will commonly use the interview to provide information about the site itself), you should also ask what your specific tasks/roles would be at the site. Will you be doing intakes, running groups, giving individual therapy? This is important information for you to know before committing to a site, so these are questions you should ask if the site does not preemptively provide this information.

It may also be beneficial to ask for more detail about the specific services that the site provides as a whole. This will show the interviewer that you want to be aware of the inner workings of the site, and it will also help you understand the site better as well. Even more specifically, do they primarily promote/utilize one type of therapy model or training program or operate from a specific faith? We know students who interviewed at a site and found out during the interview that the entire site operated from a Christian faith-based approach. Again, this information will help you determine if the site is a right fit for you.

Another big component of internships that has come up more recently has been the in-person versus online internship experience. During COVID-19, many internships provided student interns the option to work at the site via telehealth. Although the COVID-19 situation—at the time we are writing this book—has died down and most interns are primarily in person, some sites might still offer online options. If this is something that you are looking for, then this is obviously an important question to ask during your interview.

With all the information that you'll gather at the interview, we recommend that you bring something to write with and something to write on. It will help keep the information you receive organized as well as demonstrate to the interviewer that you are taking this process seriously. If you know you will be engaging in multiple interviews, just be sure to keep each site's information separate from one another—it's not quite helpful if you look back in your notes and don't know which information belongs to which site!

An interview can often be an anxiety-provoking situation for people, so we believe that mentally preparing for an interview is going to be helpful as well. If you find that the anxiety before an interview really gets to you, come up with some strategies beforehand to help keep you calm and collected during the interview. These strategies will likely differ for each person, but common ones such as taking deep breaths/doing breathwork and meditating are often helpful because they can physiologically calm the body down.

It may also help to do a practice interview with a friend, family member, or colleague. As therapy students, you are likely used to doing role-plays in class anyway, and this is really no different. Have someone else prepare some typical interview questions, and wear your interview outfit if you can to simulate the ambience of the actual interview. Through this practice run, you can get a feeling for a good talking speed and get an idea of how you might answer some common interview questions.

It may also put your mind at ease if you are able to find some colleagues who have interviewed at that particular site beforehand. We encourage students to inquire within the cohort ahead of them and see if any of those students interned at the site at which the current students are interviewing. While some things may have changed at the site since the other students interviewed, it can still be helpful to get some feedback on the experiences of the other students.

Quick Tip: Check with your school's career development office. They tend to have services and resources to help you with internship and job searching. They may even be able to do a mock interview with you and provide you with tips and pointers to help you prepare better for the interview.

Following Up

When you are done with your interview, the interviewer will usually say something like, "It was great to meet you. I am going to talk with my team, and you should hear from me in about a week or so." Depending on the site, the amount of time that they say they'll get back to you may change. Your first step is to send them a follow-up email later that day (or the next day if the interview is in the evening) thanking them for the opportunity and letting them know that you look forward to hearing from them. This shows your professionalism and appreciation of their time.

Your second step is to give each interview site the allotted time to respond (based on when they said they would reach out again). If they say they will get back to you in a week, wait a week. If they say they will get back to you in a few days, give them a few days. Now, there is no hard-and-fast rule that tells you exactly how long to wait to follow up with a potential site. Usually, in the professional world, you give someone 48 hours to respond before following up. If you have not received any communication from them by the end of their stated time, then wait another two days to reach out again. This shows courtesy to their timeline but also initiative and interest on your part. Some sites are often swamped with interviews along with normal day-to-day responsibilities. Sometimes, they may forget exactly when they said they would respond. Even if they are going to hire you, they may forget to email you because they have it in their heads that they will offer you the position. Hopefully, this will be rarer than not. However, if it happens, then it is appropriate to follow up after that two-day mark.

An email is typically the best way to contact them again, as you want to reach back out to the specific person who conducted your interview in writing. You should have been given this person's email prior to interviewing with them, as your program usually provides the list of approved sites with the contact information of the appropriate site employee. If the person who conducted your interview was not the person who is on your program's approved site list as the point of contact (i.e., the original person you would have reached out to expressing your interest), then email the point of contact. This is the specific person who handles the internship coordination at that site even if they didn't conduct your interview.

The next question you may ask yourself is, "What exactly do I put in this email so that I am showing I'm still interested without being pushy?" You basically just want to be kind, professional, and appreciative. Remind the person who you are by stating your name and the date that you interviewed with them. Let them know that you are still interested in being an intern at their site and are happy to provide any additional information if needed. Thank them again for their time and the opportunity, and state that you look forward to hearing from them.

We will address the best-case scenario first: The site(s) that you want to work at offered you an internship position! The following step is to obviously reply to this offer affirming that you'd love to accept. This one is easy—just reply to their email (they will most likely inform you of this news via email) and state your excitement, acceptance, and once again, your thanks. From there, they will probably just email you about whatever the next steps will be. For example, they may send you paperwork they need you to sign on their end or schedule a training day before the actual internship starts. In the next section, we will talk about more logistics of starting the internship after being accepted at a site.

Now, we of course hope that you get accepted to every internship that you apply to so that you can make the best choice based on your goals. We do, however, still need to go over what to do if you do not get accepted to a site. You probably guessed it, but you should reply to this email with the same professionalism and poise as you would the other emails. Thank them for getting back to you and for the opportunity. If you feel comfortable, you might ask why they didn't accept you so that you can learn for your own growth. The hope would be that they might give you feedback such as, "You didn't have X type of training" or "We are looking for someone who has Y availability." This could let you know whether you might revise your resume or change your expectations for a placement.

What Would You Do?: 2.1

You have applied to two potential internship sites. There is one that is your ideal placement based on the clientele it serves, the hours they can provide, and the supervision they supply. The other one you really do not want to do, but they are your safety outlet. The site you want tells you that you are on the waiting list, as there were a couple of other intern candidates that they have offered the placement to first. However, they will not be able to give you a definitive answer until just before the semester starts. The other placement says that they would like you to intern with them. What would you do?

Depending on how many sites you applied to, you may get an offer from sites that you are going to wind up saying no to. It is equally important to reply to these offers as well because ghosting them is not very professional. If a site offers you a position and you decide not to take it (perhaps you were offered a position at your first choice, and this was choice number two), then reply to their email thanking them for the offer and for their time and politely explain that you have accepted an offer at another site. If you did like this site but another site just worked better for you, you can even add that you will refer other colleagues to them in the future because of the wonderful experience you had with them. This once again shows your appreciation and also keeps you in good standing with this site (you never know if you might work there in the future!). Basically, simply saying, "Thank you, but I found a better site," is probably not the best move.

Tales From the Field: Intern

For me, finding an external practicum site was similar in some degree to seeking and applying for a job. Beginning in the winter term for first-year master's students, there was a virtual internship/job fair. In a span of a couple hours, site representatives presented their programs. My school's MFT department had an extensive list of participating externship sites that was provided to the students through email. This took the guesswork out of finding a site that was approved by the program. We were told that once we had an idea of the clientele we wanted to work with, we should reach out to the site's contact person through phone or email. From there, we were to receive a response from that site's contact asking for a resume and initiating the interview process.

Still early in my program, I had not been totally convinced of the niche of clients I wanted to work with. The context to my uncertainty in finding a site centered around where I was at that point with my knowledge as a student therapist and what I felt comfortable with. What potential and qualities could I provide for a site? What niche of therapy did I want to get into? What could a site provide me in experiential learning for my growth as a student therapist? Less than two months before the start of the fall semester, in which I was to start external practicum, I optimistically started reaching out to organizations around my area that specialized in couples therapy. I was open to working with many groups, but I wanted to work specifically with couples and felt drawn to understanding and helping couple dynamics. I thought to myself, "This is going to be easy to find a site." I sent several emails to several sites and awaited replies. Some never replied, and some replied once. Awaiting replies often took a week, as points of contact would be "out of the office" or on vacation. Once the organizations that were my first choices came to a dead end, I had to expand my options. The pit in my stomach started to grow bigger, heavier, and even developed a voice that would wake me out of my sleep in the morning. This was not as seamless as I thought it would be, and time was ticking one month before the fall semester. I applied to more organizations that were in my area and extended my radius, expanding from couples therapy to working with families and children. From there, I got an interview and fortunately received an offer by an organization in my area that worked with families, especially with younger children.

I had underestimated the difficulty and time it would take to find a site. Having been accepted by a site one month before the start of the semester and still awaiting background checks to clear and formal administrative tasks to be fulfilled was cutting it close. I was also surprised by the experience I had when finding a site for external practicum. When reaching out to some of the listed externship sites, not all were receptive to me as an intern looking for a placement. I had a preconceived expectation that I was going to be welcomed with open arms to the first place I applied to just because it was on the school list. This was not the case.

Fortunately, I was persistent. I had to keep applying to sites until I received acceptance. I had to find an externship site, be open to the possibility of learning in a different environment that wasn't what I envisioned, and embrace my discomfort that I would be working with a different demographic. I primarily hoped to work with couples, yet I had to adjust and expand my scope of the therapy experience I wanted. I have been telling myself that growth and self-awareness stems from discomfort and new experiences. I know now going into the site that I will have some discomfort but also a lot of new experiences that I will learn a lot from.

Sonia Burgos, MS in Couple and Family Therapy program, Nova Southeastern University

Matching

The acquisition of many field placements occurs by you reaching out to the placement, expressing your interest, interviewing with them, and having them offer you an internship opportunity. However, there are other internship experiences that happen through a **matching** process, in which you submit an application into a large (perhaps national) database and are matched. You can find the programs that have internships through your school. You would consider their location, populations they work with, specialization areas, and theoretical orientation. You would then submit your application to the database. The application will typically include your resume, cover letter, academic transcripts, and letters of recommendation. Placements will then interview their top choices to find out more about you and determine the potential fit. Then, a ranking process happens in which you will rank the sites you would like to go to and the sites will rank the potential interns. A computer program then matches people and programs based on the rankings. The results are announced on "Match Day" which, if this is the process of you obtaining a site, will be one of the most important days in your program. Once matched, you then accept or decline the offer. If you decline the offer, you would reach out to other programs to see if they have any unfilled positions.

What Happens If You Are Accepted at Multiple Sites?

Depending on your program, you may only be able to work at one site. However, other programs allow the possibility of working at multiple sites. If this is the case for you, and two or more sites have offered you a field placement position, then you will need to decide which of them to accept. There are pros and cons to having one or multiple sites. Let's quickly discuss them here.

One of the pros of only interning at one site is that you only have to learn one set of policies and procedures. Each site has their own expectations and ways of working. There are different sets of paperwork, therapy styles, and rules based on the site you are at. It takes time to learn them all. Having only one site allows you to immerse yourself in their way of working, and you don't have to become confused by having to learn a different system. Further, you will gain a deeper experience working with that placement's clients. This is also one of the cons. If that placement is very client specific (e.g., middle school students, substance abuse, people dealing with PTSD), you will get great exposure to that population. However, you will not get exposure to other populations. If you know going in that you want to specialize in that specific population, then great. This one site will be very useful for you. However, if you are unsure of a future specialty or you want to work with a general population, having one site may be a little limiting.

This is where having multiple sites might be useful. You could choose two or more sites that service quite different populations. This will give you greater exposure to the variety of populations and treatment issues that therapists work with. For instance, one site may be working with substance abusing teens while the other site works primarily with couples having marital difficulties. While we might hypothesize that these two populations are related (that the substance abusing teens likely come from families where the parents are in conflict), working with each population is quite different.

A quick word of caution here—some sites will require that you commit to interning there for a certain number of semesters. This is important information to find out beforehand if you were thinking about interning at one site one semester and then at another site the following semester, for example. We knew of a student intern who wanted to do exactly this and then realized that her first site required a two-semester commitment.

Tips From an Intern

Deciding on an internship site is perhaps one of the most important decisions you will make during your psychotherapy graduate program. This is the place (or places, if you have more than one site) where you will synthesize everything you learn in the classroom in a real therapeutic setting. This is also the place where you start to discover the ins and outs of the therapy world outside of academia.

Equally as important, this phase of researching, interviewing at, and deciding on the right internship placement is an amazing opportunity for you to be reflexive and intentional about your self-of-the-therapist development. You might have gone over this already in your academic courses, but this is basically the process of critically and thoughtfully reflecting on and intertwining your personal self (including your own outlook on life, culture, background, and more) with your professional therapeutic self. I also like the way Timm and Blow (1999) defined it:

> Self of the therapist work is the willingness of a therapist or supervisor to participate in a process that requires introspective work on issues in his or her own life, that has an impact the [*sic*] the process of therapy in both positive and negative ways.
>
> (p. 333)

In my eyes, you have to exercise this self-of-the-therapist work in order to effectively find the best practicum/internship for *you*. As we mentioned in this chapter, you have to consider the type of site (e.g., private practice, agency, school), the primary population they work with (e.g., teenagers, couples, hospital patients), the hours they can offer, and more. You then must take this information and determine how it matches up to your own background and biases as well as your hopes for your future therapy career. For me, this makes the self-of-the-therapist work integral in attaining an internship site where you will flourish. My advice is to heavily take this important developmental process into consideration as you weave through the steps we have outlined in this chapter.

What Happens If You Can't Find a Placement?

Depending on your program, the steps to gain a field placement will likely be different. Some programs will set you up in placements, but this is rare. Usually, they have a list of past sites or sites that have already been approved. As mentioned, they may also have an internship fair where representatives from those agencies come to your school (or present virtually) and are there to talk with you about their placement. This is an excellent time for you to bring your resume and your personality and make a good first impression. We know of many students who secured their placement in this manner.

However, there may be times when, for whatever reason, you do not make an agreement with a placement. What do you do when this happens? The first answer is to not give up. It is easy to get disillusioned and upset. That will likely lead you to either not try as hard or not have the positive energy and attitude that site coordinators are looking for in an intern. Rather, use this as an opportunity to upgrade your resume, work on your internship seeking pitch, and become more expansive and creative in how and where you look for a placement.

You have colleagues in your program who have gotten placements. Talk with them to see if their site is accepting any more interns. **Networking** is an amazing way to make connections and perhaps gain entry when you might not have previously. There is also someone in your department who works as the **internship coordinator** (they might have a different title than this, such as field placement coordinator). One of their main roles is to help students gain placements. Set up an in-person meeting with them (or virtual if you are a distance from them) and utilize their services. They probably have tips for you or might have just talked to a placement who is in need of someone.

Our main tip for you if you have not obtained a placement yet, despite trying, is to widen your lens of what you want and expect. Remember that this is not a decision that you have to stick with for the rest of your life. Your internship is quite time-limited. Further, with whatever placement you get, there is probably also the possibility for you to change sites if you are not having a good learning experience or you want to work with a different population.

Tales From the Field: Supervisor

Karen was eager to complete the final requirement of her academic program: a clinical internship. During her clinical psychology graduate program, she continued full-time employment, raised her two young children in a single-parent home, and successfully maintained a GPA of 3.8. She was looking forward to graduation and had already started studying for the licensure exam. She was proud to have maintained full-time academic enrollment while also being the sole financial provider for her family. She was certainly motivated and dedicated to her future career. To ensure she was on track to complete academic requirements and an on-time graduation, Karen scheduled a meeting with me, her academic program's director of clinical training. Karen's time management skills, organizational abilities, and assertiveness were clear strengths. I reviewed the internship requirements with her and suggested several potential site placements. Following the meeting, Karen felt ready to conquer this final phase of her clinical program. She didn't waste any time and soon applied to several clinical placement sites. She was pleased to accept two interviews the following week. After waiting several weeks and hearing no response from the sites, she applied to several additional sites. Just as before, she quickly received offers to interview but, to her dismay, was not offered an intern position. Karen grew more worried about the lack of internship placement with only three months to go before her proposed start date.

Karen requested another meeting with me for assistance, which was promptly arranged. I asked about how the interviews went and what questions the prospective site supervisors asked during the interviews. A common question was about her availability. Karen explained that since she worked full-time during the day, her only availability was between 6:00 and 8:00 p.m. during the week and every other Sunday afternoon. I suspected Karen's limited availability may have been the primary barrier to finding a suitable internship placement.

Karen was disappointed to hear this feedback, although she was not surprised. For the past three years, Karen was burning the candle at both ends, but it was not sustainable any longer. Karen shared that she was so close to the finish line, and she wanted to push through without thinking about the practicality of her plan. I normalized the difficulty related to attaining an internship site, even under the best of circumstances. Additional factors such as employment or other life responsibilities can add to the difficulty. I encouraged Karen to consider what aspects of her plan she valued most and what parts could be adjusted. After deep thought and additional discussion with her family and friends, Karen decided to temporarily reduce her hours at work, request a small student loan to help offset expenses, and seek out an internship placement that offered post-internship opportunities for employment. This decision allowed Karen much more flexibility with her availability, and she soon gained an internship placement. More importantly, Karen felt more rested each day and went to her internship site with the mindset of feeling "present." She realized it was not enough to "check the box" to get the internship done and move on; rather, internship was a time to learn, experience, and prepare for her future career as a counselor.

Kristi L. Mueller, PsyD, LP, Clinical Psychology, Capella University

Next Steps After Internship Acceptance

You did it, you obtained your internship site! Congratulations. The next chapter, "Getting in the Right Mindset," will be about ways to prepare for your time at your internship site. Right now, we'd like to go over some final logistical considerations that you need to have squared away so that you are officially able to work at your site.

Just because the site offered you an intern position and you emailed back accepting the position, that does not mean you are ready to go. You are doing this internship for your graduate program, so you need to get everything registered with them before you can begin working at your site.

First, practicums/internships are usually credit-based courses. This means that you will have to register for practicum or internship like you would any other class. The title of this course can range from Clinical Practicum, External Internship, Internship, etc. You need to make sure you register for this course (for the semester in which you are planning to take it) in order to count anything from your internship.

Second, you will probably need to create/sign some sort of contract between you and your site to submit to your program. While the title of the course will be something general like the ones listed in the previous section, different students will obviously be working at different sites. Psychotherapy programs usually need this contract from each student from their specific site to know that the student is officially approved to be working there. This means that you will be doing all this the semester *before* your internship actually starts. This is something that is important to be on top of because you usually need this paperwork to be submitted and accepted for you to count your hours at your site. Your program should go over all this and provide relevant timelines for everything—we just wanted to bring it up here as well to put it on your radar.

Third, complete whatever your internship site requires of you before starting. We mentioned previously that your site will likely send you their own paperwork or procedures before you begin working there. For example, perhaps they ask for you to provide your exact schedule with the hours that you are available to work there. It is also usually required that you get a background check if you do not have one already (which can be time-consuming depending on how soon you are able to make an appointment). This may be obvious, but you want to do these tasks sooner rather than later. Start off on the right foot and submit anything that they request in a timely manner so you present reliably and you don't have to worry about any logistics getting in the way.

Summary

This chapter covered aspects surrounding how you might attain an internship site. For some programs, it might not take much, as they might assign you a placement (e.g., if there is an on-campus therapy clinic at which you are required to do a practicum). For other programs, there might be a lot more onus on you to curate a site. We encourage you to be very proactive in this process, ensuring that you are professional throughout from your resume and cover letter to your interview(s) and follow up with the site. This process is an opportunity for you to sell yourself, letting them know what you can bring to the table.

Reference

Timm, T. M., & Blow, A. J. (1999). Self-of-the-therapist work: A balance between removing restraints and identifying resources. *Contemporary Family Therapy: An International Journal, 21*(3), 331–351. https://doi.org/10.1023/A:102190315503

Chapter 3

Getting in the Right Mindset

Starting a practicum/internship can naturally be both an exciting yet nerve-racking experience. Luckily, you can prepare for the start of this endeavor beforehand to build your confidence and get in the right mindset. The classes you take before beginning your practicum/internship prepare you for some of this hands-on experience, and your professors probably discussed practicum/internship-specific topics in class as well. In addition to the information you have learned from your program, this chapter addresses the depth and breadth of considerations that are helpful to make so that you feel more prepared and confident going into your site.

Myth About the Field

"I should be ready to do my best right from the get-go."

This may seem like a confusing statement to be a myth. Should your program have critically prepared you for starting to work with clients? Absolutely. But should you know how to do everything perfectly from day one? Absolutely not. Again, that is the point of a practicum/internship—to help you put into practice and refine what you know and then learn a whole lot more of what you don't. This myth is a mindset that is best to let go of before you begin your practicum/internship. It will free you up to accept your mistakes and learn a lot more than you would have if you thought everything was going to be peachy keen from the beginning.

Motivation to Become a Therapist

From when people are young, they may have a dream job. This could be a doctor, lawyer, pilot, or teacher. There are few people who, from childhood or adolescence, want to be therapists. It tends to be a career choice that people make later in their schooling (for undergraduates), or perhaps it is a second career for many others.

Some years ago, you told yourself, "I want to be a therapist." How come? What was the impetus for you to choose this path? This isn't just a throwaway question. Your motivations to become a therapist are highly related to your effectiveness as a therapist. The more you can take a hard and honest look at yourself, the more you can get into an appropriate mindset in which you are more focused on helping the client than getting your own needs met.

DOI: 10.4324/9781003433484-3

All of us in this field are here, for one reason or another, to get our needs met. There is nothing wrong with that. Corey and Corey (2020) suggested several typical needs and motivations for people wanting to become therapists:

- The need to make an impact
- The need to reciprocate
- The need to care for others
- The need for self-help
- The need to be needed
- The need for recognition and status
- The need to provide answers
- The need for control

Exercise 3.1   Your Needs for Becoming a Therapist

Take a second and see where you lie on the scale for each of these needs. Use a scale from 1 to 10 where 1 is low and 10 is high. [Now, we know that there are always biases in self-ratings. We can guess that there are a few of these needs where you will write a very low score because we are not supposed to score high in them. Challenge yourself to be as honest as you can. No one else is listening, and you are not being graded. This is just you.]

Need to	1	2	3	4	5	6	7	8	9	10
Make an impact										
Reciprocate										
Care for others										
Engage in self-help										
Be needed										
Recognition/status										
Provide answers										
Have control										

Which needs do you believe you are low on?
On which did you score high?
What do you think about the scores you put?
How would you like to score on each?

Believing in Yourself

How much do you believe in yourself? The answer to this is usually related to self-esteem and self-efficacy. **Self-esteem** is how much you prize yourself. This is a concept that you should know quite well since most of the clients that you encounter in therapy will have difficulties in their relationship to self-esteem. In essence, we might say they have low self-esteem. **Self-efficacy** is how well you think you can do something. Usually, these two are related. Someone with low self-esteem tends to have low self-efficacy. However, that is not always the case. You can have high self-efficacy in something (say being a grifter) and feel bad about yourself (low self-esteem) because you swindle people.

There will be times when you are sure this is the right field for you and other times when you feel you're not suited to be a therapist. Perhaps it has already happened. During the process of becoming a therapist, you will doubt yourself. This can be really confusing, heavy, and overwhelming. At some point, you are going to need to give yourself grace to appreciate that you are a human being. What this means is that you are continually growing. Carl Rogers, Viktor Frankl, and Rollo May were humanistic therapists who believed that all people are in a perpetual progression toward increased **self-actualization**. This process happens when we continually move forward to recognize and fulfill our potential.

One way to enhance your belief in yourself is to engage in **positive self-talk**. Many times, we might denigrate ourselves and tell ourselves we aren't good enough. This can have a serious impact on our self-esteem. Having a good self-image is an important aspect to maintaining and improving your self-esteem as well as enhancing your personal well-being. Positive self-talk may include telling yourself what you like about yourself, repeating affirmations, and giving yourself encouragement. Here are a few examples of things that you might tell yourself:

Gratitude

- "I appreciate that even though I made a mistake, I owned up to it and tried to learn from it."
- "Wow. I really went for it and committed myself to this process."
- "I am grateful that I reached out to my friend, and they were there for me."

Self-Compassion

- "It is okay that I don't know everything. I am not supposed to."
- "I deserve to be cared for by others and by myself."
- "I am not always perfect, but I am trying."

Encouragement

- "I am learning. Which means I am growing. Which means I will continue to learn and grow."
- "I got knocked down. But then I got up. That shows my strength."
- "I know that I can do this."

Affirmations

- "I am a capable person."
- "I have all of the resources that I need to succeed."
- "I choose to have a good day."

Exercise 3.2   Positive Self-Talk

For this exercise, write three responses that you can tell yourself for each category of positive self-talk.

Gratitude

1.
2.
3.

Self-Compassion

1.
2.
3.

Encouragement

1.
2.
3.

Affirmations

1.
2.
3.

Now, make sure that you tell yourself at least one of these per day. When you use these up, come back to this exercise and develop 12 more examples of self-talk. Continue doing this, and you should see an increase in your self-esteem.

Tips From an Intern

The tip that is resonating with me the most for this chapter ties back to believing in yourself. This chapter is about getting in the right mindset before starting your practicum/internship, and for me, the most helpful mindset I adopted centered around confidence. I am a generally confident person, and I discovered that this mindset and sense of self helped lessen my nerves when starting my practicums and internships, made my work at my sites more consistent and seamless, impressed my supervisors, and allowed me to stand out. Again, this does not mean I believed everything I was going to do would be perfect (tying back to the myth for this chapter). Instead, I was confident that no matter the mistakes I made and no matter what happened, I would be able to navigate any situation that I faced with a good mindset.

Perhaps some of what we mentioned in this chapter might seem like obvious points or even small things that aren't a big deal. From personal experience, I can tell you that these things add up, and it's often the small efforts that make the difference. I'm willing to bet that putting this effort into the considerations we discuss in this chapter will help boost your confidence going into your practicum/internship. Doing these things helped me feel like I had my ducks in a row, and I was able to navigate my sites with more knowledge and poise.

Imposter Syndrome

In 1978, Clance and Imes coined the term "**imposter phenomenon**" that talked about an internal experience of intellectual phoniness; in essence, the person feels like a fraud. While academics may use the phrase "imposter phenomenon," the lay public tends to use **imposter syndrome**, but it still means the same thing: The person tries to do an activity (likely a job) that they don't feel fully competent in. Further, the person thinks that at some point, those they are around and are working with will realize that they are a fraud and will expose them (Pákozdy et al., 2023).

In the field of therapy, periodic experiences of imposter syndrome are common. People are coming to you expecting you to know exactly what they should do to get better. They may think that this is an episode of Dr. Phil in which they will tell you their dilemma and you will provide specific advice that will solve their situation. When you then look at them and don't know what to do, you are likely to think that you're in the wrong field. Just know that this is probably not the case. More likely, you have the wrong template that you are using. Perhaps shift from using Dr. Phil as a guide of what to do and utilize Carl Rogers instead.

Quick Tip: When you begin to doubt yourself, take a breath, recall your motivation for going into the field, and tell yourself that you are worthwhile. Also, normalize doubting yourself (i.e., don't beat yourself up about it). It is normal in this process to be unsure of yourself sometimes while you are still finding your therapeutic groove.

Stress and Fears

When you think about your first day of your practicum/internship, what are you experiencing? Perhaps a bit of excitement but likely nervousness and anxiety as well. If you are like us and almost every other student therapist, you are probably feeling stressed to some degree. Up to 73% of psychology graduate students report feeling high levels of stress in relation to their clinical training (Stafford-Brown & Pakenham, 2012).

How do you tend to handle things when you get stressed? This is important to reflect on because it is just about a guarantee that you will be stressed leading up to and during your field experience. If you notice that you usually shut down and lose yourself a bit when you get stressed, have practices in place that will help mitigate this (e.g., take a day off, do breathwork, talk with a friend, go to your own therapy). Additionally, pay attention to the strengths that you do have when it comes to dealing with stress (as we all have them), as they can be helpful to employ at this phase in your graduate program.

We suggest that you give yourself some grace and don't berate yourself about what you are experiencing. It is very normal to feel fear and stress. We can guarantee that, regardless of their outward presentation, every other person in your program is feeling stress and fear as well. The main question is, how can you use those feelings as motivation to learn?

Tales From the Field: Supervisor

Selena was a master's-level marriage and family therapy student in her first semester of practicum. She was completing her practicum at an outpatient community mental health treatment facility working with adults, adolescents, families, and couples from the local community. Selena did not have a bachelor's degree in psychology or a mental health-related field, so she entered the program and practicum feeling less than capable of seeing clients.

Selena was very nervous when faced with the idea she would be seeing her first client on her own. When Selena talked about this in class, her voice was shaky, and she was visibly nervous. As many of my students often express, she felt like she did not have enough training or experience to help her future clients. She was worried she would make a mistake and felt like an imposter.

During the second week of class, I had Selena and the other practicum students review the basic and necessary things they should do in a first session: For example, introduce yourself, review confidentiality and informed consent, join and build rapport, and explore the presenting problem and preferred goals. Through an open discussion, Selena was able to review what she had learned in her courses and think about how she could apply this information in a clinical setting with her upcoming client. I provided Selena and the other students with some examples of how to phrase these common first-session statements. I encouraged Selena to avoid minimizing her status as a student and instead introduce herself as a graduate-level student completing the last stage of her master's degree. This allowed her to take ownership of the knowledge and experience she learned in this program and build confidence by labeling herself as a competent student clinician. I ended the class by instructing Selena and her peers to develop their own "script" of how they would start a session, practice the script throughout the week, and come to the next class prepared to practice the script in a role-play.

The following week, Selena and each of her peers took turns in a role-play being the therapist and the client. Selena was able to practice her introduction speech, and although her voice started off shaky, she slowly became more comfortable and successfully completed her role-play. Selena was then asked to reflect on her role-play and also received feedback from her peers and myself. By the end of the class, Selena felt more confident. She started to see clients on her own and reported that while she still felt nervous at times, she felt more capable because of the supervision she received.

Jessica Popham, PhD, LMFT, Assistant Professor, Albizu University

Competence

We have talked about how many people experience some type of imposter syndrome. Just remember, while you may occasionally feel like a fraud, this happens when we don't appreciate our abilities. This section talks about your competencies. You are not expected to be an expert yet because you are not a seasoned therapist. You can't rush that, as it takes experience for that to happen. You are a student and are learning what it means to be a therapist. Even so, you do know things.

Just about all ethical codes have one or more codes or statements related to competence. For instance, the American Association for Marriage and Family Therapy (2015, Standard 3.1) Maintenance of Competency states as follows:

> Marriage and family therapists pursue knowledge of new developments and maintain their competence in marriage and family therapy through education, training, and/or supervised experience.

You will be doing all three of these things: receiving the education to be a therapist, receiving training on therapeutic concepts and skills, and receiving supervision while you work with your clients.

While you are not expected to know everything right now at this stage in your career, you are also not supposed to engage in therapeutic practice that you are not competent or trained in. As an example, the American Counseling Association (2014, Section C.2.b.) New Specialty Areas of Practice holds the following:

> Counselors practice in specialty areas new to them only after appropriate education, training, and supervised experience. While developing skills in new specialty areas, counselors take steps to ensure the competence of their work and protect others from possible harm.

As we've said, you are not expected to be fully competent in all areas of psychotherapy right now, or really ever. As a field, we know that there are always new developments. This is why, to maintain licensure, you are required to obtain continuing education credits. Competence isn't something that you will fully meet but rather is a continual process (Corey & Corey, 2020).

Being Humble

Okay. So it is clear that you should be competent. Competency is both skills-based and mentality-based. The skills portion you should achieve through the coursework in your program. You are also going to improve your skills while you are at your site, as that is one of the main purposes of field placements. Mentally, as we just discussed, you should be competent in that you are present and functional when working with clients.

Let's hang out with the skills portion of competence. No matter how good you did in role-plays, how many therapy videos you've watched, or how well you understood the material in the textbooks you read, there is still a lot for you to learn. This holds for every therapist. Both of us are continually learning. Michael has been in the therapy field for over 30 years, and you better believe there is a lifetime of things about therapy he does not know. And that's okay. It's expected.

This is where humility will be useful for you. In some definitions, **humility** is not functioning from a position of pride or arrogance. The more we are prideful or arrogant, the more we think we are right and will need to do things to maintain our position. This can be problematic in that it shifts us out of a place of thinking that we have something to learn. Regardless of where you are at in your program, there is so much about therapy that you don't know yet. Embrace that.

Tales From the Field: Intern

Becoming a therapist has been my primary goal for what feels like a long time. As a master of social work (MSW) student, I've spent years studying to become a professional social worker. Now, I am in my advanced field placement—I am a social worker. I have had to work to shift my mindset towards my work in this new role. Changing my perspective from that of a student to that of a learning professional has been rather challenging at times. My internship—a runaway and homeless youth shelter—has provided me with an excellent professional space to work through this mental shift.

At the beginning of my internship, I stepped into a youth specialist role, which primarily consisted of the facilitation and supervision of the youth during their daily activities. I anticipated eventually shifting into a case management role; however, the shift was rather sudden when I was recently assigned to my first case. I had only shadowed one case management meeting with this client a couple of weeks prior when I was told that I would be taking over the case starting with that day's client meeting. I had about a ten-minute notice, so I had not had much time to prepare mentally for this shift in my role. During the meeting with my client, I found myself feeling nervous, not because I didn't know how to do the job but because I had never practiced in this role before.

This experience taught me that getting in the right mindset not only happens before you start at your placement but happens continuously throughout your placement as well. Sometimes, you will have more time to prepare; in others, you won't. In my case, I had to shift roles rather abruptly at my site and needed to adapt my mindset to provide effective services. I also find that I had to change my viewpoint to fully see myself in this professional role as a social worker in general. The preparation from my educational program and from the agency's training protocols helped me adapt. Educational programs are vital, and so is the opportunity to practice professional skills. I knew what I needed to do to have a successful meeting with my client. I was, and am, confident in my ability to be a social worker. My field placement has and will continue to offer multiple opportunities for me to practice these skills. As I continue to take on professional roles and practice professional skills, I will continue to grow in my mindset, and it will become easier over time to see myself in the role of a social work professional.

Rayna Larson, Master of Social Work student, Walden University

Online Presence

Therapists in this day and age have to thoughtfully maneuver one realm that therapists just 30 years ago didn't even think twice about—**social media**. Having an **online presence** via social media and other related avenues is something extremely common for many people, as these platforms can be a place where you are free to express yourself and connect with others. However, employers are increasingly combing through these sites to see how potential employees present themselves. The same can be the case for you as a student intern: Just because you aren't officially working as a paid employee at your practicum/internship site does not mean that your supervisor will not look you up online or scrutinize your online presence.

Because supervisors at a practicum/internship site may look you up on social media and give your profiles a once-over, it is important for you to sift through your online presence before you even apply/begin working at any site. We are not asking that you scour every last post and photo and delete anything that would be a potential concern—we understand it is important to have a balance between becoming a professional and being yourself/having the right to free speech. However, we do want to go over common red flags that turn supervisors off and that can create issues with clients along with some easy changes that can be made to make your profiles more professional.

First, we want to make it clear that every site/supervisor is different. Some people consider certain things inappropriate, and others don't. That is the way life is with almost everything, so what we say here is not a universal experience for everyone. What we have seen, though, to be two frequent areas of concern are inappropriate photos and political posts. Inappropriate photos are those that might be considered unprofessional by some individuals—for example, photos of you in a bathing suit or drinking alcohol. Some supervisors also advise against posting political content, as it can reveal your bias/opinion that a client could come across if they find your profile.

Second, now that we addressed what you might encounter as a no-no for some supervisors, we want to reiterate that you don't necessarily have to delete all such content from your profiles. What we have found is that most supervisors are okay with you (a) putting all your profiles on a private setting so that only added/following friends can see any content and (b) making sure you have appropriate profile photos on all accounts (as clients can still see those even if they are not your profile friend). Usually, this is the happy medium between being professional and still having your personal online presence.

We want to give a qualifier here, however, and suggest that you openly consult with your site supervisor. Express to them that you understand a professional online presence is important and you want to be aware of their guidelines for social media and related online platforms. This will show you are taking the initiative in being a professional and are able to have your own peace of mind regarding your social media before beginning your practicum/internship.

While you want to be intentional about your online presence to be professional for your site/supervisor, this concern should also extend to your clients. In their study on the prevalence of clients searching for their therapists on the web, Eichenberg and Sawyer (2016) found that about half of their participants tried to find information on their therapist, with about 80% of participants looking their therapists up online specifically. It is therefore not a rare occurrence for a client to come across your online profiles. This makes it even more necessary for you to make the aforementioned considerations regarding your social media/related platforms for the sake of your clients.

Getting to Know the Site

As we mentioned in Chapter 1, some practicum/internship sites may be internal to your university's psychotherapy program (e.g., a school clinic) while other sites are separate workplaces (e.g., a private practice or agency). In Chapter 2, we talked about how researching a site is an important process in attaining a practicum/internship placement. If you followed that advice and have also interviewed at the site, then it is safe to assume you have some knowledge about your practicum/internship at this point.

Learning even more about your site might be a helpful tactic for several reasons. For example, it may calm your nerves to know your stuff. Have you ever had to drive to a new place and were nervous about how exactly you were going to get there, where you were going to park, if you should take the stairs or the elevator (we could probably keep going here)? If you are like any average person, you probably have had this experience. This feeling can be present when you walk into a site without knowing as much as you could prior.

It can also happen if, like in the previous example, you have actually never been to your site before. If your interview was online (such as through Zoom, which is becoming more and more common), we recommend that you physically go to your site once before your first official day there. That way, taking a wrong turn, for example, won't throw off your mojo on the first day.

One aspect of the site that would be beneficial to know about before starting your practicum/internship is the staff. Sites internal to your university are often made up of faculty and students in the program itself. For example, in some graduate programs, the front office staff at internal clinics are students working as graduate assistants. Employees at internal sites might be people who you already know; it is still important, though, to try to know who the employees are for your own knowledge and in case clients have questions/make references to them.

Sites external to your program often have websites with a page listing their team. This team may include both therapists and administrative workers. This could be helpful to peruse to know the staff members and their roles. One time at Kayleigh's internship site, a client mentioned another staff member whom she hadn't met yet and asked a question about them. Kayleigh had no idea what that person did at the facility, let alone who they even were! Needless to say, she brushed up on her site's staff members via their website very quickly after that. (As a note, if you intern at a larger site such as an agency or even a hospital, you might not be able to know every single person who works there. Focus instead on the staff members with whom you will work most frequently/closely.)

The previous example brings up another benefit of getting to know your site—you can more easily engage with clients when they have questions. Your site has policies and procedures. When you know these, you are able to treat clients confidently, consistently, and comfortably. You will know who to go to if you don't know something, who to connect clients to, and when people will be around to make these types of connections. Further, the more confident you are in explaining the site to your client, the more they will believe in you and your competence.

Many practicum/internship sites give you some sort of manual outlining these policies and procedures. For example, in Kayleigh's school-based practicum, student therapists were given a manual that included information such as how to call clients and what to say when leaving a voicemail. While it might be tempting to just glance over it, we recommend that you take the time to fully read through the manual to become familiar with how your site operates. For some sites that don't have a formal manual, you will likely have a few days where you will train at the site either prior to the start of your practicum/internship or during the first few days/weeks there. Chances are you aren't going to remember everything that you learn in these trainings, so we recommend you keep your own document of notes (sort of like your own manual). You are then able to review your notes prior to fully working at your site; you can even continually go back to these notes throughout your time at your site when necessary.

Some things you will just need to learn once you begin training and as you work at your site. These are just some extra steps you can take prior to beginning your practicum/internship that will help familiarize yourself with your site as much as possible.

What Would You Do?: 3.1

It is your first day at your practicum/internship, and the site is starting you off with a bang! You have two clients already scheduled to meet with you. During the first session, the client is asking you a lot of questions about fees, resources, and scheduling. You hadn't previously done an orientation at the site; your only information came from the one interview you did with the site coordinator. The client is looking at you with a sense of expectation, as you have not answered any of their questions yet. What do you do? In the session? After the session? Before the next session?

Site Hours

The overarching reason behind the practicum/internship experience in the first place is to begin to learn the ins and outs of the therapy field and practice your skills as a student therapist. Because you are doing this through your program to obtain a degree, however, there are some logistics that go into your time at your site as well.

Psychotherapy programs require a certain number of hours for students to log at their practicum/internship sites. These hour requirements are based on how many hours the relevant accrediting institutions believe is necessary for students to obtain the appropriate amount of field experience in order to graduate. One of your responsibilities while engaging at your site will be keeping track of your hours.

There are different types of hours that you will count toward your degree requirements. These hours can differ depending on your specific therapy degree and your specific program. An example of one type of therapy hour breakdown is direct, alternative, and supervision. **Direct hours** are hours during which you directly worked with clients; they were in front of you—either in the same room or videoconferencing platform. **Alternative hours** are hours during which you did therapy- and case-related tasks (e.g., watching therapy videos, writing up reports, or attending trainings). For these hours, you did not work *with* your clients but did activities *for* your work with them. **Supervision hours** (you guessed it) are the hours during which you talked with your supervisor or engaged in supervision in some way. Each program may also have some differences in what each type of hour is called/what constitutes each type of hour.

We have seen students not be aware of the breakdown of these different hours, so it becomes a doozy to figure out how to calculate/categorize them appropriately. Our recommendation is that you make sure you are aware of what type of activity counts toward each hour and how many of each of these hours you need for your program. Having this understanding of the hours breakdown before beginning your practicum/internship is best, as it is one less thing you will have to worry about once you start at your site.

In addition to understanding the different types of hours, it will also be incredibly helpful to map out the hours you will need each week before you even begin working at your site. As mentioned, your program will require a certain number of hours for graduation. It is your job to make sure you obtain these hours if you want to graduate on time. This means that you will need to do a bit of math.

Basically, during the semester prior to the start of your practicum/internship, you will need to (a) determine the number of weeks in the semester during which you will be at your site and (b) divide the number of hours you need in total by the number of weeks in the semester. This will give you the number of hours per week that you will need to get on average to obtain the required hours for your program. We think it is a good idea to add an hour or two (or several more) onto this average to account for any missed days (e.g., because of sickness, vacation, or client cancellations or no-shows). We mentioned this in Chapter 2 as well: You have to make sure you attain a practicum/internship site(s) that can offer the number of hours you need. This means that these calculations will be more helpful if they are done prior to attaining a site.

Physically logging these hours is something that we have seen students fail to do time and again. Many students don't consistently keep track of their hours at their site, so when the time comes to submit their hours to their program, they have no idea how many hours they really worked and then scramble at the end of the semester to get everything in order. We would advise that you not take this approach. Instead, we have found that keeping track of your hours on a weekly basis (listing hours by date) and knowing your total amount of hours at all times is the best way to make sure you stay on top of everything. Kayleigh used both her own Excel spreadsheet and the forms that her program required. The Excel spreadsheet helped her easily add all her hours together to see how many she had in comparison to how many she still needed; the program's forms allowed her to have everything preemptively filled out so that they could be submitted quickly. Michael encourages his supervisees to input the hours each week into the university's online tracking program, if the program has one.

Curating a Wardrobe

We want to take a moment to talk with you about your appearance and the clothes that you will wear at your site. This may sound strange to get fashion advice in a psychotherapy book, but appearance does matter. Depending on your program, you might have been able to wear whatever you wanted to class. If you were in an online program, you could take this notion to an extreme: Wearing your pajamas to class, as no one was able to see you.

At your site, however, you will be contacting real people, both staff and clients. What you wear has an impact on the impression that people have about you, their reaction to you, as well as your own sense of self. Business attire is becoming more casual, and you will need to think about your specific site and what will be most appropriate.

You will likely not need to dress business formal. This might be a suit and tie or a pencil skirt/pants and blazer. It will be very unlikely you will dress this formally. However, you will likely not want to go to the opposite extreme and dress casually (such as T-shirt, shorts, flip-flops, or ripped jeans). Our recommendation to you is to think business casual. Unless you are working at a site with predominantly children or that is outside (such as an equine-assisted therapy placement), you shouldn't wear sneakers.

You also don't want to wear outfits that are too flashy. The more that the client is focused on aspects of you (such as your hair style, jewelry, or clothing), the less they are focused on aspects of themselves, which is why they are in therapy in the first place. Michael had a supervisee who, during the pandemic, would wear a face mask that had designs or sayings on it that were pertinent to them, such as "I love to rock-and-roll" or "My dog is my best friend." Wearing this in the therapy room would encourage the client to focus on the therapist rather than the reason they came to therapy. Michael asked the intern to switch to a neutral mask so that the focus of the session was on the client rather than the therapist.

At your site, you will most likely run into some therapists that dress very professionally and others that dress quite casually. It can be confusing to see so many different outfits in the same setting for the same job. At Kayleigh's nonprofit site, some therapists had small heels, black pants, and a nice blouse with a blazer, while other therapists wore staff T-shirts, jeans, and sneakers (both of which were considered appropriate for this particular site). While each site is going to look a little different, the best advice we can give is to attend to the expectations of your site while also maintaining a balance between business professional and casual, everyday clothing.

Overall, it is also important that you stay true to your own style while still presenting as a professional yet approachable therapist. For example, Kayleigh is a pretty casual person. You won't catch her wearing business formal clothing unless absolutely necessary. Many of her colleagues at her internship sites would go the extra mile and wear blazers/jackets with their outfits, but that just wasn't her (and it also wasn't required for them at those sites). Instead, she wore business casual pants or dark jeans, a nice blouse, and nice flats or low heels. This is much more her style, so she was able to look the part and present appropriately yet still feel comfortable in her clothes. Michael tends to be a bit more old-school, wearing dress pants, long-sleeved button-down shirt, and likely a tie.

Utilizing Your Colleagues

One of the things that you will learn throughout your practicum placement is that you are not alone. You'll probably have other interns at the site, perhaps from other universities or different programs. Interns find that talking with other therapists-in-training produces some of the most positive emotions throughout the whole of their placement experience (Edwards & Patterson, 2012). However, depending on the structure of your program (e.g., online, residential) you will have varying levels of connection with your fellow student colleagues. We encourage you to reach out to them. Perhaps develop a chat group with some so that you can all connect and talk with one another. The questions, fears, concerns, tips, and plans that they have you probably do as well. If you don't speak up, there will be a lot of good information and suggestions that you will never encounter. They are there for you just like you are there for them.

Transitioning Between Sites

Perhaps this is not your first practicum/internship experience. If it isn't, there is still value in this book, especially in talking about how to transition from one site to another. Even if you are at your first site and don't think you need information on transitioning between sites, we recommend you read on anyway because you may switch sites during your program at some point. For example, some programs require multiple semesters of practicums/internships, so you may want experience at one type of site one semester and then want another experience elsewhere the following semester.

If you are transitioning to a new site, we recommend you read this chapter over again. It will be important for you to consider the Getting to Know Your Site section in particular. Sites can be very different, so it will be worthwhile to acquaint yourself with the new site rather than assume everything will be the same as your previous site. With this may come changes in your required wardrobe and the amount of site hours, for example. These are all things to be considered before you simply switch to a new practicum/internship.

Your First Couple of Days

Like us, you will probably experience two related but distinct emotions right before your first day of your practicum/internship. On the one hand, you will be extremely excited! This is what you have been waiting for since the first time you thought to yourself, "You know what, I think I may want to be a therapist." On the other hand, you will be extremely nervous. Both of these emotions, and many others, will lead to stress, anxiety, and anticipation.

Most sites will not throw you in the deep end the first day you show up. Like in a lot of organizations, there will likely be an onboarding process, especially if that agency has worked with many interns in the past. You may have paperwork to do, orientation videos to watch, or shadowing. If you have never engaged in **shadowing**, it is a useful process because you will get to sit in on activities occurring in the placement without having any of the pressure of needing to do anything but watch. This allows you to learn the rules, regulations, and processes of the site to ease into it.

This is also something important to remember: Your placement is a process, where you get in and get oriented, engage in the primary learning, and then exit the site. Your first couple of days at the site will probably entail much paperwork, observation, and anticipation. While it can be overwhelming, we recommend that you take in what you can, write down whatever you can to remember it in the future, and then take a breath. The groove of everything will come as you spend more time at your site.

Tips From a Supervisor

Having supervised practicum/internship students for over 20 years, I've seen a lot of people get into their own heads before they even begin at their site. This may be because they don't believe in themselves enough and get overly anxious or they think that they are going to have the perfect experience and there won't be any issues. I had one student who, when I told her that she was going to have her first client that day, quickly developed a migraine, said that she was going to vomit, left for the day, and did not return for the next week because she was still feeling too anxious. The following week she came back to the practicum, saw her first client, and did well. This is an extreme.

My main tip is to try to be more in the middle ground. Know that (a) you know something about therapy (that you've learned from the classes that you've taken so far), (b) you don't know a lot about therapy (which is fine because you are a student therapist), and (c) this is a process that is supposed to occur where you will learn (a lot) along the way. You shouldn't be expecting yourself to have it all down the first day you go to your site. The people at your site will probably have a lot of trainings for you to do, or if not, they will try to do some type of orientation. Even if they don't, trust enough in yourself that you can be adaptable.

You are entering into a new system. Take time to learn that system. They might do things you haven't learned about. This is an opportunity for you to learn. My tip is related to that mindset—that you are doing this to learn. Look around for the various opportunities that you can learn—about therapy, about paperwork, about agency processes, and most importantly about yourself. You might even start now before you see your first client. What have you learned about yourself in the lead-up to starting your practicum?

Summary

This chapter highlighted the notion that you are the most integral component of your practicum/internship experience. This entails you getting into the right mindset. You will likely have doubts about your capabilities, especially since you are at the beginning of your therapeutic career. This is perfectly normal. However, hopefully you are focusing on more than this in that you are acknowledging and appreciating the knowledge and competence that you do have. Take time before you start your field placement and figure out the various ways you can get yourself into the best mindset possible so that you can succeed at your placement.

References

American Association for Marriage and Family Therapy. (2015). *Code of ethics*. www.aamft.org/Legal_Ethics/Code_of_Ethics.aspx

American Counseling Association. (2014). *2014 ACA code of ethics*. www.counseling.org/resources/aca-code-of-ethics.pdf

Clance, P., & Imes, S. (1978). The imposter phenomenon in high achieving women: Dynamics and therapeutic intervention. *Psychotherapy: Theory, Research and Practice, 15*(3), 241–247. www.paulineroseclance.com/pdf/ip_high_achieving_women.pdf

Corey, M. S., & Corey, G. (2020). *Becoming a helper* (8th ed.). Cengage.

Edwards, T. M., & Patterson, J. E. (2012). The daily events and emotions of master's-level family therapy trainees in off-campus practicum settings. *Journal of Marital and Family Therapy, 38*(4), 688–696. https://doi.org/10.1111/j.1752-0606.2012.00263.x

Eichenberg, C., & Sawyer, A. (2016). Do patients look up their therapists online? An exploratory study among patients in psychotherapy. *JMIR Mental Health, 3*(2), e22. https://doi.org/10.2196/mental.5169

Pákozdy, C., Askew, J., Dyer, J., Gately, P., Martin, L., Mavor, K. I., & Brown, G. R. (2023). The imposter phenomenon and its relationship with self-efficacy, perfectionism and happiness in university students. *Current Psychology*. https://link.springer.com/article/10.1007/s12144-023-04672-4

Stafford-Brown, J., & Pakenham, K. I. (2012). The effectiveness of an ACT informed intervention for managing stress and improving therapist qualities in clinical psychology trainees. *Journal of Clinical Psychology, 68*(6), 592–613. https://doi.org/10.1002/jclp.21844

Chapter 4

Navigating Paperwork

Like us, you probably decided to become a psychotherapist to work with clients and help them to live more satisfying lives. You took classes that covered the skills and theories of therapy, you watched hours and hours of therapy videos by some of the masters of the field, and you participated in lots of role-play exercises. This was all done so that you could be successful in the therapy room with clients.

What you likely didn't spend as much time learning about was that, along with the actual therapy that you do, there is a lot of paperwork that comes with it. That statement probably didn't tickle your toes or get you excited. Don't worry, you're not alone. Paperwork is one of the least positively rated events that interns have at their sites (Edwards & Patterson, 2012). It is also one of the least enjoyable aspects of a supervisor's experience. So why do we have to do it?

Paperwork is the documentation of the course of therapy. It is how we as therapists ensure that what we are doing is on point, effective, and ethical. It is an important part of the therapeutic process for your client, you, and the therapeutic community.

Myths About the Field

"Writing notes is less important than actually giving therapy."

This is incredibly untrue because our notes are a reflection and narrative of our therapeutic work with our clients. They are the history of the therapy that we give and the therapy that our clients receive. While it is true that you cannot write the note unless you give the therapy, the note is what helps the therapist encapsulate the major themes and interventions for each session. These notes can then be reflected back on throughout treatment. They also are important legal documents that represent our work and the ethical and legal considerations that we sometimes must notate.

While there will be some freedom in how you do the paperwork, as it changes from site to site, there is a philosophy and purpose to documentation. du Plessis and Hirst (2006) explained as follows:

If the counselling process is to meet its high standards of client care, recordkeeping should assist by

1. improving continuity between sessions by providing a record of the issues raised in sessions;
2. providing a record for the use of the counsellor and, on certain occasions, the client;

DOI: 10.4324/9781003433484-4

3. facilitating assessment, regular planning, and evaluation of progress;
4. providing basic statistical information for the counselling service;
5. providing detailed information:

- to account for the actions and decisions of the counsellor;
- on patterns of behaviour in a client;
- on content and process of counselling sessions; and
- or collation and investigation—this information coming from different sources regarding a client;

6. the provision of legal record; counsellors must be able to demonstrate from their records that legal obligations have been fulfilled in respect of recordkeeping by ensuring that records are kept up-to-date, clear, and complete. (p. 92)

Regardless of the formatting of the paperwork you need to write, you should keep in mind that you are doing paperwork not for busywork but to ensure high standards of care to your clients and high standards of operating in relation to the field and community.

What Paperwork Will You Come Across?

Depending on your site, you may not come across all the paperwork we are going to talk about in this chapter. Perhaps it is just because, as an intern, you won't be required to utilize some of the paperwork that a paid therapist at the site may use. For example, at some sites, interns may not technically be responsible for any of the progress or case notes that therapists keep for their clients, even if the interns sit in on sessions with these therapists and their clients. However, the primary therapist may ask if you would like to write the note for that day's session in order to get some practice with progress notes. The licensed therapist will be the one who needs to sign off on it in the end, but they can read your draft and provide you with feedback. If the therapist doesn't offer for you to write the note of your own accord, show initiative and ask if you can write the note to get the practice.

Another reason why you may not see some of the paperwork we detail in this chapter at your site is simply because sites can use different types of paperwork. For example, though all sites will complete progress notes, the type of progress note each site uses may be different. One site may use a DAP note while another site uses a SOAP note (which we describe further later on).

We are going to go over the major types of documentation that you will likely encounter in a therapy practicum/internship so you are prepared for most of what might come your way (see Figure 4.1). We do not write this section for you to have to create the form. All the forms should already be created by your site. We are presenting this because these are the common forms that you will have to navigate when at your site (and wherever you go to practice after your field placement ends). You should know about them and their importance.

The **informed consent form** is perhaps the first bit of paperwork that the client will come across and is one of the most important, especially from a legal and ethical perspective. Every ethical code speaks about informed consent since its foundation is the ethical principle of

Informed Consent	• Ensures client self choice • Gives information about the therapy process
Biopsychosocial	• Biological, Psychological, and Social aspects of the client • The history of the client
Progress Notes	• Documentation of what occurred during session
SOAP Notes	• Subjective, Objective, Assessment, and Plan
DAP Notes	• Data, Assessment, and Plan
Group Notes	• Progress notes for when you engage in group therapy
Case Notes	• Therapy-related notes that are not progress notes
Collaborative Documentation	• Completing any paperwork with the client
Treatment Plans	• Overview of the client's problems, goals, and interventions to be used
Monthly Documentation	• Required for insurance companies
Release of Information	• Allows you to talk with others about the client's situation • Allows others to talk with you about the client

Figure 4.1 As a therapist, you will have to navigate a variety of paperwork. It is important for you to know the purpose of each to properly document the process of therapy.

autonomy, in which the client has self-choice. For instance, the National Association of Social Workers (NASW, 2021, Standard 1.03) states the following:

> Social workers should provide services to clients only in the context of a professional relationship based, when appropriate, on valid informed consent. Social workers should use clear and understandable language to inform clients of the purpose of the services, risks related to the services, limits to services because of the requirements of a third-party payer, relevant costs, reasonable alternatives, clients' right to refuse or withdraw consent, and the time frame covered by the consent. Social workers should provide clients with an opportunity to ask questions.

The client should have sufficient information to choose whether to enter into the therapeutic relationship with you. The good news here is that you do not have to worry about how to word the informed consent form. That will already have been done for you by people at the site. You will just use the form they have.

However, even if the client signs the form before you begin therapy, you should verbally go over it with them to ensure they understand it, especially about confidentiality and when you may need to break it. We encourage you to start the first session by going over the form and ensuring the client signs it *before* you begin therapy. Otherwise, you are opening yourself up for possible liability in that the client can claim that they were not informed about the therapeutic process. Now, this might seem quite easy to do; however, we have seen many novice therapists get steamrolled at the beginning of the first session since the client is coming in primed to talk about their concerns. It will be important for you to ensure that before any therapy talk happens, the informed consent is signed and discussed. Perhaps you can explain to the client, maybe on the phone when you are setting up the session or when walking from the waiting room to the office, that the first few minutes of the session will be going over important paperwork. However you do it, don't get into the client's concerns until they've signed the informed consent form. Michael once supervised a student therapist who, at her first session, had a client come into the therapy room already talking about a serious emotional concern she was having that brought her to therapy. Through the one-way mirror, Michael could see that the therapist was caught up in the client's story and was not going to stop the process to ensure that the informed consent form was signed. The therapy room had a phone that he was able to call to interrupt the conversation, remind the therapist to go over informed consent, and have the client sign it before moving forward with the therapeutic talk. Yes, it interrupted the client's flow. However, it also ensured that the therapy was following ethical guidelines. This happened during live supervision. You may not have that luxury. It will be up to you to be the leader of the session. If you need to interrupt a client to ensure that everything is being done appropriately, then do so. It is your role to do so. You are the captain of the therapy ship while the client is the navigator.

The **biopsychosocial** is usually done during the intake process. Some sites have an intake that might be done over the phone. In other settings, the biopsychosocial is the intake process. At other sites, the biopsychosocial is done by the therapist after the client's initial intake. As its name implies, this form covers the biological, psychological, and social aspects of the client. It is usually done via a lengthy conversation with the client that might take one to three hours. If your site wants you to conduct a biopsychosocial, then they likely already have this form for you to use. There is not one universal form that all therapists use. However, they all cover these three factors so that you, the therapist, can gain a comprehensive view of the challenges for the client as well as their resources. Biopsychosocials tend to include identifying information, presenting problem, history of the problem, developmental history, education and occupational history, family history, social history, medical history, psychiatric history, substance abuse history and current use, legal history, diversity considerations, and your initial impressions. As you can probably see, covering all of this information can be quite daunting. Your site might have the biopsychosocial form as a template on a computer that you fill in while you are talking to the client. This can be a bit dehumanizing, especially if lasting for hours. We suggest that you try to make the gaining of the necessary information as conversational as possible, even if you have to fill out the form during the interview.

Progress notes document what occurred in session, chronicling what you are focusing on during therapy and how you are working to ameliorate the problems the client brought into therapy. There are a few formats for progress notes that we'll go over here briefly. Before we do that, just a few words of caution: Writing notes, especially when you are a novice therapist and don't have the hang of them yet, can take quite a while. For some, it might be 20 to 30 minutes per note. This sounds like a lot for one note. Now, think about your site and how many clients you are seeing in a day. Let's say you see five clients. If it takes you 20 minutes per note, and you have five clients, and our math is accurate, that's over an hour you will spend writing notes. The longer you put this off, the worse it is since you will likely forget key information and not have the desire to write the note since it will be late, you will be hungry, you will want to get home, and you will likely do a poor job writing the note. Worse, you might say, "Heck, why do today what you can put off until tomorrow?" We will give you our number one word of advice when it comes to progress notes: Do them as immediately after the session as you can. (Or do them in session, which we will talk about when we discuss collaborative documentation.)

There are many different formats that progress notes can take. Perhaps your site will let you choose how to do them, but likely, they will have a form already created. Many agencies like to use a standardized type of progress note. The two most popular are SOAP and DAP notes. We will briefly discuss each of them here. Our recommendation is, before you attempt your first progress note at your site, you ask to review several of your supervisor's progress notes. This will give you an understanding of the format, breadth, and depth of the note that they are expecting from you.

SOAP notes are perhaps the most frequently used of the formatted progress notes. The acronym stands for Subjective, Objective, Assessment, and Plan. The subjective portion of the note contains the information that the client told you. It would include their explanation of the complaints, symptoms, and concerns. In essence, the subjective portion is the client's perspective and subjective experiences. The objective portion contains the measurable information that you gather. This might be any data that you obtained (e.g., an IQ test, self-esteem assessment, mental status exam). The assessment section is your assessment of the client. This would include your impressions, conclusions, and diagnosis. Here, you are providing your understanding of the client's situation. The plan section outlines what your course of treatment is based on the assessment. Although it is not a full-blown treatment plan (which we will also talk about), it highlights the interventions you might use, the need and frequency of sessions, referrals, and other steps to be taken.

DAP notes contain the same information as SOAP notes but are formatted just a bit differently. This acronym stands for Data, Assessment, and Plan. The data section is the combination of the subjective and objective portions of the SOAP note. Here, you include what was both reported and observed during the session. The assessment section of a DAP note is similar to the assessment section of a SOAP note. You'll write about your clinical judgments, diagnoses, and formulations that you have. You might also put your assessment of the client's progress and their challenges. The plan section is the same as the plan section of the SOAP note, in which you include aspects of the treatment plan, goals, interventions, and next steps for therapy.

Group notes are basically progress notes but for group therapy. Unlike regular progress notes that have some specific formats (such as DAP notes and SOAP notes), group notes can vary in format depending on the site and/or the electronic medical record (EMR)/electronic health record (EHR) system that is used. Oftentimes, group notes have a major summary section in which you describe the group topic and the activity/intervention/discussion that occurred during the group and then accompanying sections for each individual client who attended that group. In these individual parts of the group note, you often have an area where you can detail specifics of the client's participation in the group and several boxes to check indicating their attendance, mood, participation level, and more.

Quick Tip: Do not leave your site without doing all of the progress notes for your cases that day. It is as simple as that. The closer you can do them to the time of the session (or even in the session), the better.

Case notes are basically all other therapy-related notes that aren't progress notes. For example, if you have a quick phone conversation with a client's parent outside of a session discussing their child's progress in therapy, you would need to document this in a case note. If you work at a practice that takes insurance and have to do monthly documentation for your client (which we will also discuss), then you would write a case note if that monthly documentation will be late (e.g., because of a client canceling a session). Case notes are also used to document late cancellations, no shows, and any other information that would be important to keep track of and have official documentation for.

Collaborative documentation happens when you fill out the progress note along with the client in the session. This may sound odd at first; however, many clients really like being part of the process (MTM Services, 2012). And as an added benefit, it saves you time. You don't have to do notes after the session. When you end the session, the note is already completed. Plus, the note can be used as a therapeutic tool in which it is an excellent summary for the client of what was discussed during the session and what their continued goals are. We actually spent one whole semester utilizing collaborative documentation with our clients at the on-site therapy clinic of our university program (Reiter et al., 2022). The student therapists had not been trained on it, just like you probably haven't. However, they quickly learned how they could introduce it to their clients and how they could make it a part of the therapy session. For the most part, the clients found it useful. Kayleigh's two clients in that practicum had the most extreme reactions to it. One client found it so useful that he asked for a copy of the note each session. We did so, as this became another tool that he could use to track his progress. Kayleigh's other client was not too thrilled with the process and challenged it at the first presentation. We decided we would not utilize collaborative documentation with him, and Kayleigh filled out the progress note by herself after the session.

Exercise 4.1   Collaborative Documentation

Read the article we wrote on collaborative documentation (see Reiter et al., 2022). Then, choose one client who you think would find the process of collaborative documentation to be helpful and try it out with them. Afterward, ask them what they took from this process. What did you take from it? How was it for you? How might you continue to use it in the future?

Treatment plans are documents that provide an overview of the concerns of the client, their goals, and the pathway toward those goals. If you are being asked by your site to fill out a treatment plan with your client, they will likely provide you with the template. You should construct the treatment plan with the client. They need to have buy-in for their therapy. If they are not on board with the goals of therapy, they are probably not going to attempt to complete the goals. Most treatment plans will focus on the client's goals. When filling this section out, you can use the components of **SMART goals**: specific, measurable, achievable, relevant, and time-bound. You should go over the treatment plan with the client and will refer back to it each time you are writing progress notes, as your therapy will be connected to helping the client achieve their goals.

Monthly documentation, as mentioned, is usually required when you work at a therapy facility that takes insurance, as insurance companies like to see official documents that show therapists are checking in with their clients to make sure they are receiving the appropriate level of care. Monthly documentation therefore consists of check-in-based documents. While the exact types of monthly documentation requirements may vary from site to site, a few common ones are the **TPR** (treatment plan reviews), **PWI** (personal wellbeing index), **BOR** (behavioral outcomes report) for behavioral health programs, and **BAM** (brief addiction monitor) for substance use programs. TPRs review the client's original treatment plan (denoting any additions or changes to treatment goals), the client's progress over that month in therapy, and what the client needs from therapy moving forward. Some TPRs also go over any updates related to medical, legal, educational, vocational, or other relevant topics. The PWI is a scale that asks clients to rate their satisfaction with various elements of their life (e.g., health, personal relationships), while the BOR asks questions about certain elements of the client's life over the last 30 days (e.g., how many days they were depressed, how many days they took their medications as prescribed). The BAM is geared toward those in therapy for substance use and asks substance-related questions over the past 30 days (e.g., how many days they consumed alcohol).

There are times during the course of therapy when it will be helpful for the client—or for you in helping the client—to talk to someone in the client's relational field. This might be their spouse, parent, doctor, lawyer, or other important person. However, you cannot implicitly talk to anyone because you are bound by the ethics of confidentiality. Besides, when you have to break confidentiality (e.g., because of potential harm or abuse issues), you can move around it when the client agrees to it. You would talk to the client about who you would like to talk with, the reason for this conversation, and what information you would talk about. But just getting the client's verbal "okay" is not good enough. Everything that you do with the client should be documented. In this case, the client would need to sign a **release of information form** (sometimes called a **disclosure of information form**). As with all the other forms we have talked about, you do not need to create this form. Your site will already have one for you to use. If not, then request that the site create one. Don't do it yourself, as there are legal implications with all of these forms.

Tales From the Field: Supervisor

Talia was a senior in her social work bachelor's program and requested an internship working with children experiencing developmental disabilities. She was excited when she was placed in an agency that provided home-based services. During the first several weeks of her internship, her duties consisted solely of submitting referrals, submitting insurance authorizations, and documenting assessments. In her internship seminar, she felt disillusioned as she listened to her classmates talk about their direct client interactions. She felt like a "paper pusher" and wanted more client contact.

Talia expressed her concerns to me, the field director, who also served as the instructor of the internship seminar. A meeting was scheduled with Talia, me, and the agency-based supervisor. The agency supervisor explained that because of the sensitive nature of working in family's homes, the agency took a phase-based approach to introducing interns to direct work with clients. Following several weeks of observing the paperwork and administrative aspects of care, student interns would then begin observing seasoned helping professionals. This phase-based approach would ensure that student interns felt prepared and understood the context of home-based care prior to working directly with clients. The supervisor and I validated Talia's initiative and self-advocacy and agreed that Talia was ready to move into the next phase of orientation. Within 2 weeks, Talia had observed several seasoned workers and was ready to conduct an intake herself.

After completing the intake, Talia expressed gratitude that she spent her first few weeks observing and completing paperwork because she was more confident in the terminology and requirements that she had to review with her clients. She realized that just because a task did not involve direct client contact, she was still learning. Because of her detailed orientation, she understood the scope and context of service delivery, including how the service was funded, eligibility requirements for the service, and the type of information that families must submit to obtain the services. This knowledge increased her empathy for the families with whom she worked, and she was able to help them understand services better because of her exposure to the administrative aspects of care.

Janice Nuss, DSW, LCSW, Social Work, Gwynedd-Mercy University

How Do You Fill Out All This Paperwork?

Even if you now know about the different types of paperwork and what each document includes, we still need to go over how to actually fill out this documentation. Perhaps the biggest tip that we can give you regarding filling out any paperwork is to never sign it until you have finished. We have seen many therapists actually start filling out their progress note by putting the demographics (e.g., client name, time/length of the session, date) and then going to the bottom of the page and signing the note before they have put the content on the page (this is for paper notes rather than electronic health records). The serious issue here is what happens if you have to switch to do something else. There is now an official document with your signature that someone else can fill out, and it would seem as if you have endorsed what is written. If there is ever a place for you to sign the paperwork, only do so once the form is completely filled out.

Exercise 4.2   Filling Out Progress Notes

Progress notes are an important component of therapy practice as they document what has occurred and provide a record of the quality of your work and the process of the therapy. For this exercise, choose one of the progress notes formats we presented (SOAP or DAP notes) and write a mock note. Perhaps use a session that you sat in on, conducted, or watched via videotape (you can always go on YouTube and watch Carl Rogers working with Gloria and write the note based on that). Try to be thorough without writing an essay (usually about seven to ten sentences). Then, find someone in the field (perhaps a teacher, supervisor, or more advanced therapist) who uses that note format and ask them to provide you feedback on your note. You shouldn't be able to write a perfect note. You are learning. It is important to get feedback so that you can continuously improve. [We know this won't be the most enjoyable exercise in this book, but it is quite an important one. We encourage you not to skip it over.]

Your Setting

Although you might not think about it at first, the setting in which you are filling out paperwork is going to be important. We will go over completing documentation at home versus at your practicum/internship site later on when we address the differences between digital and physical paperwork. For now, we are mainly talking about the environment around you that can influence how you fill out paperwork.

Have you ever tried writing a paper for school, for example, and your roommate (or family member, or significant other, and so on) is making a lot of noise in the background? Maybe it is preventing you from fully concentrating; maybe you read a paragraph over and realize you wrote complete nonsense due to the distraction; maybe you even wrote some of what other people around you were saying! The same thing can happen with our therapy-related paperwork. If we try to complete documentation while in a busy setting, we are more likely to make mistakes than if we are in a quiet setting. That is why you should always try to complete this important documentation in a quiet setting in which you can concentrate. We have both attempted to fill out paperwork while other colleagues were talking around us, and it usually takes us a lot longer to complete everything because the distractions slow us down and we have to think twice as hard.

In the circumstances in which you are unable to be in a separate, quiet area to complete documentation (e.g., you are in a group practicum behind a one-way mirror), do not sign the document when you are done writing. If you can, wait until you have a moment to yourself to review the document without distractions. Even if you have to get the bulk of the document done when there are other things going on in the background, take a few minutes in a more suitable setting to review the document and fix any mistakes. Don't just assume that everything you wrote is okay—always check your work before signing. This applies even when you are able to complete the paperwork in a quiet space.

What Would You Do?: 4.1

You have seen six clients back-to-back, and it is getting late. You have plans after work where people are expecting you to be on time. However, because all of your clients showed up (sometimes a rarity, which didn't allow you to have any down time), you did not have time between sessions to write the notes. It is Friday. The agency will be closed Saturday and Sunday, and you will not be back until next Wednesday. You know that it will take you 5–10 minutes per note, which could take the better part of an hour. If you did that, you would be extremely late to your affair, which might cause significant issues. What would you do? That night? To try to prevent this from happening in the future?

Wording

You may still be asking yourself, "Okay, how exactly do I word what I will write?" As you probably learned in your ethics class, the way you word things in any documentation is both an ethical and legal responsibility because these are all documents that will be a part of your client's chart/case file. Although your site should go over this information with you during your training, we want to highlight some overarching pointers about how to fill out paperwork as well.

First, the client should never simply *do* something in your notes. They should, however, certainly *state* that they do something. Look at the difference between these two sentences: "The client is annoyed with their mom" and "The client stated they are annoyed with their mom." In the first sentence, the language implies that you somehow implicitly know that the client is annoyed with their mom. In the second sentence, you are making clear that the client *told you* that they are annoyed with their mom (through the use of the word "stated") and that this statement is how you are privy to this information. We assume liability as therapists when we write the former sentences because we cannot retroactively say, "Well. the client told me this, so that's how I know." Our language does not indicate that this was conveyed to us by our clients—we need to be very specific about that.

This logic also applies not only to statements that clients make but their behaviors and actions as well. Once again, notice the difference between saying "The client cried" versus "The therapist observed the client cry." The second sentence makes it abundantly clear that you know the client cried because you observed them do so. It may seem repetitive and unnecessary for a layperson's general understanding of a note, but these are important nuances in language that can make all the difference legally.

This type of writing should be present in all paperwork. It may seem obvious to write this way in a DAP note, for instance. When you are providing the data part of the note, you might write something like, "The client stated today has been a rough week because of trouble with her partner. The client further explained that they had gotten into a fight about their career paths again." Even in the assessment section of a DAP note when providing information on how the client presented, you may say, "The client seemed to be alert and oriented" (emphasis on the "seemed to be").

You would even want to write in this way for a biopsychosocial despite this document being like an informational form about the client. When completing the client's biopsychosocial, you may ask about medical information (e.g., "When was the last time you saw your primary care physician?"). Again, instead of just filling in the form with "May of 2023," you would want to say, "The client stated they last saw their primary care physician in May of 2023."

You also generally want to avoid using client's names in some notes or documentation. Of course, there are some circumstances in which you will need to use names—for example, when filling out a release of information (ROI) form for a client's parent (as you obviously have to put in the client's parents' name to denote who the ROI is for). However, in paperwork such as case notes and progress notes, client names are not necessary. For instance, you would use phrases such as "client," "client's mom," and "client's daughter" to refer to these particular people instead of utilizing their names. This further helps to de-identify the client's information while still allowing for contextual understanding of the information in the note.

We want to be transparent here and share that we know students who encountered practicum/internship sites in which this type of writing was not required as intensely and/or consistently as we are stating it should be. If you hear something other than what we are telling you from a different site, we of course encourage you to consult with your supervisor to get their take. Overall, however, we have found that what we described previously is the most ethical and legal approach to completing documentation. It is usually better to be a bit more strict than a bit more lax when it comes to this sort of thing, so we recommend that you take the former approach to cover your bases. In the end, writing in these ways isn't "incorrect," nor should it be a problem for your practicum/internship site. It might seem like a little more work on your end, but we believe it is worth it.

Tales From the Field: Intern

I am a second-year master's student in the MS in Couple and Family Therapy program at Nova Southeastern University. I'm currently in my first semester of external practicum at a local nonprofit community mental health facility. The site primarily services children through young adults and their families, and much of the clientele I engage with are adolescents.

In our program, we first spend two semesters in internal practicum (at our school-based clinic), and during that time, we began learning the process of writing clinical progress notes for our sessions. Over the course of those semesters, I started to become familiar with how to write notes with the purpose of capturing the most clinically relevant details of the session. Until now, my caseload was very limited, and I rarely dealt with minors, so my experience with the dilemma of discerning what makes it into a note and how the note is written is limited. My external site utilizes an electronic health record system, and while it has been a learning curve to become familiar with the technical areas of the system, the steeper area of growth has come from determining what is most clinically relevant to include in a note. This largely consists of what I need to legally include in a note, especially when minors are involved. There have been multiple scenarios where these nuances have led me to seek guidance from more senior therapists and my supervisors to determine what to include and how to phrase it while maintaining the balance of client confidentiality, client safety, and necessary documentation.

For example, I had a client disclose their preferred gender pronouns that were different from their gender pronouns assigned at birth. This is a female-at-birth client who prefers we address them as he/him. However, he shared that this is not something he has discussed with his family yet. He asked me to continue to use she/her when speaking to his mother. I checked with the therapist I was shadowing because I wanted to honor this client's gender identity and the potential impact this could be having on situations related to his mental health. At the same time, I feared potentially betraying our therapeutic alliance if his mother requested to read the session notes. In fact, when I wrote my first draft for this tale, I had misunderstood client confidentiality and was under the impression that progress notes could at any point be requested and read by the client's parent/guardian. When I consulted with the therapist that I shadow with this client, I learned that this in fact is not the case. The parent/guardian can request a clinical summary; however, the exact progress note would only be subject to being read verbatim if it were court ordered, and this would be a very rare situation. The senior therapist informed me that the site's policy was to use birth pronouns in the note to keep it consistent with the client's assigned gender at birth on their medical records.

With another client, I was in a situation where I needed guidance to determine if a relapse for self-harm needed to be included only in the notes (and how to include it) or if it also required a conversation with the client's parent. This client, whose sessions I shadow, disclosed she had relapsed with regard to self-harm. She showed the wound to both the therapist and me, and the client stated that the impulse for doing so was related to feeling numb and wanting to feel something. She shared that at the current time she was not having any suicidal ideations and did not have any plans to attempt suicide or further self-harm. The wound itself was small and did not require medical attention. In this situation, we wanted to ensure we assessed the client and documented the self-harm. The therapist explained it is important to document that the client denied any current or intended self-harm and document the pertinent details noted previously that the client shared with us. If the client shared or had given us reason to believe she had an active plan to continue, then we would need to have a conversation that would include her parent. This situation brought up various dynamics relating to documentation, client safety, and how to determine when it's necessary to contact a parent/guardian.

With these cases and more, I consulted with a more senior therapist and/or my clinical supervisor. As I continue to navigate the dilemma of what to include or not include in a progress note, I also bring it into supervision so I can discuss the many layers and navigate best practices. I have found the support from working therapists and my supervisor when making document-related decisions to be incredibly helpful as a student intern. The cases I shared here will be the first few of the many I will come to them for guidance and support while traversing this responsibility we have as therapists regarding documentation.

Lauren Jordan, MS in Couple and Family Therapy program, Nova Southeastern University

Digital Paperwork Versus Paper Paperwork

In our increasingly online world, you are most likely to intern at a site that utilizes an **electronic medical record** (EMR)/**electronic health record** (EHR) system. This is an online system that consists of the workplace calendar, the clients' charts (which contains all their documentation), and more. There are different types of EMR/EHR systems, so you will learn to navigate whatever specific one your site uses. There are a few general considerations to make when using any EMR/EHR system and utilizing technology in general to access therapy-related information.

Something that you should have gone over during your ethics class are some ethical and legal practices when it comes to using technology to access client information and documentation. We want to emphasize that these are practices that you need to follow at your practicum/internship. For example, if you are using a laptop at your practicum/internship to work on progress notes and get up to go to the bathroom, you need to close your computer when leaving it unattended so unauthorized people cannot access any **protected health information** (PHI). Additionally, you should only use Wi-Fi that is password protected in order to keep any PHI secure. These are examples of important practices to review before beginning your practicum/internship.

In the rarer case that your site is old fashioned and keeps paper records, there are different considerations that we want to go over. First, write everything in blue ink (rather than black ink). This is to clearly differentiate an original of any document from a photocopy. While other colors would technically serve the same purpose, we doubt that your practicum/internship site would think that a pink ink progress note is professional. Ethical and legal practices to follow when dealing with physical paperwork include keeping paper documents locked in some sort of filing cabinet when you're not actively using them, shredding any paper documents in a locked shredder, and refraining from taking paper documents home with you.

Your site will likely go over these specifics with you during your training and throughout your time there. Still, having this background information about these online and physical paperwork nuances may help to orient you to them more easily once you begin your practicum/internship. We are providing a general guide, so it is important to check in with your site about these details and follow their specific protocol and to follow overarching ethical and legal requirements. As always, if a particular policy or procedure that your site has regarding online and physical paperwork is not sitting right with you (i.e., your ethical spidey sense is tingling), consult with your supervisor.

Tips From an Intern

The paperwork side of the therapy world can sometimes be tough for therapists, especially student therapists in training. At my practicum and internship sites, I found this to be especially true with the progress notes. I have seen that many of my peers have a smoother time in the therapy room talking with a client, as people who are drawn to being therapists tend to have these skills innately. But when it comes to putting the words down on paper (or computer, if your site uses an online therapy server) in the correct way, things are often not so smooth.

We talked about the specific considerations of progress notes in this chapter, and these are the things that people often have trouble with. For example, a peer at my internship site—who was a wonderful therapist—kept writing statements such as "Client is feeling sad today" when it really should be "Client *stated* they are feeling sad today." This might seem like a nuanced difference, but as we mentioned, it can make all the difference in the eyes of a court or insurance company as it clarifies that the client stated it rather than having a gray area that seems like the therapist inferred it.

Essentially, my tip for you is to be vigilant about the notes you write and to not rush them. Have a template of an acceptable progress note for reference; perhaps draft this note and then go over it with your supervisor and make any necessary changes. At the risk of being cliché here, practice really does make perfect. Although, I will qualify this statement a bit with another tip: No matter how many times you write a progress note, you will make mistakes here and there, and things will not always be "perfect." Double-check your work, always. These are important documents that you are writing, and it is your responsibility to review and edit them each and every time you write one so that they are accurate and consistent.

Taking Notes During Sessions

Earlier, we talked about some of the different paperwork you may have to fill out for a client. Some of those documents—including monthly surveys and treatment plan reviews, for example—must be filled out during a session with the client in front of you. This is because this paperwork contains direct questions that you need to ask a client and require the client's signature after completing them.

Other types of paperwork—such as progress notes—don't necessarily require you to write anything for them during a session. This brings up an important question: Should you take notes during your therapy session? This is one topic that therapists can be divided on. On the one hand, those who are in-session notetakers may believe it shows their care and concern to the client because they are writing important things down and it helps them more easily remember details of the session later on. On the other hand, those who are not in-session notetakers often claim that it can be a distraction to being present with your client and can detract from reflecting on the main themes by creating a hyperfocus on insignificant details. Even Sigmund Freud, who some may consider to be one of the original psychotherapeutic notetakers, cautioned against the use of note-taking specifically in session because of the previously mentioned points (Tudor & Gledhill, 2022). There is also some research on this topic as well. One of the original studies on in-session note-taking found that both prospective social work graduate students and clients perceived a session to be better when there was no in-session note-taking (Hickling et al., 1984).

Some clients are divided on this stance as well. We've both had clients who have asked us how we are going to remember everything in a session since we don't take notes (sometimes with a tone implying that we should be taking notes). We have also seen clients ask therapists to stop taking notes during a session because they think the therapist is distracted from listening to the client in the moment. We will talk more about how to handle these situations further along.

The first question you need to ask yourself when considering in-session note-taking is, "What is my purpose?" Many student therapists, whether they want to answer this question honestly or not, use in-session notes as a blankie. More specifically, the physical act of holding a clipboard or a client's file can be used as a source of comfort during a session. Have you ever felt more at ease doing a class presentation behind a podium instead of directly in front of your audience? Holding that clipboard or file in front of you is sort of the same idea. Sometimes, clients don't notice this. Other times, they will. We knew of a student intern who held a clipboard for "notes" across her chest (like she was hugging a teddy bear) during her first session. It was obvious that the clipboard was a function of comfort. If you find that this is the case when you take notes during sessions, perhaps reconsider your purpose of needing to take notes during the session.

If your answer to the previous question was, "Well, I need to take notes to remember all the important information that my client shared," we recommend that you reflect on the need for this further as well. Oftentimes, we have seen student interns write down so many notes to remember the minutiae of the session that they can't even conceptualize what the theme of the session was about. Though it may seem paradoxical, sometimes more details through the notes leads to less presence and overall awareness of the important moments of the session. In essence, less is sometimes more.

At the same time, however, sometimes you may actually find it helpful or necessary to write down certain details of a session. In your practicum/internship, you may not see clients back-to-back and thus can take some more time in formulating your note and reflecting on the session right after the session ends. Unfortunately, the real world of therapy usually does not allow for this.

For instance, you may have multiple sessions one after another in your future work setting and are unable to complete your notes in between (you may want that time to take a breath, eat a snack, or even get to the bathroom before your next client). But if something important comes up during a session that you ethically and legally must document (e.g., a teenage client tells you that their medication is not working well for them), you need to remember to put this in your note.

When working with minors, for example, we need to communicate with their guardians about medical-related topics, so this is something that you would definitely want to include in your note (both that the client told you about it and that you will be reaching out to their guardian). If you have five other back-to-back sessions for the rest of the day, it may slip your mind to include this exact detail in your notes (which isn't any fault of yours, as five more sessions produce a lot of information to keep track of).

In these situations, it is perhaps a good idea to have a happy medium and have a notepad off to the side so that it isn't distracting or front and center but is still accessible in case you need to write down important information that must be included in a note. Jotting down "Client's meds—email dad" is oftentimes all it takes to jog your memory later to include it in your note (and to also follow up with your client's dad!).

In the end, you can always talk to your client about this beforehand. Kayleigh will often describe how she does therapy with her clients during their first session and explain that on busy days, she will keep a notepad to the side in case something significant comes up but that she otherwise likes to be as present with her clients as possible. Most of the time, they will roll with whatever your approach is once you have explained its purpose to them. If you don't want to do this spiel beforehand, that is fine, too. Just be ready to talk to a client and therapeutically explain your reasoning for taking or not taking notes during a session if they ask.

Tips From a Supervisor

Having been a faculty member for 25 years, I have read my share of textbooks about therapy. While you might think you have to read a lot for classes, I can assure you that I (and your faculty members) have read a lot more. And in most of those books, very few have addressed writing and paperwork. There are a few that are focused on progress notes or treatment plans. Given this scarcity of books addressing paperwork and writing in therapy, I wrote a book about it called *A Therapist's Guide to Writing in Psychotherapy* (Reiter, 2023a). Not trying to do self-promotion (okay, maybe just a little), but that book—and the other books that focus on a specific type of paperwork in psychotherapy—are related to my tip: You are not expected to know how to do the paperwork. Doing it well is a skill. Skills need to be learned.

I recommend that you think about paperwork just like you would specific therapeutic techniques. You wouldn't expect yourself to just know how to do the empty chair technique without ever reading about it, watching it, or practicing it. I think the same holds for paperwork. You shouldn't know how to write a good progress note or treatment plan (unless you were to have read material about them and got trained on how to do them).

As with much we will talk about throughout this book, don't keep to yourself. Ask your supervisor for training and suggestions. Ask to read other therapists' notes, treatment plans, and assessments. When you write your first one (of whatever paperwork it is), immediately bring it to your supervisor and ask for feedback. This way you can quickly develop good writing habits so that your paperwork is more accurate and useful.

Summary

Whatever site you do your practicum/internship at, you will be doing paperwork. Each site may have their own unique forms or expectations of how you fill them out. Students are usually not trained in the classroom on how to fill out paperwork. Further, for many, it seems like it is a drudgery. We encourage you to take the paperwork seriously. It is not only a part of the client's official record, but it is also an opportunity to enhance the therapeutic process. Take personal agency to put yourself in a position of a learner of how you can—with each successive note, treatment plan, and assessment—become more efficient and effective at writing them, which should then lead to more efficient and effective therapy.

References

du Plessis, P., & Hirst, F. (2006). Written communication and counseling. In R. Bor & M. Watts (Eds.), *The trainee handbook* (2nd ed., pp. 91–109). Sage Publications.

Edwards, T. M., & Patterson, J. E. (2012). The daily events and emotions of master's-level family therapy trainees in off-campus practicum settings. *Journal of Marital and Family Therapy, 38*(4), 688–696. https://doi.org/10.1111/j.1752-0606.2012.00263.x

Hickling, L. P., Hickling, E. J., Sison Jr., G. F., & Radetsky, S. (1984). The effect of note-taking on a simulated clinical interview. *The Journal of Psychology, 116*(2), 235–240. https://doi.org/10.1080/00223980.1984.9923641

MTM Services. (2012). *Collaborative documentation: There's nothing basic about it* [PowerPoint slides]. https://static1.squarespace.com/static/59c005cd8a02c7dae8cd5e80/t/5c9eb982eb3931364258c4a4/1553906063959/Natcon2019+Collaborative+Documentation+-+There%27s+Nothing+Basic+About+It+-+M.+Flora+and+J.+Fruth+%28Final%29+DB.pdf

National Association of Social Workers. (2021). *Code of ethics of the National Association of Social Workers.* https://www.socialworkers.org/About/Ethics/Code-of-Ethics/Code-of-Ethics-English

Reiter, M. D. (2023a). *A therapist's guide to writing in psychotherapy.* Routledge.

Reiter, M. D., Bibliowicz, V., Sabo, K., Yu, X. C., Delgado, Y., Barrionuevo, D., & Rich, B. (2022). Collaborative documentation: Therapist experiences in jointly writing progress notes. *Journal of Systemic Therapies, 41*(2), 89–104.

Tudor, K., & Gledhill, K. (2022). Notes on notes: Note-taking and record-keeping in psychotherapy. *Ata: Journal of Psychotherapy Aotearoa New Zealand, 26*(2), 123–144. https://doi.org/10.9791/ajpanz.2022.12

Chapter 5

Knowing Yourself

At the Temple of Apollo at Delphi were inscribed three Delphic maxims:

1. "Know thyself"
2. "Nothing to excess"
3. "Certainty brings ruin"

The first of these has become the most known, sometimes attributed to being put forth by Plato, Socrates, or other Greek philosophers. Regardless of their origins, they are still pertinent these thousands of years later.

As psychotherapists, we are trained to focus on our clients, putting ourselves in their shoes, and trying to understand how they make sense of the world. We learn how to conduct assessments, diagnose, and develop treatment plans. What we might not pay as much attention to is the **person of the therapist** (also called **self of the therapist**). We are the most important therapeutic tool in the therapy room. This chapter provides you with an opportunity to know yourself on a deeper level than you do now.

Let's first take a second to explore those other two Delphic maxims, as we believe they are useful for therapists to also keep in mind. "Nothing to excess" is a different way of talking about moderation. Clients will likely be coming to therapy because there is excess in their life—excess anxiety, sadness, conflict, trauma, and so on. For therapists, using or doing something to excess tends to lead to problems. You can utilize a skill, challenge, or not challenge too much, which can be detrimental to the therapeutic process.

The last maxim, "Certainty brings ruin," is important to keep in mind as you develop therapeutic hypotheses. We don't ever know the "truth" of a situation, and that is okay. We don't have to be right, just useful. Salvador Minuchin, one of the most influential family therapists of all time, used to say that certainty is the enemy of change (Minuchin et al., 2021). As he explained, "The more clients maintain their certainty about the problem, the less open they are to viewing the situation differently, and thus they will be unlikely to alter their way of being with one another" (p. 4). The same holds for therapists. The more you maintain your own certainty about the client's problem, or what you can and can't do, the less pathways toward change are available for you (and your client).

Myths About the Field

"My personal self and my therapist self are separate entities."

DOI: 10.4324/9781003433484-5

This entire chapter is basically a culmination of information and reflections that prove this statement to be false. The mere existence of this chapter makes the previous statement a myth, as this chapter wouldn't even be necessary if it were true. If the personal self and the therapist self did not influence one another, then every therapist coming out of the same psychotherapy graduate program would practice therapy the exact same way because they got the same training. It is our personal self—which itself is shaped by our culture, family of origin, religion, personal beliefs, age, hobbies, goals, and more—that makes us unique therapists. And it is our duty to learn how our personal self plays a role in our therapeutic uniqueness.

Self-of-the-Therapist

Have you ever had anyone tell you that you were biased? You had to have, just as we have, many times. And you know what? That person was right. You were biased (but maybe not in the way that they thought). They were biased as well. They couldn't help it, and neither can you. We are human beings, and we each have a way of viewing the world. Unfortunately, the word "biases" has a negative connotation. Not too many people want to be viewed as being biased. Usually that is associated with having a flaw or, even worse, being discriminatory.

If we switch out **bias** for **viewpoint**, then perhaps it is more palatable. You have a way of viewing the world in which you think some things are good and some things are bad. For instance, most people in the United States have been raised and socialized to think that monogamy is "good" and polygamy is "bad." There are only a few times when we can accept that it is okay for someone to play the field, such as when we watch a season of *The Bachelor*. But in the end, the bachelor or bachelorette is supposed to find one person whom they love. Our viewpoint that people should try to find one person is a bias. And we are not trying to change your belief on this issue, whichever way you fall. What we are trying to do is get you to think about what your belief is on this topic and just about every other topic. This is because these beliefs will eventually seep their way into the therapy room, and you need to be conscious of this. The more that you are aware of your beliefs, the more you can think about them before they infiltrate themselves into your comments and questions in an unhelpful way (such as by making judgments about or implications to the client).

Your Values

We have a huge dilemma as therapists. Our ethical codes hold that we should not impose our values on our clients. However, our values are one of the primary motivating factors for our behaviors. So how do we become aware of our values and respect our clients' values?

One way to prevent the imposition of your values on your client is through **ethical bracketing**, which is when the therapist attempts to put aside their own values to engage in ethical practice that respects the client's values (Kocet & Herlihy, 2014). The way to do this is to really put your values in your foreground. When you try not to think about them, they will wind up influencing your beliefs and behaviors without you realizing it. Functioning in the background, they become your lens to take in and give out information.

However, when you place your values in your foreground, you are better able to tell yourself, "Hold on a second. I know that I believe that people should be monogamous. But not everyone has this same view. Let me try to put this to the side and really understand where the other person is coming from." Ethical bracketing is not agreeing with another person but rather seeing how their viewpoint makes sense for them without you trying to tell them how they should think, feel, or behave. Corey and Corey (2016) explained the difficulty of this when they stated, "Even if you think it is inappropriate to impose your values on clients, you may unintentionally influence them in subtle ways to subscribe to your values" (p. 43). But keep in mind there is a difference between imposing your values on your client and talking about values in a way that gets the client to make their own choice of what they believe and how they want to act. One value that you should almost always abide by is that people should have autonomy and make their own choices.

Tales From the Field: Supervisor

Madison started her internship at a local community mental health center, where she would be working with adults with co-occurring disorders. She was excited to get started because it allowed her to work with the population that she was most passionate about serving. It was at this new site, where she was given the opportunity to provide individual therapy, as well as co-lead groups, for adults with co-occurring substance use and mental health disorders. This was very different from her practicum experience, where she had worked with adolescents in a sub-acute psychiatric inpatient hospital. Although she enjoyed her time at the hospital, she really wanted to gain experience working with adults with co-occurring disorders.

During her first week at the community mental health center, Madison spent much of her time onboarding and observing individual and group therapy sessions with her supervisor. This was hard for Madison because she was eager to engage and interact with clients. After discussing this with her site supervisor, Madison was given the opportunity to lead the individual check-ins for one of the groups the following week. The check-ins, which occur at the beginning of each group session, went without incident until a male participant disclosed that he was going through some difficult times. Upon concluding his check-in, Madison said, *"I understand what you're going through; thank you for sharing."* The male participant then inquired, *"You do? Are you in recovery?"*

Madison, startled by the participant's question, was unsure how to respond and immediately glanced toward her supervisor. Madison's supervisor quickly interjected and reminded the participants about the group rules/expectations, as well as the importance of respecting and maintaining healthy boundaries. The supervisor successfully redirected the focus of the discussion and then gently prompted Madison to continue with the next participant's check-in. Immediately after group, Madison felt discouraged and asked to meet with her supervisor. They spoke briefly; however, her supervisor encouraged her to discuss the situation with me (faculty supervisor) and that they could discuss her concerns in supervision, which was scheduled later in the week.

Madison and I met later that afternoon for supervision, and she explained how the client's question had caught her off-guard, and as a result, she didn't know how to respond appropriately. To complicate things, Madison also disclosed that she was, in fact, a person in long-term recovery, but she'd always been very guarded in revealing this to others (mainly because of the stigma associated with these conditions). She felt a tremendous amount of internal conflict that day; part of her felt that she would be validated by the group if she disclosed that she was in recovery, but part of her felt exposed, insecure, and vulnerable. I thanked her for her openness and honesty, and then we spent the remaining time exploring some very important yet difficult topics, including the ethics of counselor self-disclosure (e.g., risks and benefits), therapeutic boundaries, as well as the importance of self-awareness.

Throughout our supervision that day, as well as in subsequent supervision sessions, Madison and I focused much of our attention on exploring her sense of self (both personally and professionally). I encouraged Madison to explore her concept of self by comparing her view of self now to her view of self throughout other times in her life, a process akin to temporal self-comparison/reflection. By doing this, Madison recognized that her self-concept and identity were rooted, and deeply connected, to her role as a former patient (and person in recovery) rather than identifying as a counselor-in-training. This revelation helped Madison strengthen her sense of self (self-clarity and self-efficacy) and identify more as a counselor-in-training. The proceeding supervision sessions were critical to Madison's development and professional identity. She also gained a better understanding of the importance of continuous self-development, as well as the advantages of self-reflection, especially regarding the interpersonal, intrapersonal, and clinical issues that influence her work now as a counselor-in-training and throughout her career.

Ben Wilson, PhD, LMHC, LCAC, NCC, Department of Counselor Education, Adams State University

Triggers

The last 5 to 10 years have seen an exponential increase in the public's discussion of triggers. This concept was once reserved for the substance abuse field, in which therapists worked with clients dealing with addictions so that they would reduce and avoid those things that triggered them to want to drink or drug. Nowadays, the concept of triggers is used for things that make people upset. We now have trigger warnings. And each person is triggered by something unique.

A **trigger** is something that impacts a person to lead them to have a reaction. We almost always view triggers as something that brings a negative response or leads to emotional or physical symptoms. This section is not about the triggers that your clients may have. They will have a lot of them, but that is part of the therapeutic process. We won't get into what to do when your client has triggers. That's a conversation for you and your supervisor. What we do want to talk about are *your* triggers. You have them, and they impact you. Just like your biases, it is important to know your triggers so that you can prevent them from having a negative influence during sessions.

Corey and Corey (2020) provided several types of clients that may pose a challenge to you; that is, they might be triggering. These include the following:

- Involuntary clients
- Clients who are withdrawn and silent
- Clients who talk excessively

- Clients who overwhelm themselves
- Clients who often say "Yes, but . . . "
- Clients who deny needing help
- Clients who manifest passive-aggressive behavior
- Clients who rely primarily on their intellect
- Clients who use emotions as a defense

This is not an exhaustive list. We know therapists who have been triggered by clients who stay in abusive relationships, have overbearing in-laws, are know-it-alls, and do a plethora of other things.

Exercise 5.1   Thinking About Your Triggers

All people have triggers. For this exercise, write down a few of the primary triggers that you experience.

1. Trigger:

   - Your reaction:

2. Trigger:

   - Your reaction:

3. Trigger:

   - Your reaction:

4. Trigger:

   - Your reaction:

5. Trigger:

   - Your reaction:

While we tend to think of triggers as something problematic, they do not need to be. You can be triggered in positive ways. Think about things that other people do that lead you to feel closer to them. These can be classified as triggers. What might clients do to trigger you to feel more connected, caring, or attracted to them? Knowing these positive triggers is equally as useful as knowing your negative triggers, as both lead you to behave in certain ways with your clients.

The Personal and the Professional You

In your personal life, you have a certain style. This comes through in many ways, including the words you use, your body language, and your choice of clothing. The question is, how do you maintain your style while functioning in a professional setting?

The big thing to address here is personality. It is important to not be a completely neutral blob during sessions to the point where your clients don't feel like they can even relate to you as a fellow human being. On the flip side, you also have to regulate your personality to some degree so that it doesn't interfere with the therapeutic process.

For example, Michael had a practicum student who had a very boisterous, confident personality. This was important for her to bring into the therapy room in some ways as it distinguished her as a human being and allowed her client to laugh and relate to her when appropriate. However, there were times when her personality would become the dominant force of energy in the sessions and would detract from the client's own personhood. There were important therapeutic moments that required more seriousness or even silence, and this was difficult for the student therapist. Michael had to work hard with her to be genuine yet professional and therapeutic in the therapy room. Another example involves cursing—for instance, we both curse quite freely in our personal lives, but we don't usually curse in sessions unless our clients curse as well. It is about meeting clients where they are at and attending to each client and each session.

We already talked about curating a therapy wardrobe in Chapter 3 to help prepare you to present professionally at your practicum/internship site. Here, we want to further highlight how the personal you plays a factor in this wardrobe. Once again, the specifics of what is considered to be appropriate clothing may change based on each site—one may expect more business casual (which often means no jeans), while another site may be more casual and allow you to wear jeans, for instance. This is what you must consider first and foremost. You must then decide which aspects of your personal style are appropriate at your site and which aspects are not. For instance, we knew of a student intern who frequently wore T-shirts with numerous rhinestones and busy prints. This was definitely a part of her personal style; however, these tops weren't really appropriate for therapy (even with a cardigan or blazer over them) because they were quite flashy and distracting.

You have learned many microskills of therapy (e.g., paraphrases, reflections, reframing, questions). These do not just happen. They are utilized by a person. You are important! Otherwise, we can program computers or have artificial intelligence provide therapy and do the skills better than any of us. However, there is something magical when two people have an encounter with one another. You cannot help but use yourself in the therapy room. The question becomes, how much do you do so consciously and purposely? Aponte and Carlsen (2009) stated, "Personally, all therapists use themselves within the relationship with clients to establish trust with clients, develop empathy for them, and implement their interventions" (p. 35). Thus, therapy becomes the combination of the professional (e.g., the therapeutic techniques) and the personal (e.g., your personality).

Tips From an Intern

I will not lie to you; you may battle with your sense of identity during your practicum/internship. Perhaps you have already experienced this even through your classes in the program. You are going to be inundated with so much information and so many opinions about therapy (e.g., theories, techniques, case conceptualizations, opinions on disclosure) and even the logistics behind therapy (e.g., administrative tasks, documentation) that it can oftentimes be hard to stay on course with your own approach. It can sometimes feel like a tug of war but in all directions.

We have addressed several considerations and tactics to help you know yourself and stay true to yourself through your practicum/internship experience. I have another specific tip that I used throughout my practicum/internship experience (actually, throughout the whole graduate experience in general) that may be helpful. I kept a journal with each page split into two columns—one side was titled "Things I Like" and the other side said, "Things I Don't Like." I basically put the relevant information into each column as I experienced it during therapy. For example, a lot of therapists use the word "homework" when they want clients to do something at home outside of therapy. That word never really sat quite right with me as homework is something that can be graded and done correctly/incorrectly. I don't necessarily think that it encourages the client's own resources or the spontaneity of the therapeutic process, so I put that in the "Things I Don't Like" column. I put "experiments" in the "Things I Like" column because experiments imply an ever-evolving process in which you can learn valuable information even if they do not go as planned. In my mind, they give the client more room to play with them and not feel like they will fail.

For me, this journal helped me sort through everything I was learning at my practicum/internship site. While it may seem somewhat binary to only "like" or "not like" something, it was just an easy way for me to reflect on different therapeutic styles, interventions, and approaches without it becoming overwhelming. It allowed me to be purposeful even about the little things and make sense of them within my own developing therapeutic approach. This journal provided a comprehensive list of the nuts and bolts of what I didn't particularly resonate with and, even more importantly, what I did resonate with as a therapist. Even if you don't use this exact strategy, keeping some sort of reflective journal such as this may help you stay in touch with both your personal and professional identity throughout your practicum/internship process.

Genuineness

A natural part of the practicum/internship process involves learning from other therapists and incorporating certain models of therapy and their accompanying philosophies and techniques into your work with clients. This is all about testing what you are learning, so it is expected that you will go through trial runs with different theories and ways of being as a therapist. We will talk more about the ins and outs of this process in Chapter 7.

Just because this process is expected, however, doesn't mean that it is necessarily going to be easy. Sorting through all of what you have learned in the classroom and the feedback you will be receiving from on-site therapists and your supervisor is no small feat. We fully expect that this will be a confusing experience at times. That is why we want to talk about genuineness.

Genuineness is the noun version of genuine, which has a few definitions in *Merriam-Webster*'s online dictionary. The one we want to focus on is the following: "sincerely and honestly felt or experienced" (Merriam-Webster, n.d., Definition 1c). When describing genuineness, *Merriam-Webster* states that synonyms for genuineness include sincerity, honesty, integrity, and truthfulness.

Being genuine is one of the core conditions put forth by Carl Rogers, who also talked about this concept in terms of **congruence** (Rogers, 1961). His thoughts were that when you, as therapist, were real with your client, they were more willing and able to be real. As he explained,

> It has been found that personal change is facilitated when the psychotherapist is what he *is*, when in the relationship with his client he is genuine and without "front" or façade, openly being the feeling and attitudes which at that moment are flowing *in* him.
>
> (Rogers, 1961, p. 61)

This will be something that will change the course of your therapy. You are allowed to bring your personality into the room. It is the person-to-person encounter that is at the core of therapy. That happens when you are yourself while also using all of your therapeutic skills.

Throughout your journey of navigating the feedback from your supervisor/other therapists and the knowledge you have obtained from your classroom studies, we also believe it is necessary to consider your genuineness as a person and as a therapist as well. You need to be truthful and honest with yourself about what feedback or theories resonate with you because—spoiler alert—not all of it will resonate with you. You have to be sincere with yourself and hold onto your integrity. Essentially, you need to stay true to yourself in the midst of the learning and information/opinion overload that you will experience at your practicum/internship site.

We want to give an example of the genuineness that we are talking about. We knew a practicum student who went into the therapy room and was professional but too professional. She never brought *herself* into the room. She could perform all of the skills of therapy and she could conceptualize the case, but what she was not doing was being a human being who was in contact with another human being while in the therapy room. She believed she had to behave in the role of a mental health professional. Unfortunately, she had forgotten one of the important parts of being a therapist: Whatever skills and models you use have to come through you. You are the most important therapeutic tool. It took her a while to shed the misconception that you couldn't be you in the therapy room. When she did, she was able to relax, and the skills flowed more smoothly through her, and her therapy improved.

While you should change some of your behaviors when you go into the therapy room, you don't need to change your personality. If you are humorous, you can continue to be this way. You just might tone it down a little bit when in the therapy room, especially with some clients who won't appreciate it at that moment. We want to make it clear: There is a difference between your personality and the presentation of your personality. Allow your personality to come through in therapy while appropriately monitoring the behaviors of how you are doing so. Context is important. How you are with your parents, partner, friend, and client will be different. Yet you should still bring yourself to every one of these encounters.

Tales From the Field: Intern

The process of knowing yourself as a therapist while you are a student intern is as if you are a tadpole seeing all the other metamorphosed creatures wading through the water with acute agility and confidence. As a tadpole, you start to look at your lack of limbs and fin and feel less than, as if you will never be able to transition to a frog. But I am here to assure you that it's all an illusion. Confidence and agility will naturally come with time, but ultimately, the more I practice therapy with clients, the more I realize that a core element of it is just being a genuine person with other human beings. I have found that being present and authentic with your clients will earn you a one-way ticket to their inner world and to your understanding of yourself as a therapist.

This authenticity has also helped clue me in on the more specific elements of therapy (e.g., my preferred therapeutic model) that I align with. I discovered that I am able to determine a lot about who I am as a therapist by the way I run group sessions, for example. I tend to focus heavily on having discussions, building rapport, and creating connections rather than always abiding by a structured and activity-driven session. As a result, most of my current clients want me to guide their group therapy sessions because I allow them the space to be themselves while still tying it back to a therapeutic topic. This is not to say I do not involve any interventions but rather that I enjoy implementing them in a seamless manner so the teenagers I work with feel a sense of ease, comfort, and understanding. Meeting clients where they are at and working with what they enjoy doing can be more therapeutic than using a worksheet they will often throw away immediately after a group session. I have found that this genuine approach I have as a person has informed the way I am as a therapist.

Connected to this concept of being authentic with clients (and with myself) is the concept of self-reflection. I can sometimes get in my head about whether I am in the right field, whether I am doing the right thing in the therapy room, and so on. This leads to a lot of questioning about who I am as a budding therapist. Getting feedback from supervisors and peers, however, gives me insight into what I am doing well and what I can improve on. Having a supervisor "hype" me up is riveting and reinstates my drive to continue helping and doing the work that I do. It is a positive way to use self-reflection in the pursuit of knowing my personal and therapeutic selves better. Overall, knowing yourself as a therapist is a never-ending journey, but I have found that being your genuine self and tapping into the feedback and support at your site are steps that make the process easier and more meaningful.

Alexandra Pestano, MS in Counseling program, Clinical Mental Health Counseling concentration, Nova Southeastern University

Personal Therapy

The first formal model of therapy was psychoanalysis. When therapy started, with Freud's approach of psychoanalysis, training was needed not only to learn how to do therapy but for the therapist's personal growth as well. Psychoanalysts had to go through their own analysis. This was partly to ensure that they did not engage in **countertransference**, in which their own issues might find their way into the therapy room and negatively influence what was happening. Based on this notion of decreasing chances of countertransference, many psychotherapy training programs had a mandate that student therapists had to go for their own therapy. In recent years, this obligation has decreased. However, we think that if you are not or have not gone for your own therapy, you might consider doing so.

There are several benefits to going to your own therapy as a student therapist. First, you could potentially resolve many of your own issues that might negatively impact the therapy you provide to your clients. Second, you could get to know yourself better. Last, being a client provides you—as a therapist in other contexts—a better appreciation of the experience of the people with whom you work. You get to see what it's like being on the other side.

Personal therapy for psychotherapists can be considered a form of professional development as it increases the person's self-awareness, self-reflexivity, and self-knowledge (Moe & Thimm, 2021). Another benefit for you of being a client is that you get to see what things are like on the other side of the therapy room. When you are the therapist, you are in the power position of the therapeutic relationship. When client, the conversation is all about you and your growth as a person and problem resolution. This focus is impactful. Being the client allows you the experience of your current and future clients. You can see aspects of therapy that you like and don't like, which can inform how you are with your clients when you are in the therapist role.

For instance, as a client, your therapist might start each session with ten minutes of deep breathing together. You then determine whether you like this or not. If not, you probably won't do this practice with your own clients. Further, you might start your sessions by asking your clients how they would like to begin rather than imposing how you want to start.

Here are a few questions for you to consider when thinking about whether you will go for your own therapy:

- What would I like to change about myself?
- How might going to therapy be useful for me as a therapist?
- What are a few of the triggers and/or biases that I find myself experiencing?
- What do other people say about me and my ways of interacting that they think I could improve on?
- How can I explore aspects of myself that I'm not fully aware of right now?

We understand that, if you are like we are/were in graduate school, finances can be an issue. And therapy, at least if you go to private practice, can be quite expensive. There is likely good news on this front. Your university should be like most universities in that they have a student counseling center. Here is an opportunity for you to receive free therapy services (we are not guaranteeing that every university provides free therapy for students, but more and more are doing so as they see the benefit of positive mental health for their students). Even online universities tend to have programs that will connect you to therapy services. Depending on your university, you might have limited or unlimited sessions. We know some universities specify ten sessions while others provide as many as you want. Given that you most likely have free access to therapy services, our question to you is, what is stopping you from going online, finding the phone number or online registration form, and making an appointment?

Self-Compassion

As a therapist, you learn how to think about other people not as problems but as human beings who are struggling to deal with the contexts of their lives. You develop compassion for other people. The person that you might have the least compassion for is yourself. Another way we can talk about this is giving yourself some grace. **Self-compassion** is a recognition of our humanity in which not only do we accept our experiences as they are, but we also engage ourselves with warmth and tenderness (Neff, 2015). Self-compassion is difficult since most of us tend to utilize self-criticism as a primary way of self-engagement (Schwartz, 2015).

One way of engaging in self-compassion is going for your own therapy. Other ways include prioritizing self-care, challenging negative self-talk, and appreciating various aspects of yourself. Depending on your connection to yourself, you may be more quickly able to practice self-compassion. One recommendation is for you to think of it as a skill. As we know, skills take time and practice to build up.

Quick Tip: When you find yourself chastising yourself for making an error, take a second and change your self-talk. Think about what you would say to a close friend if they were experiencing something similar and say that to yourself. You are likely to be much more forgiving and compassionate to yourself that way.

Knowing Yourself While Giving Co-Therapy

We noted in Chapter 1 that depending on your practicum/internship site, you might be working with another therapist in some scenarios. For example, perhaps you shadow a licensed therapist or you conduct sessions or groups with another student intern. Lagogianni et al. (2023) discussed that co-therapy can be a therapeutic resource in and of itself as it allows therapists to model positive behavior to their clients, bounce ideas off one another, and grow together during sessions. Lagogianni et al. also addressed the challenges that often accompany co-therapy, such as when each therapist is trying to gain control and practice therapy their way (as each clinician is different in their approach, both in terms of preferred theory and personality).

This brings up the necessary task of presenting as a team to your clients while still staying true to yourself. One way to do this is to establish trust with your co-therapist (Lagogianni et al., 2023). When this is the foundation of the co-therapist relationship, it is much easier to talk with one another about how each person wants to approach the session. Even if you both usually utilize different models, for example, you can openly discuss your hopes for the session beforehand and ask your co-therapist to work within a certain model that you think may be appropriate and helpful for your shared client.

Another common concern that comes up with co-therapy is when one therapist has a more outgoing personality and the other therapist has a more reserved personality. When there is an imbalance, the therapist who is more outgoing tends to dominate the sessions compared to their more reserved counterpart. This creates a skew in the co-therapist relationship, and clients often notice this and perceive one therapist as the leader. How does knowing yourself come into play here? It is your responsibility to notice this imbalance happening in the therapy room, know what type of person you are, and then talk openly with your co-therapist about this. It is partially your responsibility to regulate yourself a bit: If you recognize that you are speaking over and interrupting your co-therapist because you are usually the leader in situations, then it is important for you to scale back. Inversely, it is also your co-therapist's responsibility to then insert themselves into sessions more.

Family-of-Origin Work

Who you are now is the amalgamation of the whole of your life. However, much of it was formed early on while you were growing up. As family therapists, we can't help but think that your **family-of-origin** was the medium through which you began to learn about who you are. These early attachments and dynamics helped to shape the construction of your personality. Taking some time to explore your family of origin can be useful for you to understand how you currently engage with people. Let's rewind the clock and trace the roots of your current you.

A great way to do this is through a **genogram**, which was a key conceptualization tool in Murray Bowen's work (see Kerr & Bowen, 1988; McGoldrick et al., 2020). You may have learned about genograms in your coursework. As a refresher, a genogram is essentially a family tree/map that allows someone to visually see the network of one's family, including deaths, marriages, divorces, relationship qualities, and more. Through the analysis of your own genogram, you can reflect on your family patterns and relationship dynamics to increase your understanding about your current self and even your relationships outside of your family-of-origin. This insight can also apply to how you operate as a therapist in the therapy room. What dynamics are you paying the most attention to? What biases do you notice are coming up based on your own family history/dynamics? What role are you playing in the therapy room, and how does that role relate to the role you played growing up in your household? This process of exploring your family-of-origin takes a lot of time but can be quite valuable for you to see your role in the various relationships you have, even including those with your current clients.

Countertransference

Therapy is for the client, and the therapist's "baggage" should not negatively impact the client. Ethically, you are responsible to ensure that you are doing well enough to provide competent services. For instance, the American Counseling Association (2014, Section C.2.g.) states as follows:

> Counselors monitor themselves for signs of impairment from their own physical, mental, or emotional problems and refrain from offering or providing professional services when impaired. They seek assistance for problems that reach the level of professional impairment, and if necessary, they limit, suspend, or terminate their professional responsibilities until it is determined that they may safely resume their work. Counselors assist colleagues or supervisors in recognizing their own professional impairment and provide consultation and assistance when warranted with colleagues or supervisors showing signs of impairment and intervene as appropriate to prevent imminent harm to clients.

You can see it is extremely important for you to ensure that not only are you functioning well but that your colleagues are as well.

However, sometimes we are not impaired but are negatively impacted by our contact with clients. We usually refer to this process as **countertransference**. Countertransference was first coined by Freud, who explained that it was the therapist's unconscious reactions and unresolved conflicts that were triggered by the client. This has now come to be called classical countertransference. For the most part, psychoanalysts hold that countertransference happening in the therapy room is not good. Conversely, for that model, transference is very good and should be utilized. **Transference** is when the client transfers past unfinished business with a significant individual onto the therapy/therapist. The therapist then helps the client work through the transference. This is beneficial for the client. Countertransference does not include the client but rather is the therapist's unfinished business from past relationships that is impacting the current therapeutic relationship. However, today, countertransference is used a bit more generally, where it refers to the therapist's psychological and emotional reactions to the client (Reiter, 2022).

What Would You Do?: 5.1

You are working with a client where, just before each session you are to have with them, you find your gut tightening up. You are feeling apprehension, and there is a part of you that would prefer not to work with that client. There is not something that the client has overtly done to you, but you are not excited to work with them like you are all your other clients. What would you do? Whom might you talk with about this? How might you change your experience of working with that client?

Now, not all countertransference negatively impacts the therapy. But it can, and if it does, it is your responsibility to address it outside of the session. How do you know if the countertransference you experience is detrimental? Corey et al. (2019) explained, "Destructive or harmful countertransference occurs when a counselor's own needs or unresolved personal conflicts become entangled in the therapeutic relationship, obstructing or destroying a sense of objectivity" (p. 52).

One of the things that can help you deal with countertransference is being more aware of and conceptualizing it (Cartwright et al., 2018, 2021). Reading articles or book chapters or attending workshops related to countertransference can be useful for you to better understand the process. You might also engage in reflective practice. Cartwright et al. (2021) developed a five-component model of countertransference that included origins, triggers, manifestations, effects, and management. The student therapists that they studied used a variety of management techniques when dealing with countertransference, including self-talk, mindfulness and calming strategies, session-specific interventions, and supervision. This last one is extremely important. While your supervisor is not your therapist, having an open conversation about what is happening in the therapy room for you helps bring awareness of this process to you. You may then be better able to manage it or to decide to meet with a therapist to address your past so that it doesn't play such a powerful role in the present during your therapy sessions.

Tips From a Supervisor

Most of the supervisees I have worked with think that there is something wrong with them if they have negative feelings towards a client. This goes beyond not liking what a client has done, such as my supervisees who worked with child sexual abusers or domestic violence perpetrators. You should not like what these people have done. It is bad and wrong and shouldn't be endorsed or accepted. However, they have done these things, so you will have to think about the present and future more than the past.

My main tip here is for you to really try to embrace Carl Rogers' notion of **unconditional positive regard** (Rogers, 1961). What Rogers was talking about was that everyone we come in contact with is worthwhile given that they are a human being. It is respecting them as a person who, if presented with the right conditions, can strive for being better—moving closer to self-actualization. Again, it is not about accepting the thoughts and behaviors that someone has but rather accepting that they are a human being that has thoughts and behaviors, some that we deem socially acceptable and others not. It is also about believing that people can continually grow.

When you can engage a person from a place of unconditional positive regard, you provide them with a safe space to be able to risk exposing themselves to you and to themselves without thinking that they will be judged or chastised. While I am writing this, I am thinking of how easy it is to write it but very difficult to enact because we all have our own lens of morality. It is difficult to not try to change a person who is doing something that you think is very harmful to others. My tip here is to try to embrace engaging people from a place of unconditional positive regard while also being comfortable in challenging their behavior. Most people want to be a good person. It is perfectly fine to use a confrontation in which you show them the discrepancy between their self-concept and their actions. When they are the main ones upset with their behaviors, they will be more likely to change.

Summary

In your therapy program, you have learned about many models and techniques of therapy. However, the most important tool that you have available to you is yourself. It is important for you to be able to know yourself. This comes from engaging in self-of-the-therapist work in which you address who you are, know your biases, and strive to grow. This process of self-improvement will be a key component on your path to increasing your skill as a psychotherapist. There are many ways for you to engage in self-of-the-therapist work, such as exploring your values and triggers, participating in personal therapy, engaging in family-of-origin work, and addressing any countertransference that arises during your work with clients.

References

American Counseling Association. (2014). *2014 ACA code of ethics*. www.counseling.org/resources/aca-code-of-ethics.pdf

Aponte, H. J., & Carlsen, J. C. (2009). An instrument for person-of-the-therapist supervision. *Journal of Marital and Family Therapy, 35*(4), 395–405. https://doi.org/10.1111/j.1752-0606.2009.00127.x

Cartwright, C., Barber, C., Cowie, S., & Thompson, N. (2018). A trans-theoretical training designed to promote understanding and management of countertransference for trainee therapists. *Psychotherapy Research, 28*(4), 517–531. https://doi.org/10.1080/10503307.2016.1252071

Cartwright, C., Hayes, J. A., Yang, Y., & Shires, A. (2021). "Thinking it through": Toward a model of reflective practice for trainee psychologists' countertransference reactions. *Australian Psychologist, 56*(2), 168–180. https://doi.org/10.1080/00050067.2021.1893599

Corey, G., Corey, M. S., & Corey, C. (2019). *Issues and ethics in the helping professions* (10th ed.). Cengage.

Corey, M. S., & Corey, G. (2016). *Becoming a helper* (7th ed.). Cengage.

Corey, M. S., & Corey, G. (2020). *Becoming a helper* (8th ed.). Cengage.

Kerr, M. E., & Bowen, M. (1988). *Family evaluation*. Norton.

Kocet, M. M., & Herlihy, B. J. (2014). Addressing value-based conflicts within the counseling relationship: A decision-making model. *Journal of Counseling & Development, 92*(2), 180–186. https://doi.org/10.1002/j.1556-6676.2014.00146.x

Lagogianni, C., Georgaca, E., & Christoforidou, D. (2023). Co-therapy in open dialogue: Transforming therapists' self in a shared space. *Frontiers in Psychology, 14*, Article 1083502. https://doi.org/10.3389/fpsyg.2023.1083502

McGoldrick, M., Gerson, R., & Petry, S. (2020). *Genograms: Assessment and treatment*. Norton.

Merriam-Webster. (n.d.). Genuine. In *Merriam-Webster.com dictionary*. Retrieved April 13, 2023, from www.merriam-webster.com/dictionary/genuineness

Minuchin, S., Reiter, M. D., & Borda, C. (2021). *The craft of family therapy: Challenging certainties* (2nd ed.). Routledge.

Moe, F. D., & Thimm, J. (2021). Personal therapy and the personal therapist. *Nordic Psychology, 73*(1), 3–28. https://doi.org/10.1080/19012276.2020.1762713

Neff, K. (2015). The 5 myths of self-compassion: What keeps us from being kinder to ourselves? *Psychotherapy Networker*. https://self-compassion.org/wp-content/uploads/2017/08/The_5_Myths_of_SelfCompassion.Psychotherapy.Networker.Sept_.2015.pdf

Reiter, M. D. (2022). *Therapeutic interviewing: Essential skills and contexts of counseling* (2nd ed.). Routledge.

Rogers, C. (1961). *On becoming a person: A therapist's view of psychotherapy*. Houghton Mifflin.

Schwartz, R. (2015). Facing our dark side: Some forms of self-compassion are harder than others. *Psychotherapy Networker*. www.psychotherapynetworker.org/article/facing-our-dark-side

Chapter 6

Navigating Telehealth

Telehealth—therapy sessions conducted electronically through phone call, video, or text message—has become an increasingly common way of providing therapy services, especially since the start of the COVID-19 pandemic (Richartz et al., 2021). Telehealth can provide individuals seeking therapy with the care they need even if they are not able to make it to a physical office location. For example, clients who live in a rural area or who don't have a car often rely on telehealth as their medium through which they are able to see a therapist. Even if clients don't have consistent telehealth sessions, telehealth presents an easy switch from going to the office if the therapist or client is sick or out of town yet still wants to have the session, for instance.

Myths About the Field

"Telehealth sessions are easier than in-person sessions."

We have heard from many beginning therapists that telehealth seems like the easier way to give therapy. You can do it from the comfort of your home instead of coming into the office. You can wear a nice shirt on top and sweatpants on the bottom (another myth that we'll address later), and you don't have to "do" as much because the client isn't there in front of you—you just have to talk. We have seen this is actually the opposite in many cases. For example, a lot of client—especially kids and teens—are actually much harder to keep engaged over telehealth because of other distractions (e.g., we've seen in the reflection of their glasses that they are also playing video games while talking to us). You also have to rethink some interventions that you would have used in person (e.g., a sculpt) and deal with any technical issues that will inevitably happen during some sessions.

Exercise 6.1   Your Beliefs About Telehealth

Telehealth was a fringe medium for psychotherapy before 2020, but the COVID-19 pandemic changed the therapy world, making videoconferencing for therapy sessions much more accessible and accepted. However, it changes some of the vibe of the therapy process. In this exercise, consider your own reactions to telehealth.

DOI: 10.4324/9781003433484-6

1. What are your initial impressions of providing telehealth?
2. What similarities and differences do you see between a therapy session conducted in person or via telehealth?
3. How comfortable and functional are you when using technology?
4. What can you foresee as some potential difficulties when conducting telehealth?
5. What are some potential benefits of therapy via telehealth?

Benefits of Telehealth

Before the COVID-19 lockdown, most therapists were against or apprehensive about conducting sessions via telehealth. One of the arguments against it was that it would not be as effective as in-person sessions. However, recent studies are showing that telehealth is an effective delivery system for psychotherapy (Springer et al., 2020). We already mentioned the convenience of telehealth and the ability of telehealth to provide therapy services when in-person sessions aren't an option.

There are many other benefits of telehealth. Botaitis and Southern (2020) provided several of these benefits:

- Identifying a compatible therapist
- Avoiding a sense of stigma or personal failure
- Maintaining privacy and confidentiality
- Avoiding multiple or conflicting relationships or roles
- Solving logistical problems with time/place
- Reducing financial costs or losses

In terms of ethics, Stoll et al. (2020) explained that the top five ethical arguments for telehealth included (a) increased access, availability, and flexibility of services; (b) therapy benefits and enhancements in communication; (c) client characteristics—especially those who are homebound and mobility impaired; (d) convenience and comfortability; and (e) economic advantages.

Challenges of Telehealth

While our field is finding more and more benefits of telehealth, challenges also come from this type of medium. Some of these challenges are related to the logistics of telehealth. For instance, we have both had telehealth sessions in which either our or the client's Wi-Fi wasn't working. In these situations, we often have had to spend a good chunk of the session rejoining the session/restarting our routers or repeating what we said so the other person could hear us.

We also mentioned the increased distractibility that can result from telehealth sessions. We have found that clients are more likely to engage in normal life tasks when they do therapy via telehealth versus in person because they have access to these tasks. Kayleigh once had a client join their scheduled telehealth session while she was actively working as an Uber driver! Needless to say, Kayleigh did not allow the session to happen until the client was alone and parked somewhere safe.

Stoll et al. (2020) also provided several ethical arguments against telehealth. The top five included (a) privacy, confidentiality, and security issues; (b) therapist competence and training; (c) communication issues, especially the reduction of nonverbal cues; (d) research gaps, as telehealth is quite a new phenomena; and (e) emergency issues, including crisis issues such as threat to self or others.

Tales From the Field: Intern

At first, when I was introduced to the idea of doing practicum virtually via offering telehealth to clients contacting the Community Counseling Service at Our Lady of the Lake University, I was thrilled. I thought about all the positive aspects. As a student, this included avoiding a long commute to the clinic, allotting more time for studying, and learning how to manage a therapy session through a medium that is becoming widespread. It was not until the practicum started that all the pros I thought about telehealth got clouded by the cons. I felt I lacked control over the many variables that could present in each therapy session, including being in different settings, missing non-verbal cues, and running into language barriers (as I am an international student whose first language is not English).

Just imagine what a surprise it was to hear some clients joining me on Zoom to say, "I am not going to turn on my camera" or "I am dropping off my child, but we can start. I am driving, but I am almost there." On other occasions, the conversation during the session turned into "Can you hear me?"; "I cannot hear you, my phone has a bad connection"; "Can you wait? I need to answer this phone call"; "Can you repeat? I cannot understand you well—there is background noise, and you have an accent." Prior to the start of the scheduled appointment, I found myself hoping that the client is safe at home, is using the computer rather than the phone to avoid getting disconnected, and is going to turn on their camera. This way, I can gain more information about the client, making it easier to match words to lip movements.

Of course, I had to come up with a strategy to navigate these challenges that could show up during telehealth sessions. The first thing I started to do was change my mindset and adapt. With practice, I became comfortable with asking questions such as "Are you in a safe place?"; "Could you park the car in a safe spot?"; "Can you join the virtual therapy session when you are safe at home?"; or "Do you prefer to reschedule?" Still, the main challenge remains in meeting a client that refuses my invitation to turn on the camera and leaves me having to talk to a black screen, especially when it is a new client. Not being able to give a face to a voice and not having cues of any sort besides changes in the client's speech (e.g., speed, pitches, word repetition) became an interesting hurdle because the main risk for me was making assumptions. To address this, I found a technique to improve my listening skills. I started to simply listen to the video recording of other therapy sessions while blindfolded. This allowed me to practice and become more confident in my listening skills, perceptions, and language.

I still vividly remember the most challenging session I had with a client that I will name Stu. It was a rainy Tuesday evening, and I was already trembling because it was my turn to see the client. I was going over the repertoire of things that could happen and prayed for them not to occur. I guess it was not my lucky day, or at least that's what I thought at the beginning. Stu's name appeared in the bottom left corner of my screen, but I could not see anything. So I said hello, introduced myself, asked the client about their preferred name, and then with crossed fingers I asked, "Stu, can you turn on your camera?" With a soft voice, Stu stated, "I'd rather keep it off." I answered that it was okay, and I tried my best during the joining portion of the session to make him feel comfortable and to build a therapeutic alliance so that he could trust me and maybe turn on the camera later. We chatted for a bit about his interests, his job, family, and friends, prior to asking what brought him to therapy now and what he hoped to gain from the session. His tone of voice became even lower, and he started to talk about his medical condition, his problematic relationship with his father, and his depression. There were long pauses, and I was paying attention to each silence but also to his voice changes and if there was some sobbing. Because in front of me, there was just a black screen, and I did not want to dismiss Stu's emotionality. Each time there was a long pause, I would acknowledge the situation, giving a reflection prior to asking a question. It was almost halfway through the session that I got the courage to ask Stu if what we had talked about so far has been helpful, and to my surprise he answered something along the lines of, "Yes, I feel listened to. Usually, people get annoyed and make assumptions about me. The truth is that I am confined in bed and in pain, and I did not want to get judged by my appearance or status." Stu then added, "You did not bombard me with questions, and you gave me time to be myself. You were open and understanding, and you did not cut me off as my dad does when we talk on the phone." The counseling session went on until the time was up. Prior to saying good-bye, Stu had decided to turn on the camera, allowing me to see him. Looking back at that session, I think that practicing with the recording provided me with confidence in my listening skills. Observing my colleagues during their telehealth sessions and attempting to see how clients could react gave me the opportunity to improve my soft skills as a psychologist in training.

Grazia Raineri Acosta, PsyD Counseling Psychology program, Our Lady of the Lake University

Telehealth Sessions

Your Setting

Sometimes you may conduct telehealth sessions while being physically located at your practicum/internship site. There are times when in-person clients call last minute and request a telehealth session (because they are sick or running late, for example). There are also times when you have a telehealth session in between in-person sessions and have to be at your practicum/internship site anyway. There are other times, however, in which you are going to conduct telehealth sessions from the comfort of your own home.

Usually, we would not invite a client to our house (although Freud's office was in his home, and other therapists do have a special therapy office in their house). However, when the video camera turns on, the client now has potential information about you that they would not have if the session were in a standard office. Given this, we'd like to take a few moments to talk about where you are conducting the telehealth session from and ideas for you to consider based on your location.

You have the option to have your normal background or a virtual background. There are pros and cons for either. If you decide to use your normal background, consider what the client will see. We recommend that you ensure that they cannot see certain areas of your home such as your bed or your kitchen. Seeing your kitchen may be a little too informal, and seeing your bed may lead them to think about you being in that bed, which can bring up relational dynamics that you do not want. Try to find a neutral area. However, it will also need to be an area that will not have any human traffic in it (we will discuss ethics related to telehealth later on).

When using a virtual background, choose one that is professional. Perhaps you can find a background that looks like a business office to try to approximate a typical session. Just a note of caution here: Some people think that the virtual background will prevent the client from seeing what is behind the person on the screen. This is not always the case. One of Michael's supervisees utilized a virtual background, but when she moved, the computer program would lose the background, and her real background became visible. The client was then able to see the student's unmade bed.

While people may commonly use virtual backgrounds in an effort to hide their actual background (which, as we mentioned, we caution), they can sometimes get in the way of the therapeutic process. For example, you may do an intervention that requires you and your client to stand up, or you may want to pick something up and show it to the client (e.g., a worksheet). If your virtual background is on, it will be unlikely that the client will be able to clearly see whatever it is you are doing/want to show them. This brings up two main points: (a) Make sure you are familiar with the telehealth platform you are using to turn off the virtual background when necessary and (b) make sure you are not using the virtual background to hide your actual background. You don't want to get stuck not knowing how to turn off a virtual background in the middle of a session and wind up wasting session time trying to figure it out. Additionally, as we mentioned, the client should see a clean, neutral space behind you if you turn that virtual background off during the session.

Another point to consider when using virtual backgrounds is how they can make the person on the screen seem unreal. We can usually tell when someone is using a virtual background (besides that we know they are not standing in front of a mountain or the Golden Gate bridge). Movements come across differently as the distinction between the person and the background, depending on the quality of the computer and the program, becomes blurred.

Not only does the background of your screen during a telehealth session need to be professional, but your clothing does as well. During the pandemic, you may have heard or known of some people being able to work online from home in their pajamas (maybe we are referring to you right now!). This was considered a silver lining for some during the pandemic. However, you need to present professionally in terms of your wardrobe even from the comfort of your own home. Now, we know what you might be thinking: "I will just wear a professional top. I can wear comfy pants because no one will see the bottom half of my body on the screen." We regret to inform you that this is probably not a smart move.

For example, we both utilize an experiential technique called a sculpt in which—when using it with individuals—the therapist stands up, has the client stand up with them, and then instructs the client to put themself in a physical pose that represents their current experience. We have used this technique through telehealth, so that means the majority of our bodies become visible on the screen. This would be an awkward technique to engage in if we were wearing a nice button-down shirt or blouse but had gym shorts on instead of work pants. If you decide to utilize a movement-based technique (or if the therapist with whom you sit in on sessions decides to use one), then you are going to find yourself in a pickle if you aren't dressed appropriately. Just save yourself the trouble and dress as if you were going in person to your site.

Tips From a Supervisor

In my experience, telehealth is a bit deceptive. You are not going into an office, so you think that you don't have to set the stage like you do in person. I've seen some student therapists come to their telehealth sessions in a button-down shirt, tie, and jacket. There is something that seems a bit off with such formal dress for telehealth, whereas it would seem okay for a face-to-face session. However, I've also seen things go quite the other way. Some of my supervisees, when I was doing live supervision on telehealth, would enter the meeting wearing quite casual clothing, such as a sweatshirt or T-shirt. Just like I've done in the university clinic, I told them they would not be going into the therapy room dressed so informally. In live sessions, I've given an extra polo shirt I had to a therapist dressed in a T-shirt. The benefit of telehealth is the therapist can take just a minute and go to their closet and change. By dressing professionally, you put yourself into a more professional mindset. My tip is this: Don't think that just because you are doing telehealth that all the rules that you had in the clinic change. Prepare yourself as you would normally, including your hair, clothing, and attitude.

Navigating Different Telehealth Platforms

The boom in utilizing telehealth as an option for conducting therapy naturally came with a boom in the telehealth platform options that therapists can choose from. While the choices can seem overwhelming at first, there are a few tips we want to go over to hopefully provide some ease and clarity.

Your practicum/internship site likely has a telehealth platform that they already utilize. This means you won't have to worry about picking a telehealth platform at all. You will simply need to learn how to use their chosen platform. It might be a familiar platform such as Zoom or Microsoft Teams. It might also be a telehealth platform internal to the electronic medical record (EMR)/electronic health record (EHR) system that your site utilizes to electronically access each client's chart (which contains consent forms, progress notes, the calendar, etc.).

Now, as we will detail further in Chapter 10, you might come across a situation in which your site is not using a confidential telehealth platform. While we hope this does not happen to you, it is important to address it here anyway in case it does. If you find out or believe that the telehealth platform your site uses is not Health Insurance Portability and Accountability Act (HIPAA) compliant (PHIPA in Canada), talk to your supervisor about it. Consult with them first to determine if the platform is actually HIPAA compliant or not. If you both determine that it is not, then you will obviously consult further with your supervisor about what to do next. Again, we will use Chapter 10 to give a more in-depth explanation on what these next steps may look like. We wanted to bring this point up here in order to stress the importance of utilizing HIPAA-compliant telehealth platforms.

Navigating the Technology Behind Telehealth

It is obvious that in order to engage in telehealth sessions with our clients, we need to use technology. Michael was a supervisor, and Kayleigh was a student intern in his practicum when telehealth really took off because of the COVID-19 pandemic, so we both had to—in some ways—relearn how to engage in therapy through the use of technology. The specifics of the technology you may use (e.g., Apple versus Microsoft products) are beyond the scope of this book; however, we do want to comment on some general uses of technology that may help if your practicum/internship site utilizes telehealth sessions.

This one may seem obvious, but we recommend that you keep a charger next to your device when you conduct telehealth sessions. We both know several students who didn't realize that their computer was low on battery, and their laptop died in the middle of session. While mistakes happen, it is better to get out in front of one that is easily preventable to present as professional and prepared as possible.

Before beginning any telehealth sessions, it is also important to make sure both your device and the specific telehealth application you will be using are fully updated. We can't tell you how many people we know (including us) who have logged into a meeting at the time of the session only to see that they needed to update Zoom and then ran a few minutes late. Again, it seems like a small thing, but it's something that you can prevent from happening beforehand.

This brings up another good point: Familiarize yourself with the telehealth platform before using it for a session. Some of the techniques you will use via teletherapy will be different from in-person therapy; for example, you would probably use the telehealth platform's whiteboard function (if it has one) instead of a physical whiteboard in an office. It is going to be helpful to know these functions of the platform beforehand, and you might even come across situations in which the platform does not have a particular function you were banking on it having. You'll then have to rethink the logistics of some interventions. Additionally, you want to be able to know how to change a background, let someone in the meeting, direct message someone, or whatever else the platform offers. This will prevent you from being flustered and wasting session time if you wait to figure it out during a session.

No matter how much you can prepare, there are going to be hiccups that you can't avoid when utilizing technology. You can still have a plan set when these issues happen during your therapy sessions, however. Some practicum/internship sites will have a plan in place for any technical issues that occur. For example, if either the client or therapist gets disconnected during the session, the site may have a policy in place that if the client or therapist doesn't log back on within five minutes, they would call one another to figure out a game plan from there.

Ethics of Telehealth

There are a few ethical considerations regarding telehealth sessions that are helpful to be aware of before starting your practicum/internship. The first relates back to your physical setting during a telehealth session: Confidentiality needs to be maintained whether you are doing an in-person session at the office or a telehealth session at home. Sometimes, we can't help certain things about our home setting (e.g., living with another person). What we can help is how we maintain the confidentiality of our sessions even if they are conducted via telehealth with these extra factors in play.

First, make sure you do the session in a separate room with the door closed. You can't be conducting a telehealth session in your living room with your partner visible in the kitchen making dinner. Second, get a sound machine. Your site should have these as well, as they create background noise that prevents others from hearing you and your client talk even behind a closed door. Put this sound machine outside of the room in which you are conducting the session. Third, let anyone you live with know when you will be doing sessions. This way, they know that they need to keep it down while you are in session. It also lets them know that they cannot enter the room you are in while in session.

If these actions can't realistically be put into place in order to maintain confidentiality, then you might unfortunately have to reconsider whether it is appropriate for you to conduct telehealth sessions at home. For example, there are some student interns who have children and cannot prevent their children from coming into a room if there is no other adult home to watch them (as locking the door with no child supervision is unsafe). While it may be an inconvenience to have to go into the office for telehealth sessions (and hire a babysitter), it is something we need to take seriously as therapists and make the appropriate sacrifices for if necessary.

As therapists, we also have to determine if telehealth is even appropriate for our clients. This is a part of the varying ethical guidelines in each of the differing mental health field standards, including American Association for Marriage and Family Therapy (AAMFT) (2015, Standard 6.1), the American Counseling Association (ACA) (2014, Section H.4.c.), and the American Mental Health Counselors Association (AMHCA) (2020, Standard 6c). While telehealth practices are not addressed in the American Psychological Association's (APA) Ethical Principles of Psychologists and Code of Conduct, they are addressed in their Guidelines for the Practice of Telepsychology (American Psychological Association, 2017).

There are certain factors that we need to consider when making this determination, such as the client's need for telehealth, potential for harm to self or others, and client engagement and distractibility. For example, as mentioned, adolescent clients (or really any client) can sometimes struggle with staying engaged through a computer screen and are commonly on screens for a good chunk of the day anyway. In these scenarios, it is likely to be more therapeutically beneficial for them to come in person. If they are able to make it in person (i.e., there is not an explicit need for telehealth), these types of clients should probably physically come to the office. The same goes for a client who has suicidal ideation—these are usually more intense cases that require in-person therapy.

These are considerations that need to be made if a client at your site is asking for telehealth or is currently a telehealth-only client. If you are wondering about the appropriateness of telehealth for a client, talk to your supervisor about it and refer to your field's ethical guidelines for telehealth.

For student interns and those in pursuit of full licensure, there are laws that outline the legality of engaging in telehealth as well. For example, we are both located in Florida where the law stipulates that registered interns are able to provide telehealth services by themselves if they have certain precautions in place, such as having a safety plan and telehealth protocol, being able to contact their supervisor if needed during a session, and determining that telehealth is appropriate for the client. These are laws that you need to review for your state. Your program most likely discussed these laws in whatever ethics course they provided. If they didn't, you need to research them.

Overall, you should continuously consult with your supervisor about what we have listed previously. These telehealth considerations can be confusing for new therapists in training, so asking questions and consulting is one of the best ways to stay informed and be sure you are conducting yourself in an ethical way. In addition to consulting with your supervisor, you also have to be knowledgeable on the laws in your particular state. We have provided examples from the perspectives of Florida-based therapists. Unlike Florida, however, some states do not even allow for student interns or registered interns to engage in telehealth sessions. We are also writing about these ethical considerations at a certain point in time—the laws that go behind some of these ethical considerations may change by the time you even pick up this book.

Tales From the Field: Supervisor

In the realm of telehealth, where therapists like Dana connect with clients through screens and communicate via text, Dana faced a common yet sometimes complex dilemma that tested her abilities as a therapist. This tale underscores the nuanced challenges that therapists are more frequently encountering when seeing clients online.

Dana had been diligently working with her client, Phil, a middle-aged man navigating the turbulent waters of a breakup. Through solution-focused brief therapy, she had been helping him regain a sense of direction and hope for the future. However, a persistent issue had emerged—Phil's habit of texting Dana between sessions with personal reflections, self-help articles, and emotional triggers. Despite Dana's boundaries to reinforce appropriate technological communication between therapy sessions (such as confirmation of appointments or schedule changes via text), Phil continued to cross them.

During a supervisory session, Dana and I, her faculty supervisor, recognized that the telehealth setting amplified this issue. We talked about how the lack of physical proximity was most likely part of what prompted Phil to reach out more frequently and intensively. When a client does not see their therapist in person, it can sometimes create an unspoken expectation from the client that they are able to reach out to their therapist in between sessions more frequently. Additionally, even though texts in between sessions may not technically be full telehealth sessions, therapists now often face that technology-based boundary crossing that texting commonly allows for. We understood that this dynamic between her and Phil could potentially lead to miscommunication and harm if left unaddressed, especially given the challenges some clients face in adapting to the technology and the potential for it to be misunderstood and misused.

With this in mind, we approached the situation with sensitivity and decided that a clear conversation with Phil about the boundaries in their therapeutic relationship was needed. We explained to Phil that his messages, while well-intentioned, were not appropriate for the outpatient care he was receiving, even if this care was through telehealth rather than in person. Phil, seemingly understanding, agreed to comply. Dana was further tested in the future when Phil left her a voicemail a bit later into treatment. Again, the boundaries of this action were clearly discussed with Phil, and

Dana made sure to not waver in these boundaries. It can become quite easy for therapists to immediately respond to their clients' technology-based communication. It is important that therapists—especially student therapists entering into this world—slow down, take a breath, and think through their communication with their clients to establish clear boundaries. These were all decisions that tested Dana's resolve as a therapist and reminded her of the complex nature of her profession, specifically in navigating telehealth.

Limor Ast, DMFT, LMFT, Department of Couple and Family Therapy, Nova Southeastern University

Navigating the Therapy Part of Telehealth

One thing that we've experienced and heard from other therapists is that, during telehealth, they find that there are more potential distractions. Pruitt and Glennon (2023) explained that there are three areas of distraction during telehealth: clinician, client, and technology. **Clinician distractions** are when there are things that happen to you, the therapist, that impede the therapy to some degree. This might be your lack of technology skills, distractions occurring in your home (or wherever you are providing therapy), attempts at multitasking (such as looking at other websites or reading and responding to emails), and screen time fatigue. **Client distractions** occur when the client has a lack of technology skills or there are distractions in their locale, such as phone calls, other people in the house, or even pets (yes, we've seen a lot of times when dogs or cats would try to jump on the client in the middle of a session or start barking). **Technology distractions** happen because of you and/or the client not having high-speed internet, the Wi-Fi going out, or one or both of you not having the technological skills to navigate the platform. Any and all of these distractions create difficulties during a session.

We have already addressed how to prevent/mitigate these distractions when they are the result of the technological hiccups of telehealth. We also want to talk about how to navigate a therapy session when a client gets distracted. There are some scenarios that we have mentioned (e.g., a client playing a video game in the background) that may be easier to handle. A lot of the time, it just takes a quick comment (or even a joke) to bring the client back on track: "I see you are trying to outrun those Creepers in Minecraft. I think they might catch up to you since you are trying to get away from them and listen to me at the same time. Do you mind pausing the game until we finish our session?" Kayleigh is a fan of Minecraft and has said something along these lines to a client before. The client (a teen) laughed and then paused the game and brought her focus back to the session.

There are other times, however, in which a more direct therapeutic conversation may need to happen if the client's distractions are impeding the therapeutic process. Kayleigh once had a client who joined their telehealth sessions from a new location almost every session—for example, outside a library, inside a movie theater, and while driving. While there are some locations (like an empty park) where it is more acceptable to do a telehealth session (after you have documented in your notes that your client stated they are in a confidential spot), there are others (like driving as an Uber driver with a passenger in the car, as mentioned before) that are just not appropriate to conduct a session. Since this client continually puts herself in situations where distractions were abundant and confidentiality was compromised, Kayleigh had a conversation with the client about the importance and necessity of being in a private space moving forward.

One suggestion is for you to learn what the standards of communication are when communicating via telehealth. **Netiquette** is the concept that there are norms and etiquette when interacting online. For instance, DON'T WRITE TO SOMEONE IN ALL CAPS!!! This means that you are yelling at them. Also, think about how close or far you are from your camera as well as how bright the light is in your room. We've seen some therapy sessions where the sun was coming through the window into the therapist's room in such a way that we had to squint since it was so bright. But we've also seen a couple of times when the room was so dark that you couldn't see the details of the therapist's face, similar to what you might see when someone is trying to catfish you and not show you their true appearance. But perhaps our biggest netiquette tip for telehealth is to never conduct therapy with a client while they are driving (or when you are driving). Therapy is a very serious endeavor, likely exploring sensitive and impactful topics. We don't want what we are doing with the client to impact them so they are not focusing on the road, which may potentially lead to an accident that could be life-threatening.

Tips From an Intern

One of the toughest things about doing telehealth for me is not multitasking. I am a multitasker in all aspects of my life—it's not rare to find me doing the dishes while actively cooking and watching TV. Naturally, this habit tries to find its way into telehealth sessions as well. You will see that it becomes very easy to slyly check your email, for example, while you are talking to a client. You have so much in front of you to become distracted by, and the urge to do something else on your computer while you are in a session is going to be present at some point.

My tip consists of two parts. First, give yourself grace when this happens. I think we need to be honest with ourselves here and admit that most therapists (if not every single therapist) have had at least one instance during a telehealth session when they became distracted and multitasked in some way. This does not mean you are a bad therapist; things like this will happen. Second, you then also need to take responsibility for moments like this and take necessary actions to prevent it from happening again. Put your notifications (on both your phone and computer) on Do Not Disturb, close out of or minimize your email and any other open tabs, and keep the telehealth platform in front of you during the entire session. Think about other things you can do that will make it easier for you to not succumb to the temptation to do something else discreetly while in a telehealth session. Keep yourself accountable and be present with your client.

Therapeutic Presence Online

One aspect of therapy that is important is **therapeutic presence**, which is when the therapist is fully engaged in the session and in the here and now. This can sometimes be more difficult when conducting therapy via telehealth, as there are many distracting factors and lack of in-person connections. It will be important for you to think about, before you have your telehealth session, how you can increase your therapeutic presence.

Geller (2021) provided several tips for cultivating therapeutic presence online. First, think about how you can create safety. This includes ensuring that you are utilizing a HIPAA-compliant program and that you are psychologically present when you go online. Second, think about your setup and consistency. Try to maintain the same locale when you meet with your clients, ensuring privacy and minimization of distractions. Third, figure out what the optimal distance is for you as well as your client. You'll want to be far enough away from the screen and camera that you are not filling the client's screen but not too far away that you seem distant. Also, try to look into the camera or very close to it. To do so, move the client's video box as close to your camera as possible so you can see the client's facial features while having it seem like you are giving direct eye contact to the client. If you are taking notes on your computer, have them as close to the camera as possible, so when you look at them it looks like you are looking at the camera. You might consider letting the client know that you will be taking notes, especially if you have a keyboard that makes noise when you type. Michael was supervising an intern who liked to take notes during telehealth sessions. She had the word processing document open on the lower left of her screen, and Michael, as well as the client, could see her eyes frequently move to that location, demonstrating she was paying attention a bit more to the notes than the client. Further, she had quite a loud keyboard (or she typed quite hard) so that even during conversation the keys could be heard being tapped. If you didn't preface this so that the client expected it, they might think that you were online doing something else besides working with them.

A fourth way to enhance therapeutic presence online is to think about the lighting (Geller, 2021). You'll want to move your computer, open or close the blinds, or bring in a lamp so that you are bright enough to be seen but not too bright that it is visually oversaturated. You can encourage the client to do the same. Michael was supervising a telehealth session during which the therapist had their blinds open. It was during the day, and the sun was in just the right position where this aura was behind the therapist's head. It was difficult for the client (or supervisor or other therapists who were watching the session during the team supervision) to look at the client's screen because it was too bright. The last tip Geller (2021) suggested is to dress professionally. Dress as you would if you were to go into the office.

What Would You Do?: 6.1

You are working with a 27-year-old male who is very depressed. He had a suicide attempt one year ago and has been making progress. However, during this week's telehealth session, he tells you that he is psychologically struggling. You begin to do a suicide assessment; however, five minutes in, you notice something strange. Your client hasn't moved in the last couple of minutes. They haven't said anything either. You realize that they are frozen, or really, that something happened to their internet connection and their picture is frozen. After a few more moments, the client is no longer in the session. What do you do?

Telesupervision

The COVID-19 pandemic sparked a switch to the cyberworld for anything that could realistically be accomplished online. That trend has stuck even as we have come back to a mostly pre-COVID lifestyle. This goes for supervision as well—many psychotherapy programs made the switch to online supervision permanent even when regular classes went back to being in person. This is mostly for the convenience of both the supervisors and students.

That means that it is not unlikely for your supervision experience during your practicum/internship to be online at some point. This may be especially true if your supervisor is not affiliated with your site. If your program involves receiving live supervision at your school's therapy clinic, then your supervision will be in person (assuming you are also giving therapy in person at this clinic). However, if you engage in a practicum/internship external to your university, then your supervisor will likely not have direct ties to that site and thus won't be in person at that site. If this is the case, you will probably do supervision via telehealth so you and your supervisor don't have to meet up in person. The good news is that most supervisees find telesupervision to be acceptable or even highly acceptable (Thompson et al., 2022).

Aviram and Nadan (2022) provided three primary challenges of telesupervision: technological skillfulness, scheduling, and limiting intervention. We have already discussed the technological side of telehealth. We will reiterate that it is important for you to know how to navigate online videoconferencing platforms both for when you work with clients but also when you have telesupervision. In terms of scheduling, be mindful of boundaries. Being able to meet virtually sometimes is too great a flexibility in that the workday is not as concrete. Be mindful of your supervisor's schedule. Lastly, as with telehealth, telesupervision isn't able to include as many communication cues, as you are likely seeing only the upper half (or less) of your supervisor (and they you). You will miss out on some nonverbal communication as well as the energy that may be present in in-person supervision.

Self-Care and Telehealth

Being in front of a screen all day sucks. You are sitting and not moving, which is not good for our circulatory systems. Further, you are staring at a screen and could get eye strain or other maladies. In face-to-face sessions, you walk from your office to the waiting room, greet the client, walk them back to your office, have the session, walk them back to the waiting room, and then walk back to your office. There is movement built into this process. In telehealth you sit, click a button to let the client into the videoconferencing platform, have the session, and then click a button to end the therapy. Unfortunately, there is a lack of movement built in. It will be important for you to maintain awareness of yourself during your telehealth sessions to ensure that you are functioning at your peak capacity.

One way to do this is to schedule movement breaks for yourself. At the end of each session, get up and walk around the room or your home for a few minutes. Close your computer as well—get as much time away from the blue light as you can. If you have a longer break in between sessions, we recommend that you don't do any other work on your computer if you are able to help it. Close your eyes, go outside, play with your cat. Just do something else for a bit of time, especially if you have a long day with multiple telehealth sessions. Reflect on and implement any other habits you think would be helpful for you to avoid the often draining nature of technology. If you find that you need more than this, you might consider personal therapy, even personal teletherapy (yes, you need a break from your computer, yet this is a very different context than providing therapy). Botaitis and Southern (2020) view personal telehealth therapy for therapists as a form of self-care as well as career development.

Exercise 6.2   Chair Yoga

A great way to keep your body limber and your blood flowing while doing telehealth sessions is chair yoga. In addition to being a therapist, Kayleigh is also a yoga instructor, so she is going to give you a quick and easy chair yoga lesson for you to do in between telehealth sessions.

1. Sit comfortably with your feet grounded on the floor and your hands in your lap.
2. Start to relax your muscles and take a few deep breaths through your nose. Use your exhales to help release any parts of the body that are tense.
3. Start to make small, slow circles with your head to stretch out your neck. Flow with the breath and go at the speed that feels best for you—listen to your body on what feels good.
4. Bring your head back up to neutral, take a deep breath in, and lift your arms up above your head. Take a few deep breaths here, reaching your arms up high while keeping your shoulders relaxed.
5. Drop your right hand down to grab the seat of your chair, then bend into your right side of the body for a side stretch. Your right elbow will bend a bit, and your left arm will curve to the right as you lean to the side. Take a couple of breaths.
6. Lift everything back up to neutral (i.e., both arms above your head and your torso straight), and then drop your left hand down to grab the left side of the chair and do the same side stretch. Take a couple breaths again.
7. Lift everything back up one more time (arms above your head), and then bend straight forward and reach your arms down to the ground. Don't worry if they can't touch—just hang passively and let your back and neck relax. Take a few breaths.
8. Inhale and slowly roll the spine back up to a regular seated position.

Quick Tip: If you are doing telehealth, make sure you are not doing back-to-back sessions that are 60 minutes in length. Ensure that between each client you have 5 to 15 minutes that, given your physical capabilities, you can stretch, move around, and get your blood pumping.

Summary

In all likelihood, you will be engaged in at least one session of telehealth during your practicum/internship. Even if you are not, it is becoming more and more common in our field. It will therefore be quite useful for you to begin thinking about what the benefits and challenges of telehealth provide for you and your client. In this chapter, we gave some tips to help you navigate the various aspects of conducting telehealth sessions. Hopefully, you will be able to successfully navigate them to provide ethical and effective services for your clients.

References

American Association for Marriage and Family Therapy. (2015). *Code of ethics*. www.aamft.org/Legal_Ethics/Code_of_Ethics.aspx

American Counseling Association. (2014). *2014 ACA code of ethics*. www.counseling.org/resources/aca-code-of-ethics.pdf

American Mental Health Counselors Association. (2020). *AMHCA code of ethics*. www.amhca.org/events/publications/ethics

American Psychological Association. (2017). *Ethical principles of psychologists and code of conduct*. www.apa.org/ethics/code/ethics-code-2017.pdf

Aviram, A., & Nadan, Y. (2022). Online clinical supervision in couple and family therapy: A scoping review. *Family Process, 61*(4), 1417–1436. https://doi.org/10.1111/famp.12809

Botaitis, N., & Southern, S. (2020). Telehealth therapy for therapists: Barriers and benefits. *The Family Journal, 28*(3), 204–214. https://doi.org/10.1177/1066480720934269

Geller, S. (2021). Cultivating online therapeutic presence: Strengthening therapeutic relationships in teletherapy sessions. *Counselling Psychology Quarterly, 34*(3–4), 687–703. https://doi.org/10.1080/09515070.2020.1787348

Pruitt, D. K., & Glennon, A. S. (2023). Self-care for clinicians during remote sessions: Adapting to the new world. *Journal of Human Behavior in the Social Environment, 33*(5), 633–646. https://doi.org/10.1080/10911359.2022.2077499

Richartz, J., Smith, N., Sabo, K., & Mejia, M. A. (2021). Teletherapy in training: A trying and transformative experience. *Journal of Systemic Therapies, 40*(1), 36–51. https://doi.org/10.1521/jsyt.2021.40.1.36

Springer, P., Bischoff, R. J., Kohel, K., Taylor, N. C., & Farero, A. (2020). Collaborative care at a distance: Student therapists' experiences of learning and delivering relationally focused telemental health. *Journal of Marital and Family Therapy, 46*(2), 201–217. https://doi.org/10.1111/jmft.12431

Stoll, J., Müller, J. A., & Trachsel, M. (2020). Ethical issues in online psychotherapy: A narrative review. *Frontiers in Psychiatry, 10*, Article 993. https://doi.org/10.3389/fpsyt.2019.00993

Thompson, S. M., Keenan-Miller, D., Dunn, D., Hersh, J., Saules, K. K., Graham, S. R., Bell, D. J., Hames, J. L., Wray, A., Hiraoka, R., Heller, M. B., Taber-Thomas, S. M., Taylor, M. J., Hawkins, R. C. II, Schacht, R. L., Liu, N. H., Schwartz, J. L., & Akey, E. H. (2022). Preferences for and acceptability of telesupervision among health service psychology trainees. *Training and Education in Professional Psychology, 17*(3), 221–230. https://doi.org/10.1037/tep0000415

Chapter 7

Applying Classroom Learning

So far in your clinical program you have read many books and articles, engaged in hours upon hours of discussions about the material, written many papers and assignments, and perhaps taken a few too many tests. These were all designed to prepare you for the next step—work with real clients. Your academic experience and your clinical experience should not be mutually exclusive. What you learned in the classroom should be pertinent to what you do in the therapy room. Otherwise, why pay all that money, spend all that time, and write all those papers and tests if there isn't a direct connection between the learning that you do in both settings? Dale Carnegie once said, "Knowledge isn't power until it is applied." In this chapter, we discuss how you might think about applying what you learn in class into therapy.

Myth About the Field

"I already learned it in class and did well. That means I know it."

You've probably conducted a bunch of role-plays during your training so far. These are quite useful to get you to start practicing how to apply what you are learning. However, they are done in a controlled environment. You knew that the "client" was your classmate, who was probably making up a problem. This simulated experience was important, but it didn't have the gravitas as a real client does when they are sitting across from you, desperate, expecting you to know what to say and do so that their life is manageable. The application of your class learnings at your practicum/internship, therefore, is likely going to be and feel different.

Microskills

Regardless of the field that you are going into, the foundation of all of therapy is the **microskills** that we use for active listening. These are the skills of paraphrasing and reflecting that are the hallmark of Rogerian person-centered therapy. However, they are also the foundation of every single model and approach of therapy, even if you are not doing therapy but are doing testing or an intake. Let's take a few minutes to go over those skills so that you can better apply them with your clients.

The primary microskills can be found in the **issue cycle** (Reiter, 2022), which comprises a door opener, minimal encouragers, paraphrases, reflections of feeling, reflections of meaning, questions, and summary (see Figure 7.1). The better that you can do them on paper, the

DOI: 10.4324/9781003433484-7

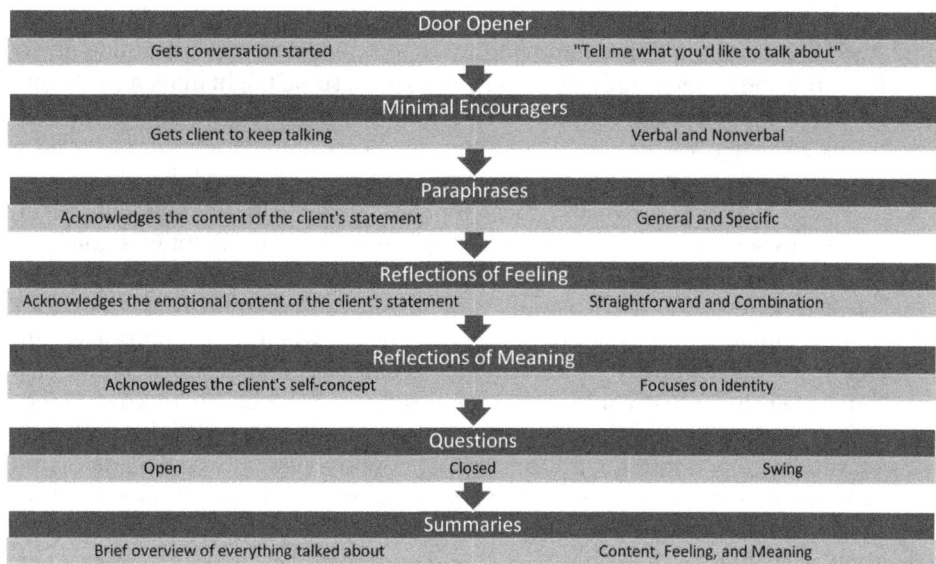

Figure 7.1 The components of the issue cycle are the main microskills that therapists from all fields using any model tend to utilize as the foundation of their work.

better you can think quickly and do them in a real session. Here is your chance to review them one more time.

Door openers get the conversation started. This may be for the whole of the session or for a particular topic. To start the session, your door opener might be, "Tell me what you'd like to talk about today" or "Last week we left off talking about your relationship with your mother. What further thoughts did you have about that?" Many beginning student therapists tend to start their sessions with an opening that we really don't suggest: "How was your week?" There are a few reasons we think this is problematic. First, it is a bit weak. It is as if you are unsure of what to say. Second, there is no direction to the question. It is not related to the therapy process that has already happened. Third, because it is not clearly related to the therapy agenda, it encourages a therapy that doesn't end. The client is always going to have a week. If this opening is continually used, therapy then becomes talking mainly about what happened during the client's week. It will probably be more content than process driven. Our suggestion is to start your door opener, for at least second and subsequent sessions, with some connection to the previous session or the themes you've been highlighting in the therapy. Or if you want to have it a bit more general, then do as the solution-focused therapists do and start your sessions with, "What was better this week?" (Berg, 1994).

Minimal encouragers are small things that we do to let the client know to keep talking in the direction that they are talking. They can be either verbal or nonverbal. If a door opener is the first big push when spinning a basketball on your finger, minimal encouragers are the tiny taps to keep the ball spinning. **Nonverbal minimal encouragers** include eye contact, head nods, and hand motions. **Verbal minimal encouragers** can be as simple as "Mhm" or "Okay" or a bit more lengthy such as "Can you talk more about what it was like when you first realized that this wasn't what you wanted?" You've done verbal and nonverbal minimal encouragers millions of times throughout your life, so it is not a matter of learning the skill. The trick with them is when to use them and when to not. Overuse of them (and any of the microskills) can come across poorly for some clients (e.g., some might think it a bit repetitive if you are constantly nodding your head up and down to everything they say).

Paraphrases are when we let the client know we heard the content of their statement. There are two types of paraphrases. **General paraphrases** wrap everything up as a whole. They are so general that you can use them for most content that clients tell you. These include comments such as: "Wow, that was really rough for you," "A lot was going on," or "That must have been difficult." As you can see, you don't know what the therapist is referring to. This is a benefit of general paraphrases, as you can come up with a slew of them at home and use them with just about all of your clients, when it is appropriate. **Specific paraphrases** let the client know you heard the important parts of their story. Some examples include, "You went home early and found your partner in the bed with your friend. You told them they could have one another and that you were through with both of them" or "This week you failed one test, got a B on a paper, found a new job, and made plans for a vacation." As you can see, you can't preplan your specific paraphrases. They come from the details of what the client says.

Reflections of feeling let the client know you heard the emotional content of what they said. Even if the client isn't overt, every statement they make has an emotional undercurrent. Sometimes hearing their emotionality is quite easy, especially when they say, "I'm so mad" or "I was so sad." Other times you will have to **listen with the third ear**—to hear the unsaid and reflect that to the client. There are two types of reflections of feeling: straightforward reflections and combination reflections. **Straightforward reflections of feeling** just reflect back the feeling. To do them, you can use the cheat sheet: You feel _____. They are quite easy to do: "You feel happy," "You feel sad," "You feel hopeful," "You feel mad," and so on. **Combination reflections of feeling** combine the emotions with the content they are related to. The cheat sheet for them is: You feel _____ because _____. Examples of these include: "You feel angry because your partner cheated on you," "You feel happy because after all of your hard work you passed the course," or "You feel excited because you are going to start college."

Reflections of meaning let the client know you are hearing how what has happened is related to their self-identity and self-concept. This is where the real meat is of the issue cycle, as it is on the level of identity that significant movement happens for the client. Out of all of the skills in the issue cycle, this is the most difficult because it requires that the therapist really gains the depth of the client's experience as to why the situation they are talking about is so important to them. Just like with reflections of feeling, there is a cheat sheet for reflections of meaning: You feel _____ because _____. You're probably saying to yourself, "Hey, that's the same cheat sheet for combination reflections of feeling." You're right. And wrong. The difference comes in what is put into that second blank. Instead of content, it is about identity. This may be about the person's role or self-concept. Some examples of reflections of meaning include: "You feel disappointed because you view yourself as an honest person, yet you find yourself lying to your spouse" or "You feel confused because you want so much to be a loving daughter, but you don't want to be around your mother."

Questions are multivarious and have many purposes throughout the therapeutic process. Questions can take three forms: open, closed, and swing. **Open questions** prompt the client to answer in a lengthier format. They will usually start with "How," "What," or "Why." However, we recommend removing why questions from your repertoire. Why would we say this?

Because the use, and likely overuse, of why questions may lead the client to feel defensive (e.g., "Why do you feel this way?" can seem more like a challenge than a curiosity-based question). Further, clients likely don't know why, which is why they are in therapy. **Closed questions** ask for a specific answer. They usually start with "Is," "Have," "Are," "Do," "Does," "Did," or "Has." For the most part, you should stay away from closed questions because their overuse can feel like an interrogation. Further, if you have a client who may not really want to be in therapy, they may take you up on the closed question and give you a closed answer. After a few minutes, you'll feel like you are pulling teeth. Take the following interchange as an example:

Therapist: Have you decided what to do?
Client: No.
Therapist: Do you have a timeframe for when you want to decide?
Client: No.
Therapist: Is this important to you?
Client: Yes.

After just three interchanges, you are probably already frustrated. So is the client! There are times when asking closed questions is fine (e.g., "Do you have any siblings?" or "Where were you born?"). Then, once they answer, follow it up with one of the other microskills or an open question. **Swing questions** are technically closed questions but are intended as open questions. They tend to start with "Could," "Can," "Will," or "Would." For example: "Could you explain your decision-making process?" or "Will you tell me about what it was like growing up in your house?" The client could answer with "Yes" or "No" but would likely give a lengthier explanation.

Summaries take everything that has been talked about and present it as one package. We recommend that you frame your summary. One way of doing so is: "I want to take a few moments to go over what we talked about to make sure that I have it right." The summary isn't about bringing in any new information but more about presenting the conversation as a whole. The summary has three components: content, feeling, and meaning. It will usually be about five sentences long in which the first two sentences highlight the content, the next two sentences highlight the emotions, and the final sentence focuses on the meaning.

Exercise 7.1   Practicing the Microskills

For the following exercise, insert an appropriate therapist response based on the microskill that is being asked for. Do this exercise twice so that you have more practice developing each skill.

Therapist: (Provide a door opener)
Client: I am really anxious. I am in a relationship, and I don't know if it is right for me or not.
Therapist: (Provide a minimal encourager)
Client: We've been together about a year now, and they are wanting to move in. Not only that, I know that they would want to quickly get married. I like them, but I'm not sure I'm ready for that intense of a commitment.

Therapist: (Provide a general paraphrase)
Client: Yeah. I think we are on two different tempos. I want to be in the relationship, but not if there is going to be so much pressure.
Therapist: (Provide a specific paraphrase)
Client: This is just too much. My last relationship was similar. They kind of smothered me, and I felt like I couldn't breathe.
Therapist: (Provide a straightforward reflection of feeling)
Client: Yes, there are times I want freedom. But I do want connection. I feel lonely when I'm not with someone.
Therapist: (Provide a combination reflection of feeling)
Client: It has been like this for my past three relationships.
Therapist: (Provide an open question)
Client: I don't know. Sometimes I feel like there is something wrong with me that I want to be connected to someone, but I don't like to be too connected. It's like I'm not a good enough partner for someone.
Therapist: (Provide a reflection of meaning)
Client: I haven't fully thought of it like that. But that makes sense.
Therapist: (Provide a summary)

We have presented the skills in this order. You could do it like this in a session, but you don't have to. That is the thing about all of the skills you are learning—they are not just these ones we demonstrated. They are all tools in your therapeutic tool belt. The craft of therapy comes in you figuring out when to bring out each tool and then using it properly. We find this ordering, generally, works well as you move from less intense to more intense information about the client's story. These are the foundational skills. You can use all of them regardless of the therapeutic model you are using or the specific technique such as thought stopping, empty chair, enactments, and more.

Tales From the Field: Supervisor

In our marriage and family therapy program at Our Lady of the Lake University, we embrace Harlene Anderson's (1997) collaborative stance with clients. This form of dialogical practice encourages a conversational partnership or shared inquiry, which Anderson (1997) describes as "an in-there-together, two-way, give-and-take exchange" (p. 112). Regardless of the circumstances, we approach our clients from a curious and not-knowing stance.

How I like to introduce a not-knowing or collaborative stance is by asking the class to raise their hands if they have had some experience of "anxiety." Normally, all students will raise their hands, and we all agree that "anxiety" is a common occurrence with similar characteristics. That is, this is the case until I go around the room (one by one) and ask each student what "anxiety" means to them. We soon realize that "anxiety" has a wealth of different descriptions, meanings, perceptions, and functions. How "anxiety" is understood by one student is often different from how it is experienced by others. This conversation then segues into the idea of a "diagnosis" and how the diversity of lived experiences and meanings of a "diagnosis" may vary across clients.

During a team pre-session at our university clinic, one of my supervisees, Sofia, expressed her concerns with her client's information on his intake form. The client shared that he had a diagnosis of bipolar disorder, which included detailed descriptions of what he identified as "intrusive thoughts, insomnia, and depression." Sofia mentioned that she had never worked with someone with bipolar disorder, so she felt unprepared and questioned her capabilities.

I wondered if Sofia could embrace a collaborative stance and approach this conversation like her other therapeutic conversations from a not-knowing and curious standpoint. If so, what could be her initial inquiry? Sofia mentioned that she was curious about what her client wanted to focus on. During her first session with him, after some initial small chat, Sofia asked him, "What do you hope to get out of this conversation?" The client shared that work had recently become overwhelmingly stressful, which was affecting his mood and sleep. Their conversations mostly revolved around exploring different relaxation exercises to enhance sleep. Although he did bring up his diagnosis, the client's goals and concerns were like many of our other clients who have a wide range of difficulties affecting their well-being, regardless of a diagnosis. This was quite a learning experience for Sofia. She realized that her pathological understanding of bipolar disorder initially overwhelmed her curiosity about her client's unique experiences and personal goals. However, Sofia discovered a practical use for her classroom learnings and discussions. Her ability to embrace a not-knowing stance facilitated a co-construction of the client's desired goals and outcomes. Sofia also realized that intake forms don't tell the full story. They can oftentimes mislead our assumptions and curiosities about our clients.

Carlos Ramos, PhD, LMFT, Marriage and Family Therapy program, Our Lady of the Lake University

Book Learning to Application

You have read thousands of pages describing case conceptualization, clinical issues to think about, and skills to utilize. You have written papers about this material, had class discussions, and even taken tests to demonstrate that you know it. That is all well and good. Being a good therapist on paper is one thing. Now, in your practicum/internship placement, it is imperative that you can apply your classroom learning. Otherwise, your client won't be helped.

However, you might have read so much that it all jumbles together. For many of us, we read and study so that we can succeed on a paper or a test, and then that material seems to magically evaporate from our brains. Yet we don't know that we don't really know it anymore. Now, it is not really that we don't know it but that we don't have a direct pathway of accessing the material. Just like in therapy where one of the primary therapeutic tools is repetition, the same can be said for how you can apply your book learning to your clinical work. Going over something once will likely not provide sufficient depth for you to really understand and remember that material. Thus, it is imperative that you read the material and then reread the material and perhaps read it again. We know what you are going to say: "I hardly had enough time the first time I had to read it, let alone time to reread it." Yes, and how can you find the time? Where might you be able to sneak 5, 10, or 20 minutes in to read? Might you record yourself reading the material the first time and then listen to that recording while you are cooking, cleaning, or driving?

Whatever field of therapy you are studying, there are certain models of therapy that you have been learning about. Your field placement is the opportunity for you to connect the microskills that all therapists utilize with the specific models of your discipline. You may have learned the terms of the model but haven't had to implement them yourself. Now, during your practicum/internship, there is that expectation. This will be a challenge for you. How do you enact the theory in your style? Many therapists can use the same model but will do so differently since the most important tool in psychotherapy is the self of the therapist. Yet having a thorough grasp of the model you will be using is important.

Our tip for you is to use the various resources of your program to help you gain a better depth of your chosen theory. Check with the library to see if there is an online video library that might have a repository of therapy videos you can watch. For instance, if you want to practice client-centered therapy, then watch Carl Rogers. If you are planning to use structural family therapy, watch Salvador Minuchin. Or if you are going to use cognitive behavioral therapy, watch Aaron Beck, Albert Ellis, or Donald Meichenbaum. But don't just watch the session. Go over the theory first and take notes on the process of the model, the main techniques, and the primary objectives. Then watch the session and try to identify each of these. This should help you gain a more in-depth understanding of the model and provide you with a guide for when you try to implement the model.

Tales From the Field: Intern

When I enrolled in a master's program for marriage and family therapy, I only had fuzzy memories of what it was like to be in school. At the time I finished my undergraduate degree, Bill Clinton was still Arkansas's governor. It was a close friend who prompted me to look closely at two therapeutic models that were in demand at the time: Emotionally focused therapy (EFT) and eye movement desensitization and reprocessing (EMDR). My friend, a graduate of a similar MFT program, told me these two evidence-based treatments were forms of therapy that clients were seeking out by name. The demand for EFT and EMDR caught my attention, but at the time I didn't understand that dozens of other therapeutic models existed as well.

In my first few classes, narrative therapy immediately intrigued me. At the same time, Bowen intergenerational family therapy fell in line with how I looked at my own family and also piqued my interest. However, the more I read about EFT, the more I realized that it was a model that fit my style. I knew I wanted to work with couples, and my friend recommended attending an in-person training for EFT simultaneously with my master's program. I will admit it sounded ambitious. Actually, if I'm being honest, it sounded crazy! How would I fit something extracurricular into an already demanding graduate program? I checked the website for ICEEFT, the certification organization for

EFT, and found a four-day, in-person workshop nearby. Still wondering if I was biting off more than I could chew, I signed up for the workshop.

To my surprise, the additional educational experience actually enhanced my understanding of several crucial things. It was the theoretical equivalent of taking a semester abroad. By immersing myself in one theory, I gained the ability to have deeper conversations about how couples interact and to understand how EFT is different from other models like Gottman and solution-focused therapy. It helped me grasp other theories better as well and set me up to feel surer of myself in the therapy room at my internship site.

After the four-day workshop, I signed up for the next round of training: Core Skills 1–4. Currently, I am on track to graduate from my MFT program and become licensed in the state in which I practice. I am able to market myself as "EFT trained," and shortly after becoming fully licensed, I will also have my EFT certification. If I had not listened to my friend's suggestion, I am uncertain I would have had the same confidence at the start of my internship. Most of the guidance I received from school was "pick a model that speaks to you" and explore it. I don't think that's enough of a push. I think that taking the deep dive into a specific model while I was still in school truly rounded out my education and made a difference in the therapy I gave at my internship.

Chris Cantergiani, MS in Family Therapy program, Capella University

Exercise 7.2   Applying Classroom Learning

We've mentioned that having knowledge in your head but not allowing it to come out in the therapy room doesn't help your client. For this exercise, instead of looking toward the past or the present, we want you to look to the future. Think about a technique that you have learned about in one (or more) of your classes that you have not tried yet. Reread about that technique so that you think you have a good understanding of it (and make sure that it is a technique that you don't need specialized training on). Perhaps it is the use of thought disruption, deep breathing, or sculpting (or a variety of other techniques). Then, choose a client that you think that technique would be useful for and use it. See what happens. Make sure you work closely with your supervisor when doing this, going over what you want to do and then how you think it went after using it. How much did it occur similarly to what you read about it? What was different? What could you do differently the next time you use that technique so that it is even more effective?

Tips from an Intern

For me, one of the hardest parts of the practicums/internships I engaged in was the smooth integration of what I learned in the classroom with what I did as a therapist in the therapy room. In the classroom, you learn about the different theories of approaching therapy; the various diagnoses, life transitions, and other relevant background information about your clients; the myriad of ethical and legal considerations that you need to be aware of at all times, and more. This is all incredibly difficult to seamlessly synthesize while you are finding your footing as a therapist.

For example, as a marriage and family therapy student, I learned about the many theories that make up our field (e.g., solution-focused brief therapy, experiential family therapy, structural family therapy). Part of my program involved seeing which of these theories resonated with us most in order to have a foundational theory from which we base our philosophy of change and interventions in the therapy room. This was incredibly challenging to do—sorting through and trying out several different theories to see which one fit while seeing clients for the first time was an overwhelming process.

I'm going to let you in on a little secret: It is not going to be perfectly smooth. In Chapter 12, we will talk about learning from your mistakes. This implies that mistakes will be made: This is an innate expectation for your practicum/internship and even beyond. Specifically, you will make mistakes related to applying classroom learning. You will mess up an intervention from a particular theory, you may not catch every single ethical consideration at first, you will likely forget to consider all parts of the client's context. Accepting all of these things beforehand—without throwing caution to the wind and acting without purpose—is going to be helpful so you don't beat yourself up and are able to refine the classroom learning that you do apply.

Common Factors

We don't have enough space in this book to describe how everything you've learned in your classes was taught to you because your faculty believed that it will help you to be of service to your clients. There is a lot of specific information about specific theories and techniques that you have learned that can assist you in the therapy process. We want to be a bit more general and talk about, regardless of therapeutic model, some of the common factors of therapy. As you read about these (hopefully you have learned about them previously), you can use this classroom learning to then apply them to your specific therapeutic context.

There are multiple models of common factors, yet we want to highlight our personal favorite, which focuses on four common factors: extratherapeutic factors, therapeutic relationship, model and technique factors, and hope and expectancy (Lambert, 1992; Lambert et al., 1986). These common factors work in combination to lead to positive therapeutic change (see Figure 7.2).

Extratherapeutic factors account for 40% of therapeutic change. These factors are predicated on the client's resources, resiliencies, and characteristics. We might think of them as the client's motivation and commitment to change as well as their ability to make change. These are things that the client brings with them to therapy and don't really involve you. However, they are ripe for you to access in therapy. For instance, solution-focused therapists focus on exceptions, or times when the problem could have happened but didn't (Berg, 1994). By highlighting a client's strengths, you can enhance the significance of extratherapeutic factors. When going into a session, you can make sure that, to some degree, you pay attention to these client factors.

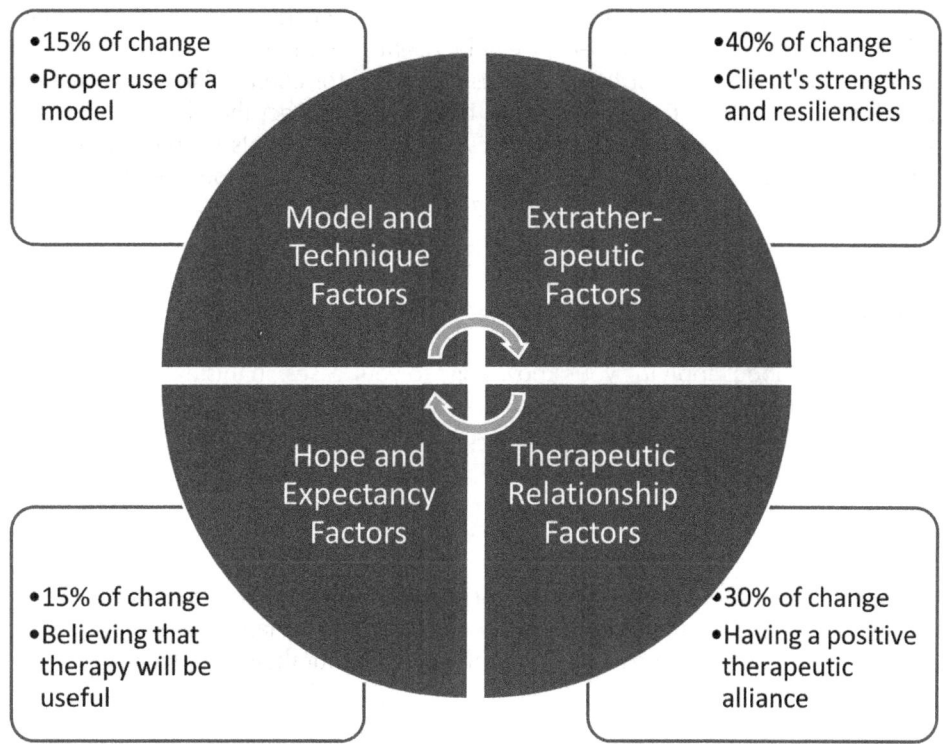

Figure 7.2 One model of the common factors of therapy demonstrate that, across all models, certain factors contribute to lead to positive client change.

The **therapeutic relationship** accounts for 30% of positive therapeutic change. When clients are asked what was useful in therapy, they tend to say things such as, "My therapist was nice," "She really understood me," or "I got along well with him." Knowing this, you can first focus on joining with your client. However, keep in mind that joining is not a static event that you do at the beginning of therapy (i.e., "Tell me a little about yourself") but is something that occurs throughout the whole of therapy. Minuchin et al. (2021) explained, "Joining is not a skill or a technique. It's a mindset constructed out of respect, empathy, curiosity, and a commitment to healing" (p. 4). This lets you know that from your first encounter with the client until the last, what should be primary in your mind is, "How do I maintain connection with the client?"

Model and technique factors account for 15% of therapeutic change. What this means is that the therapist has a clear conceptualization of the case and operates through that conceptualization. However, what we know is that no model of therapy is more effective than any other (Miller et al., 1997). Having a model is important, and who is utilizing that model is important as well, as there are differentials in therapist effectiveness. What this common factor should let you know is that you should have a thorough understanding of at least one model and be able to accurately impart that model (what we call fidelity). Once you have the facility of one model, you can then incorporate aspects of other models to be more integrative.

Hope and expectancy factors also account for 15% of positive therapeutic change. The more that the client believes that therapy will be useful, the more likely they are to change. Just being on the waiting list for therapy leads to change for clients. This common factor is enhanced the more that you, their therapist, believe and expect the client to change. The good news is that you can help foster a sense of hope for clients by presupposing positive change. As Reiter (2010) explained, "By helping to generate hope, the therapist is also increasing a client's sense of expectancy" (p. 135).

Exercise 7.3   Applying the Common Factors

This chapter is about applying your knowledge to your cases. In this exercise, we want you to take the knowledge just presented and apply it to one of your current cases. Choose a case that you've seen for several sessions and answer the following questions about your work with that client.

Extratherapeutic Factors

1. What are three strengths that your client brought with them into therapy?
2. How did you focus on each of these strengths to try to enhance them?
3. How might you have a discussion with the client about their resiliencies?

Therapeutic Relationship

1. How would you describe the therapeutic alliance?
2. What have you done to join with your client?
3. What other ways can you strengthen your connection with your client?

Model and Technique Factors

1. What therapeutic model are you utilizing with this client?
2. What techniques have you used? Why did you use them?
3. How are you maintaining theory fidelity (that you are ensuring you are accurately following the protocols of the model)?

Hope and Expectancy Factors

1. What change is your client expecting to come from therapy?
2. What change in your client are you expecting to see?
3. What have you done to ensure your client that you believe therapy will be useful for them?

Quick Tip: Check in with your clients at the end of each session to get feedback from them about what they found to be useful during the session and what they didn't. In the next session, do less of what didn't work and more of what did from the previous session.

Working With a Co-Therapist

We have already introduced the possibility that you may conduct co-therapy during some of your time at your practicum/internship site. We addressed how this comes into play in knowing yourself as a therapist (i.e., Chapter 5), and now we want to talk about it again when it comes to applying classroom learning.

We mentioned previously that even if you and your co-therapist come from the same program, you may each have different preferred models of therapy and different personalities that change how you engage with your clients. One way to bridge your viewpoints is to focus on what you have learned in the classroom and discuss this with your co-therapist. By going over the same material, it will be easier for the two of you to be on the same page (hopefully from the same textbook!).

Now, applying classroom learning can seem more discrepant when you and your co-therapist are from different psychotherapy graduate programs. Your site may have interns that are marriage and family therapy students, mental health counseling students, clinical social work students, and/or clinical psychology students. Each program's curriculum is going to vary in some ways, such as clinical psychology emphasizing diagnoses and the individual more while marriage and family therapy focusing more on the system and context. We will be honest with you and say that this may sometimes make it tough to do co-therapy because the two therapists have different epistemologies and approaches to problems and change. For example, Kayleigh had a mental health counseling student intern sit in on sessions with her at her job. Kayleigh had her write the client's progress note for practice, and the intern wrote about the client's "cognitive distortions," whereas Kayleigh tends not to use that conceptualization or terminology as a systemic therapist. Kayleigh viewed these thoughts that the client shared as normal given her context.

The important thing here is to have discussion with your co-therapist about where you are coming from. Be honest and intentional with one another when conceptualizing cases and applying techniques. Recognize that the other person isn't necessarily doing something wrong even if you don't vibe with their approach. There are many different approaches to therapy that can all be effective if applied the right way by the right person. In the previous example, Kayleigh simply had a discussion with the student intern about their different field's ways of conceptualizing things. Kayleigh explained she changed the wording in the note to match her language since Kayleigh is the therapist who signs off on the note.

What Would You Do?: 7.1

At your site, you are paired up with another intern to do co-therapy. The two of you are from different programs and have never met before. The first time that you do meet is five minutes before the session that you are to be co-therapists. You find that not only is your conceptualization different but so are your personalities. They are quite the opposite of you, which you would probably be okay with; however, they are also quite controlling. During the session, they try to take over, not giving you much room to say anything and even interrupting you and contradicting what you are saying. It is an extremely unpleasant experience for you. Yet the agency expects the two of you to continue to be co-therapists. What would you do?

Tips From a Supervisor

I am not only a supervisor but a faculty member as well. Further, I have written 15 books about psychotherapy, many of them teaching skills and theories with the intent that the reader (you) would learn them but more importantly apply the information. This chapter is extremely significant for me as it is the overlap between my two main work roles: teacher and supervisor. With the hundreds of supervisees I've had, many of them see their schoolwork as separate from their field placement. For me, this is perhaps their greatest error.

My main tip for this chapter is to really embrace the idea that what you have been learning about in all of your courses will play some role in your practicum/internship. This is your chance to put into practice everything you've taken the time to learn. This is something I encourage my supervisees to do, sometimes even giving them an assignment to take a concept they've learned and use it with at least one of their clients. For instance, we might review what they've learned about enactments and then they pick one client family and try the enactment with them.

My one caution for you here is to just make sure that you understand the technique. It might be useful to, before you try it with your client, review it with your supervisor to ensure that you can effectively operationalize it. Your supervisor and/or faculty member can help you prepare to use the skill/technique. Just imagine what would happen if you do this every week of your placement. What might your therapeutic tool belt look like once you finish your practicum/internship? How many more options will you have of what you could do with your clients?

Summary

This chapter encouraged you to make the connection between your classroom learning and the work that you are doing at your field placement. The intent of your faculty members has been to present you with information in class that will assist you in your work with clients. However, for this to happen, your active involvement is key. How are you intentionally thinking about what you have learned through readings and classroom discussions and how that information is playing out in your practicum/internship? We will end this chapter with one last thought: Information is useless if it is not applied.

References

Anderson, H. (1997). *Conversation, language, and possibilities: A postmodern approach to therapy.* Basic Books.
Berg, I. K. (1994). *Family based services: A solution-focused approach.* Norton.
Lambert, M. J. (1992). Psychotherapy outcome research: Implications for integrative and eclectic therapists. In J. C. Norcross & M. R. Goldfried (Eds.), *Handbook of psychotherapy integration* (pp. 94–129). Basic Books.
Lambert, M. J., Shapiro, D. A., & Bergin, A. E. (1986). The effectiveness of psychotherapy. In S. L. Garfield & A. E. Bergin (Eds.), *Handbook of psychotherapy and behavior change* (3rd ed., pp. 157–211). Wiley.
Miller, S. D., Duncan, B. L., & Hubble, M. A. (1997). *Escape from Babel: Toward a unifying language for psychotherapy practice.* Norton.

Minuchin, S., Reiter, M. D., & Borda, C. (2021). *The craft of family therapy: Challenging certainties* (2nd ed.). Routledge.

Reiter, M. D. (2010). Hope and expectancy in solution-focused brief therapy. *Journal of Family Psychotherapy, 21*(2), 132–148. https://doi.org/10.1080/08975353.2010.483653

Reiter, M. D. (2022). *Therapeutic interviewing: Essential skills and contexts of counseling* (2nd ed.). Routledge.

Chapter 8

Navigating Ethical Dilemmas

When you enter into a therapeutic relationship with a client, you do so primarily with the ethical value of beneficence—to do good. We trust that you came into this field because you want to help people. You want the outcome of your engagement with them to be for their betterment. And no matter how intent you are to do this, there will be many ethical dilemmas that present themselves over the course of your placement. In this chapter, we discuss how you can navigate these ethical dilemmas. It is not the case of whether you will *have to* make ethical decisions but rather *how you will react* when ethical choices inevitably present themselves to you.

Myths About the Field

"I will know exactly how to handle each ethical dilemma."

Our lives would be much easier if this were true, but alas, this is not the case. While there are certainly federal and state policies for dealing with certain ethical and legal situations, knowing exactly when to employ these procedures can be difficult at times. Not every ethical dilemma has clear delineations, as the specifics of the context can sometimes create a gray area rather than present as black and white. When this is the case, the answer on how to handle these situations may not be staring you in the face. Let's slow down a little and go over some of the primary ethical values that you should be thinking about whenever you work with a client.

Ethics

All psychotherapy fields are predicated on the notion of ethical responsibility. It is expected—and mandated—that you will engage with your clients in a professional, competent, and safe manner. **Psychotherapy ethics** "pertains to the beliefs we hold about what constitutes right conduct" (Corey et al., 2023, p. 13). We know that you've already had an ethics course in your program, as almost all psychotherapy programs require completion of the ethics course before students can begin their practicum or internship. Much of this information should therefore be a review. However, when you are covering it this time, think about what is happening for you at your site and how these ideas might come into play during your field placement.

DOI: 10.4324/9781003433484-8

Ethics can be mandatory or aspirational (Corey et al., 2023). On the one hand, **mandatory ethics** are the musts of the field, the minimum expectations of the therapist. For instance, you must provide your client with enough information for them to make an informed consent for treatment. Also, you must hold confidentiality for your client (within reason—see further along for when we must break confidentiality).

Aspirational ethics, on the other hand, are the highest standard that we would *like to* achieve. They go beyond mandatory ethics and focus on the benefits of one's actions. The push for therapists to operate from a place of social justice, for example, is more in line with aspirational ethics. For instance, you do not have to get politically involved and try to promote legislation that you believe is beneficial for your clients (and people in general). However, most ethical codes encourage you to do this, but you wouldn't come under scrutiny by the ethical body overseer if you didn't.

Let's switch to talk about, regardless of ethical body, the primary ethical values and principles that all psychotherapists operate from. There are six primary ethical values and guiding principles that all therapists, regardless of their field, are expected to follow. These include beneficence, nonmaleficence, fidelity, justice, autonomy, and competence (see Figure 8.1). We will briefly present each of these and provide an example from various ethical codes

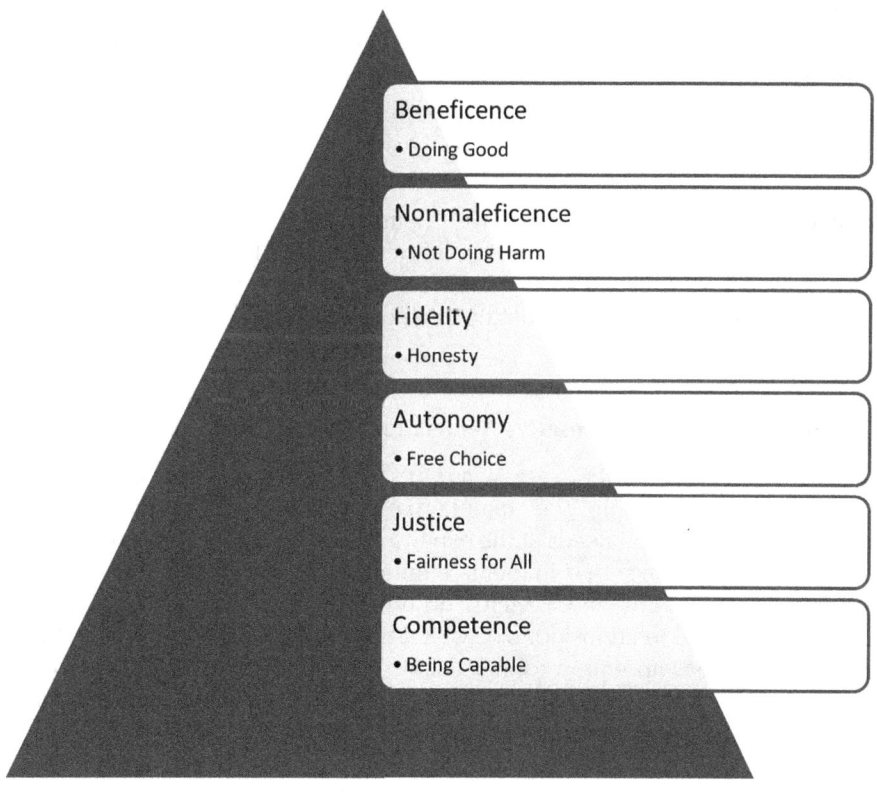

Figure 8.1 Regardless of field, there are six guiding ethical principles.

regarding them so that you can come in contact with the variety of ways that different fields talk about these concepts.

Beneficence means doing good so that the client is in a better place from having contact with you. When you create a treatment plan with your client, beneficence is seen when the goals are to increase self-esteem, increase positive interactions with others, decrease anxiety, decrease depression, and so on. This guiding principle is really why you came into the field—you want to help people. A clear focus on goals and checking in with clients about their progress toward those goals falls under the principle of beneficence.

What Would You Do?: 8.1

Put yourself into the shoes of one of Michael's supervisees during a live team therapy/supervision, which happened at a university therapy clinic. The student therapist went to the waiting room to get the clients (a mother and her 16-year-old son) for the first session, where they had been filling out the intake paperwork. When the student brought them back to the therapy room, she began to go over the informed consent. She explained confidentiality and the times when she would have to break it. Upon hearing that confidentiality would be broken in cases of imminent self-harm, the mother asked to have the paperwork back so she could take suicidal thoughts off of the list of symptoms/concerns she had checked for the boy. The mother said that the therapist should disregard that she had marked it, and she didn't want their visit or what they talked about to be disclosed to anyone. What would you do?

Nonmaleficence means not to do harm. In medicine, there is the Hippocratic Oath (although it is more than do no harm). You shouldn't intentionally try to harm your client. We expect this to be the case for all therapists. However, sometimes we unintentionally harm our clients. This leads us to always be on the lookout for the impact that our interactions with the client have on them or others.

American Mental Health Counselors Association (2020) Code of Ethics

Exploitive Relationships CMHCs are aware of the intimacy and responsibilities inherent in the counseling relationship. They maintain respect for the client and avoid actions that seek to meet their personal needs at the expense of the client. a. Romantic or sexual relationships with clients and their immediate family members (i.e., parents, children, and partners) are strictly prohibited. CMHCs do not counsel persons with whom they have had a previous sexual relationship. b. CMHCs should not knowingly enter into a romantic or sexual relationship with a former client. If a CMHC chooses to enter into such a relationship, the burden to demonstrate that neither coercion nor harm to the client has transpired is on the CMHC and not the former client.

We could harm our clients if we focused more on what *we* are getting out of the therapeutic relationship than *them*. If you continue to see your client because you need to accumulate clinical hours even when they are not benefiting from the therapy, you are engaging in maleficence. While a majority of clients, even with good intentions from the therapist, improve in symptomatology, approximately 10% get worse (Okiishi et al., 2003). It is important for you to pay attention to whether your contact with the client is helping or harming them.

Fidelity is related to the notion of trustworthiness. This mainly comes into play with aspects of confidentiality, that the client can trust us not to disclose our conversations with them to others (except when there is justification, but even then, we should have made this clear to the client during the informed consent process and then again when we have to break confidentiality).

American Psychological Association (2017) Code of Ethics

Principle B: Fidelity and Responsibility Psychologists establish relationships of trust with those with whom they work. They are aware of their professional and scientific responsibilities to society and to the specific communities in which they work. Psychologists uphold professional standards of conduct, clarify their professional roles and obligations, accept appropriate responsibility for their behavior, and seek to manage conflicts of interest that could lead to exploitation or harm. Psychologists consult with, refer to, or cooperate with other professionals and institutions to the extent needed to serve the best interests of those with whom they work. They are concerned about the ethical compliance of their colleagues' scientific and professional conduct. Psychologists strive to contribute a portion of their professional time for little or no compensation or personal advantage.

You will likely want to have your client feel good about you and the work the two of you are doing together. While there might be times that you don't tell the truth (e.g., perhaps you fabricate a story about another client to use as a therapeutic story), you should always tell the truth when it comes to policies and procedures. Further, you shouldn't make guarantees that you can't back up. Michael has seen several novice therapists tell clients that things are definitely going to get better. This is a guarantee they cannot ensure. While it is the goal of therapy, the therapeutic process is too complex for us to know that it will definitely happen. Rather, you can tell your client, "Our goal is to get you to that place. Let's work together to see how that might happen."

Clients have the right to **autonomy**. Essentially, we do not make decisions for them. Our job as therapists is always to try to increase client personal agency so that they are making their own choices. We might talk with them about what we believe the potential consequences are for their actions, but it is always ultimately up to them. This is why we go over informed consent with clients. It is their choice to enter into a therapeutic relationship with us. We try to give them enough information about that relationship for them to choose whether to engage with us or not.

American Counseling Association (2014) Code of Ethics

A.2.a. Informed Consent Clients have the freedom to choose whether to enter into or remain in a counseling relationship and need adequate information about the counseling process and the counselor. Counselors have an obligation to review in writing and verbally with clients the rights and responsibilities of both counselors and clients. Informed consent is an ongoing part of the counseling process, and counselors appropriately document discussions of informed consent throughout the counseling relationship.

Fortunately, over his 30 years of therapy and supervision, Michael hasn't seen many therapists try to control clients' lives. However, there have been a few of his supervisees that have had a tendency to try to get clients to make certain choices. You will likely feel this when you have a client who is dating someone that you think is toxic, a person that you would forbid the client to be with if the client were your family member. In therapy, we can't talk to our client like we would our family member. It is their choice whether to be with the person or not. However, we can talk with them about the impact that the relationship is having on them. We can talk with them about their rationale for staying in the relationship. But we would (just about) never say, "You need to leave this person" (if there is a very unsafe domestic violence situation, however, we might push for this option).

Over the last several decades, psychotherapists have put more of a focus on justice issues. **Justice** means being fair to all people. You'll see this guiding principle at the beginning of most ethical codes when they talk about therapists not discriminating against clients based on race, age, gender, sexual orientation, religion, or any other characteristic/social location factor. Justice is also about ensuring that people who have been marginalized are able to receive therapy services. Thus, the mandatory ethics regarding justice include not discriminating against anyone, while aspirational ethics may be providing pro bono services to clients who cannot afford your services.

American Association for Marriage and Family Therapy (2015) Code of Ethics

Standard 1.1 Non-Discrimination. Marriage and family therapists provide professional assistance to persons without discrimination on the basis of race, age, ethnicity, socioeconomic status, disability, gender, health status, religion, national origin, sexual orientation, gender identity or relationship status.

You probably view yourself as someone who wouldn't ever discriminate against a therapy client. We hope this is the case. We also know that we all have biases (remember in Chapter 5 we talked about this in terms of viewpoints). We all have a unique viewpoint, and our viewpoints were developed based on our race, age, ethnicity, socioeconomic status, sexual orientation, past experiences, and other contextual factors. They shade the area that we see, which is why in many of the diversity-based classes in various therapy programs, part of the curriculum is designed to help you to start to widen your viewpoints. When your viewpoint is shaded, you may not be able to see another person's unique experience, which could lead you to, inadvertently, treat them in a way based on some aspect of their life.

Competence refers to your capabilities as a therapist. It is understood that, at this stage in your career, you are not supposed to be as competent as someone who is a seasoned therapist. That is okay. You are learning. The competence here is partially viewed from a developmental level. Are you competent for someone just starting out? And because we know that you are not supposed to know everything, this is why you have a supervisor and need a certain number of supervised clinical hours to become licensed in your field. However, even though you are early in your career, you should not enter the therapy room psychologically or emotionally impaired. Also, you should not be trying to do interventions that you have not been trained for.

National Association of Social Workers (2021) Code of Ethics

1.04 Competence (a) Social workers should provide services and represent themselves as competent only within the boundaries of their education, training, license, certification, consultation received, supervised experience, or other relevant professional experience. (b) Social workers should provide services in substantive areas or use intervention techniques or approaches that are new to them only after engaging in appropriate study, training, consultation, and supervision from people who are competent in those interventions or techniques. (c) When generally recognized standards do not exist with respect to an emerging area of practice, social workers should exercise careful judgment and take responsible steps (including appropriate education, research, training, consultation, and supervision) to ensure the competence of their work and to protect clients from harm.

Here, the field encourages you to try to take what you are learning in the classroom and apply it in the therapy room (see Chapter 7). What you are not supposed to do is engage with clients when you don't think you are in the right mental space. If something happens to you, such as a death in the family or another traumatic event, our field encourages you to not see your clients but rather to focus on yourself. However, we need to be professional about it—as early as possible, contact your client to reschedule the session, work with your supervisor to help you navigate the practice-based situation, and work with a therapist to help you work through the personal/psychological situation.

Tales From the Field: Intern

I am a master's practicum student seeing clients at a community counseling center in Nevada. There, we work with clients from diverse backgrounds and with diverse struggles. I had been seeing a client for a few months, but she hadn't been very consistent in coming to therapy until the last month before this experience. She had recently decided she needed to make therapy more of a priority in her life and had been attending her weekly appointments. She is a cisgender female and is married with two younger children. She was coming to see me to process some childhood trauma as well as work on her self-esteem, anxiety, and parenting issues. We had only ever met and done sessions together on a telehealth platform.

During the first couple minutes into one of our sessions together, she mentioned struggling with her two children at the grocery store. She explained that when they got home, she "beat them each with a belt one time." Immediately, when she said this, alarm bells went off in my head. I was frantically trying to stay present with her and figure out the best thing for me to do at that moment. Should I stop her and ask questions? Should I stop her and let her know that, as a mandated reporter, I was going to need to report this to child services? Should I let her continue to talk and figure out what to do after the session? Well, I decided to do the latter. This client is a talker and doesn't leave much room for my input sometimes. At that moment, I chose to continue with the session and not interrupt her. This was my first time having a situation with a client in which I was questioning whether I needed to make a call to the Department of Children and Family Services (DCFS).

After our session was finished, I immediately called my supervisor and explained what had happened. She advised me that we are mandated reporters, and as such, I should probably make a call to DCFS. She also explained that I should call the clinical director of the program and get her thoughts on the matter as well. I called the clinical director at my site, and she advised me to call DCFS, too. She reminded me that we are mandated reporters, not investigators, and our job is to report even *suspected* situations of child abuse. It is not our job concerning what happens from there. I did as I was advised to do and made the report to DCFS.

The day after I made the call, I was in supervision and was speaking with my supervisor about how I was feeling. I know I am a mandated reporter, but I was struggling not to think about all the possible things that could happen because of the call I had made. My supervisor helped me see that I did what I was supposed to do and that there is a reason why we are mandated reporters. It is not my job to investigate the situation, just to report what I know. Also, because of how little information I had, there was a good possibility nothing would come of it. I was also feeling that I needed to reach out to my client and let her know what I had to do, even though I did not want to do that. I want to be a therapist that is open and honest with my clients, so I felt I needed to call my client and notify her of the situation. My supervisor advised me to get off our Zoom call, call my client, and come back to supervision so we could process the call. I was nervous about talking to my client, but I knew it was the right thing to do for myself and for her. I took my supervisor's advice and called my client. I let her know that being a mandated reporter, I had to place a call to DCFS because of her statement about hitting her kids with a belt. I expressed that I understood if she didn't feel comfortable coming to me for therapy anymore but that I would be happy to continue working together and process this further. She said she would let me know and that she had to go.

After the call, I was able to get back on the Zoom call with my supervisor and process the conversation. I was feeling better that I had told her about what I had to do, but I was also feeling anxious about what was going to happen next. I knew that I did the right thing in telling her the truth about what had happened. I was also battling feelings that if I would have never told her, she most likely would not have known about the call to DCFS at all because they most likely wouldn't have contacted her. It was frustrating having those thoughts because I was thinking that if I hadn't shared this with her, I could have gone on seeing her as a client and hopefully helped her with her anxiety, parenting, and all the other reasons she was seeking treatment. In the end, my supervisor helped me talk through the feelings I was having and struggling with, and I knew that I had done what I needed to for myself and my client.

My client ended up texting me later that day and said she could no longer continue therapy with me. I understood, and I was okay with that. Even though our therapeutic relationship ended, I sincerely hope that she will seek out help from someone else. I learned a lot about myself, my relationship with clients, and the kind of therapist I have to and want to be through this experience.

Aubrey Glover, MS in Family Therapy program, Touro University

Ethical Decision-Making Models

As you know, ethics are not black-and-white. They are usually gray, requiring you to critically think about the situation and make tough decisions. This is why you need to have an **ethical decision-making process**. It is not just that a situation happens and you react. Careful thought is needed to ensure that you are adhering to all of the values and principles of the field (and just keep in mind that what was previously presented are just the primary principles and values). Please ensure you closely look at your field's ethical codes to see the wider range of expectations of proper clinical work. In this section, we will cover a few of the more popular ethical decision-making models.

Corey et al. (2023) proposed eight steps to thinking through an ethical dilemma. First, you should identify the problem or dilemma. Sometimes it is quite clear that a problem/dilemma has occurred while other times you don't know until someone else has complained (and probably complained about you). Depending on the situation, you might talk with your client and/or your supervisor to determine whether there is a problem.

Second, identify the potential issues that are involved. Here, think about each person's responsibilities and rights. Who is supposed to do what? What cultural contexts might be at play? What might be safety and/or welfare concerns that are coming up? How do the six values and principles (presented earlier) apply in this situation?

Third, you should review the ethical codes that are applicable to you. While most ethical codes of the various fields have a high level of overlap, there may be small distinctions between them. A good perusal of your organization's ethical codes may help you to determine if they help point you in a productive pathway. If you are stumped, you can consult other people such as your site supervisor, faculty supervisor, other licensed professionals, or even a representative from your professional organization who can give guidance on the ethical codes.

Fourth, besides knowing the relevant ethical codes, you should also know the pertinent laws and regulations for your area. Just as each field has its own ethical code, each state (and country) has its own laws and rules. You are subject to follow the laws in the state that you are currently practicing. This is why we are not presenting any information here that is state specific as we wouldn't want you to think that it would then apply to you. We recommend that you bookmark on your computer not only your professional organization's ethical code but your state regulatory body's website as well.

Fifth, it is important to get consultation. This should be easy for you as you will have at least one supervisor. You might even have more than that, such as a site supervisor and a faculty supervisor. Besides your supervisor, you can consult with other licensed professionals or even colleagues (just ensure that you are maintaining confidentiality for the client). However, it is better to operate based on feedback from licensed therapists rather than fellow students. But the more voices that you seek, the more potential pathways toward the ethical dilemma's resolution you might obtain.

Sixth, based on everything that you learned and explored with consultation, laws, and ethics, you should think about what your possible courses of action are. This might be to do nothing, talk with the client, break confidentiality, or talk with your state's licensing board, among other options. Based on the situation, you might go over these possibilities with your client and/or your supervisor.

Seventh, before you do anything, consider what the consequences might be of these various courses of action. One thing that you could do here is to scale the potential course of action (Caldwell & Stone, 2016). These authors used the following scale to assess how the ethical decision holds in relation to the main psychotherapy values of autonomy, beneficence, nonmalfeasance, justice, and fidelity:

2: Likely to uphold this value in an exceptional manner.
1: Likely to meaningfully uphold this value.
0: Neutral in relation to this value, or has little related impact.
—1: Likely to run counter to this value in a minor way.
X: Likely to run counter to this value in a significant way.

You would scale the possible course of action for each psychotherapy value, giving you a range of −5 to 10. The higher the number on the scale, the more likely it is for you to take that course of action. It is recommended that if you score an X on any of the values, then that course of action should not be taken.

The last step of Corey et al.'s (2023) ethical decision tree is to, based on everything you've evaluated, make a choice of what you are going to do. This choice will not be reactionary but based on a careful consideration of the standards of the field along with the wisdom of all significant parties involved in the process of thinking through the situation. Whatever you choose to do, make sure that you are documenting this process.

Exercise 8.1   Ethical Case Example 1

For the following case scenario (based on a case Kayleigh had), use Corey et al.'s (2023) eight steps to use when thinking through an ethical choice to determine what you would do in this situation.

Suppose you have a new adolescent client (16 years old), and she discloses to you that she occasionally smokes cannabis. Upon asking her to tell you a bit more, she says she smokes every other weekend or so with friends. She recently went through a surgery for her ACL and says that smoking helps with the discomfort. After curiously asking if her mom (dad is out of the picture) knows about the smoking, the client said that mom has caught her a few times and is aware but doesn't love that the client smokes. What ethical considerations do you need to make in regard to the client's safety and potential need to break confidentiality? How would you handle this situation using the eight steps discussed previously? What number on the scale developed by Caldwell and Stone (2016) would your ethical decision be?

We spent some time going over Corey et al.'s (2023) suggested process since it is one of the more popular ones. However, it is not the only way that you can go about making ethical decisions. Here, we very briefly present a couple of other models. Pope et al. (2021) proposed 17 steps in ethical decision-making:

1. Clearly state the dilemma
2. Anticipate who will be impacted
3. Determine who the client is
4. Assess your areas of competence
5. Review ethical standards
6. Review legal standards
7. Review relevant research
8. Assess whether your personal bias is impacting your ethical judgment
9. Assess whether cultural considerations impact the decision
10. Consider consultation
11. Determine possible courses of action
12. Consider the consequences of these possible courses of action

13. Socially decenter yourself so that you can see how each person involved will be impacted
14. Make a decision and follow through on it
15. Document the ethical decision-making process
16. Be accountable for your actions
17. Learn from this process so that you might prepare and/or prevent situations from happening in the future.

Katafiasz et al. (2020) proposed a recent model for ethical decision-making that they call the **Butterfly Model**. Utilizing Bronfenbrenner's Ecological Systems Model (Bronfenbrenner, 1979), the Butterfly Model focuses equally on the client system and the therapist system. The therapist considers the ethical dilemma and its relation to the various systems of client and therapist (i.e., microsystem, mesosystem, exosystem, macrosystem, and chronosystem). If you don't know Bronfenbrenner's model, please explore it, as it helps you understand a person within context (see Figure 8.2).

We will also very quickly go over it here. First, we have the individual. They are housed in the microsystem, which includes the individual's immediate environmental setting, such as their family, work, school, and friends (Bronfenbrenner, 1979). The mesosystem includes the interactions between the people in the microsystem. For instance, this would be a child's parents talking with their teacher or a person's spouse interacting with their friend. The exosystem includes formal and informal structures that indirectly influence the individual. This would be the neighborhood, social media, a parent's job, or a spouse's friends. The macrosystem explores how cultural elements impact the individual. This would include economic and political systems, culture, and social norms. The last level is the chronosystem,

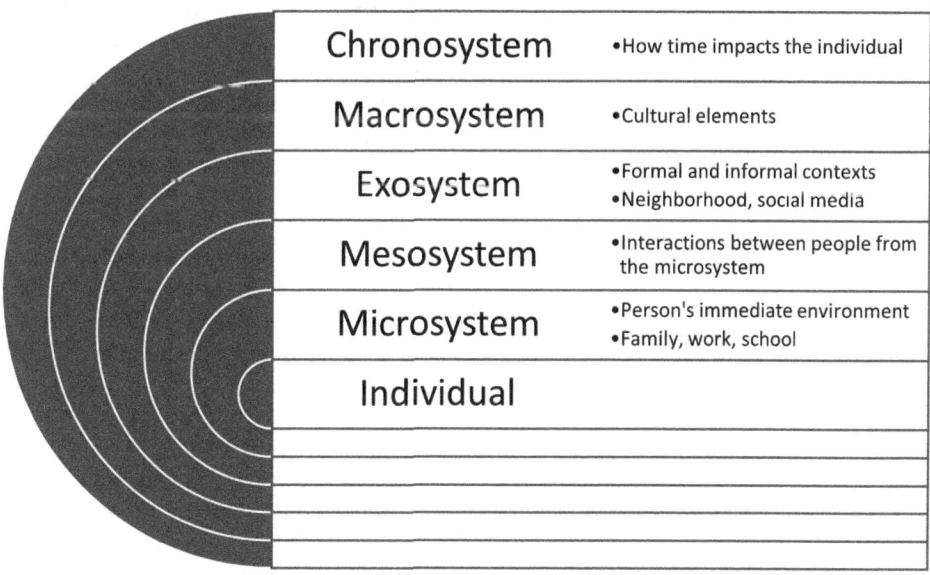

Figure 8.2 Bronfenbrenner's ecosystemic model helps us understand the individual within the various contexts of their life.

which describes how time influences changes in the individual, perhaps through human development or social change.

There are six steps that Katafiasz et al. (2020) identify in the butterfly model: (a) identifying an ethical dilemma, (b) identifying possible courses of action, (c) evaluating the consequences of those courses of action, (d) choosing and implementing a course of action, (e) evaluating the results of that course of action, and (f) feeding back the information learned from this process into future ethical situations.

Exercise 8.2: Ethical Case Example 2

For the following case scenario, apply the Butterfly Model to make a determination of what you might ethically do in this situation.

You are working with a husband and wife who have two children, 7 and 5. Over the course of a couple of months, their arguments and contempt for one another grow to the point that they decide to divorce. A nasty custody battle then ensues. One of the partners asks you to write a letter explaining how it would be better for them to have custody since the other partner has not been as engaged with the children. You now have to decide what you want to do in this situation.

As you can see, there is quite a lot of overlap between ethical decision-making models. You don't need to specifically use one. However, you should be thoughtful about how you are going about this process. People's careers and lives can be on the line. We don't want to scare you, but we do want to express the seriousness of this process. While a client can try to sue for any reason, as long as you follow standard therapeutic protocol (and document these decisions), you are usually in good shape. The more that you don't, the more you open yourself for liability. Utilizing an ethical decision-making model and documenting your steps is a standard process designed to help you to make the best ethical choice for you and your client, protecting both of you.

Tips From an Intern

My experience in the therapy field has taught me that there are going to be ethical dilemmas in every therapy setting. This has been the case for me thus far, and I have interned/worked at five different therapy settings at the time I am writing this. I will admit that I was slightly unprepared for this as a student intern, as learning about the ethical considerations in a classroom is not the same as encountering ethical dilemmas in your therapy practicum/internship. As a result, the first part of my tip is emphasizing that you *will* encounter ethical dilemmas at your site. The knowledge and acceptance of this fact beforehand will, I think, help you handle these situations better.

The second part of my tip surrounds how to handle these situations. We discussed the specifics of how to navigate ethical dilemmas in this chapter, but I want to stress the general importance of listening to your gut during these ethical dilemmas. As a student therapist at a practicum/internship site, you are learning the ropes and are not expected to know exactly how to deal with every situation that comes your way. Still, you will probably have an intuition that will put certain situations on your "Hm, I probably need to do something about this" radar. (We referred to this in a previous chapter as an ethical spidey sense.) These are often the ethical dilemmas we talked about in this chapter. I have seen too frequently that some student therapists discredit this intuition because they are beginners; if they don't see another registered intern or licensed therapist do something about it (which may not always be the right call), they won't do anything about it.

I cannot stress enough how it is better to be safe than sorry. If your gut is telling you that something may need to be addressed (and it's not being addressed by other official staff members), bring it up with your supervisor. Your supervisor should welcome these conversations, as supervision is the space for you to consult about what is going on at your practicum/internship site. So as a recap: Expect ethical dilemmas and listen to your gut. If this gut instinct is telling you to do something, don't shy away from reaching out to your supervisor first. If the situation winds up not being an issue, then that's great. But if it is an important concern, you will be happy you brought it up.

We have mentioned many times throughout this chapter that you will have to make many ethical decisions throughout your career. Those decisions start now in your practicum/internship. You cannot avoid them, and you shouldn't want to, as going through the ethical decision-making process leads you to think about how you situate yourself in your work and makes you a better therapist. It is going to be a little nerve-racking, especially when the situation is quite significant. However, the best news for you, at this point in your therapeutic career, is that you are not alone. The primary tip that we have for you is to ensure that you are consulting with your supervisor regarding the situation. You are not supposed to know what to do for all situations. Your supervisor is there to help you process your ideas and to more effectively navigate the ethical dilemma.

We presented several ethical decision-making models since you will need to make choices every time you meet with a client. We know the ones we've presented have a lot of steps. You don't need to memorize them all. You can always come back to this book or, better yet, go to the sources which we got them from. But we want to end this section making it a little easier on you. Moffett et al. (2014) presented a checklist that you can use to help you understand the hierarchy of concerns when making an ethical decision. They use the acronym DCBA:

D leads you to examine issues of danger, duty, and documentation.
C addresses consent, confidentiality, competence, and consultation.
B pertains to boundaries.
A is about applying a decision-making model, acting on it, and assessing the results.

You should start with the D, thinking about issues of danger and/or duty. These come first. You need to ensure that your client is safe. Whatever choices you make here, please ensure that you are documenting them (see Chapter 4). Once you have dealt with D, think about C, then B, and then A.

> **Quick Tip**: Remember that you are not alone. When there is a significant ethical dilemma that you are trying to navigate, you should not make it on your own. Consult your supervisor. Further, ask more people about it so that you get a variety of ideas. If you have a site supervisor and a faculty supervisor, talk to both of them. You are not expected to know what to do in every situation. Text, call, pass by the office, or, if the ethical dilemma is not life-threatening, wait until the next scheduled supervision session to bring up the dilemma and collaborate on the best possible path for you to take. We have mentioned this tip several times in this chapter because we think it is the number one thing that you should do when there is an ethical situation.

Tales From the Field: Supervisor

Briana started her first therapy practicum knowing she wanted to work with teenagers. She had prior assessment experience with children and adolescents in her master's program and came from a family of mental health professionals. In the therapy practicum, she had completed the parent portion of an intake interview and then begun the intake interview with the client, a 15-year-old teenage boy. He had requested therapy to explore his sexuality, so his mother sought services from a local community mental health center.

During his portion of the intake interview, the client revealed to Briana that he was engaging in unprotected sex with adults he sought out. He disclosed he thought this was the best way to determine if his sexual interests were merely curiosity or genuine interest. At the end of the intake interview, the client asked Briana, "This is between you and me, right?" He was essentially asking if the information he revealed about his sexual encounters with adults was confidential. Briana was caught off guard but felt the need to align with the client and honor his confidence given the depth of information he had revealed. She quickly responded "Yes" and escorted him back to his mother.

Briana had supervision with me, her practicum supervisor, later in the week. Briana brought up the question the client had asked about keeping information confidential, as she had felt uncomfortable answering the client in the affirmative knowing he—as a minor—was engaging in unprotected sexual activity with adults. During supervision, I talked with Briana about the limits of confidentiality and the need to keep minors safe. I reminded Briana about state statutes regarding reporting and the conversation she had with the client's mother about the limits of confidentiality. Ultimately, Briana talked with the client about the limits of confidentiality and the need to break confidentiality surrounding the unprotected sexual activity with adults. The client agreed to disclose his sexual activity to his mother, and Briana followed up with the mother to verify the information the client disclosed to her.

Yukari Tomozawa, PsyD, Clinical Psychology program, Nova Southeastern University

Suicidality

Perhaps the area that new therapists are most fearful about is when a client is potentially suicidal. You've probably covered this topic in one or more of your classes but probably not in depth and most likely not in the depth needed for you to feel comfortable in assessing for suicidality. Mental health care providers tend to believe that their training and education were not sufficient for them to have a good understanding of ethical issues when related to care for a suicidal client (Montreuil et al., 2021). What this means is that you should go above and beyond your classroom learning to be more comfortable in assessing and working with clients who are potentially suicidal.

In 2021, about 48,000 people in the United States completed suicide (Centers for Disease Control and Prevention, n.d.). This is only a small portion of the 12.3 million adults who had suicidal thoughts, 3.5 million who made a suicide plan, and 1.7 million who attempted suicide. You will almost certainly encounter a client who is having suicidal thoughts, let alone who is planning or actively attempting suicide. Thus, you need to be prepared.

Ethically, you have a **duty to protect**, which means it is your responsibility to protect your client from potential harm. In this case, it would be them harming themselves. We won't go into detail about how to assess for suicidality or what to do with the client when that potential is increased. We encourage you to read more about it. A few of our recommended sources are Flemons and Gralnik (2013), Alonzo and Gearing (2018), and Bell (2021).

We want to take a second for you to think about the impact that working with a suicidal client might have on you. You don't only have to think about what happens in the therapy room but also how your client's actions will impact you. This is especially the case if your client actually completes suicide. (We just want to make a note here of our field's move from talking about committing suicide to completing suicide. The word "commit" often has a negative connotation, such as committing a crime, and this casts a bad light on individuals who are dealing with this in their life.) Being exposed to a patient who completes suicide or engages in suicidal behaviors can be quite stressful and traumatic, potentially leading the therapist to experience posttraumatic stress disorder (Leaune et al., 2021). Michael has had several supervisees who had clients complete suicide during the supervisees' practicum/internship experience. This wasn't just another day at the office for these therapists. It was quite traumatizing.

Once you become aware that a client is having suicidal ideation, you will probably experience a lot of anxiety trying to figure out how to ensure that they do not make an attempt.

Many years ago, it was standard practice for a therapist to have the client sign a **no harm contract**. This contract stated that the client would not harm themselves and instead would contact either the therapist or some crisis personnel (perhaps 911, a mobile crisis response team, or other hotlines or entities). One of the things that was realized was that this contract was not that useful for the client. Instead, it was a CYA (cover your ass) tool for the therapist.

Currently, no harm contracts have gone out of favor, and safety plans are more preferred. **Safety plans** are used when the client is at risk for suicide and/or self-harm (Ferguson, 2023). The plan includes triggers and warning signs, internal coping strategies, external coping strategies, emergency services, restriction of access to means of self-harm, and reasons for living. The safety plan provides the client, when they are away from the session, with guidance on how they can stay safe when they are feeling distressed. In comparison, the no harm contract is only an agreement that they won't self-harm.

As with almost every ethical dilemma we have talked about in this chapter, you are not operating in isolation. You have one, if not more, supervisors available for you to consult. You should never be left on your own to make a determination whether it is safe for a client to leave your office if there is concern around suicidality. Involve your supervisor. Call them up and have them come to your therapy office so that they can talk with the client and provide a second opinion about the severity of the suicidal ideation. One recommendation is for you not to leave the room if you have significant concerns that your client may engage in self-harm. If you leave the room, they may harm themselves while you are gone, or they may take that opportunity to leave the office. Ensure your supervisor is involved in your therapeutic decisions when it concerns a suicidal client.

Ethical Dilemmas in Supervision

So far, we have mainly been talking about ethical dilemmas related to the therapy you will give and the clients you will interact with at your practicum/internship site. We have encouraged you to work closely with your supervisor to consider the ethical dilemmas and go through an ethical decision-making process. However, there are also ethical dilemmas that might be present in the supervision you receive (either with the supervisor at your site and/ or the faculty supervisor within your psychotherapy program).

The various codes of ethics and guidelines for each therapy field collectively address multiple relationships in some sense in relation to both therapists and their clients and supervisors and their supervisees. Lee and Nelson (2022) specifically discuss how multiple relationships can potentially become an ethical dilemma between supervisors and their supervisees. For instance, your program supervisors are oftentimes also your professors. It would be unethical, therefore, if your supervisor/professor were to give you an extension on a classwork assignment just because you are their supervisee as well. While this technically benefits you, it is your professional duty to be aware of, bring up, and rectify any ethical dilemmas that are related to multiple relationships such as in this scenario.

Power and hierarchy are also important factors between supervisors and supervisees that can become an ethical dilemma if mishandled (Lee & Nelson, 2022). A supervisor has some inherent level of power and a higher hierarchical position in relation to their supervisee, as the supervisor is the teacher providing guidance while the supervisee is the trainee receiving guidance. The supervisor will likely fill out an evaluation for you at the midterm and/or end of the semester. However, an abuse of that power dynamic from the supervisor is obviously an ethical dilemma. For instance, your supervisor is probably overstepping that line between power and collaboration if they didactically teach you and tell you that you have to do therapeutic interventions their way only. This impedes your ability as a student therapist to learn and practice multiple ways of giving therapy.

With many situations that we have presented through the chapters thus far, we have suggested that you go consult with your supervisor about it. So who do you talk to if your supervisor is the one who is creating an ethical dilemma? Well, that depends. If it is a small enough issue that you think your supervisor may be unaware of and you feel comfortable bringing this up with them, then you can certainly talk with your supervisor first. Sometimes your supervisor may not realize they are forcing their way of doing therapy upon you, for instance, and you kindly and professionally saying something really does help them realize this tendency.

If you encounter an ethical dilemma related to your supervisor that you are not comfortable talking to them about, then you should go to the next trusted person in the chain of command. If it is an issue with your site supervisor, perhaps you can consult your university program supervisor. If it is your program supervisor, then bringing this up to a trusted professor or administrator (e.g., the Program Director) would be the next best step.

We recommend that you bring up any important ethical dilemmas that involve your supervisor sooner rather than later, especially if it is affecting you and/or your clients. We knew of supervisees who encountered an ethical dilemma with a supervisor in which, among other things, the supervisor would write down inappropriate information (e.g., the supervisees' personal vacation plans) during supervision and make inappropriate comments about the supervisees' personal finances. The supervisees simply wanted to complete that practicum without causing an uproar, but when they shared these experiences with their new supervisor in the next practicum rotation a couple months later, the supervisor recommended that the students report that behavior to the clinic's director because it could affect future students as well.

Tips From a Supervisor

We have presented the primary ethical principles that all therapists follow. We have also presented a few situations that will arise for you. However, we couldn't ever get close to providing you with the myriad of scenarios that you will encounter not only in your practicum/internship but in your career. There are just too many that will come about. So my main tip here is to do a little projection into the future. Think about what *might* happen.

You have probably heard the saying that "preparation is the key to success." Your coursework has been preparing you for your practicum experience. The more ingrained your coursework was (the more prepared you were), the more successful you are likely to be during your field placement. A related saying to this is, "Success is where preparation and opportunity meet." During your therapy sessions, you will definitely have the opportunity to address ethical dilemmas. The question now is, how prepared will you be?

I recommend that you engage in various thought exercises in which you think about, for each case that you have, several potential ethical dilemmas that might arise. Once you do, you can think about how you would handle them (similar to what you did in the various exercises and What Would You Do? scenarios presented in this chapter). The more prepared you are for a potential ethical dilemma, the more likely you will successfully navigate that dilemma.

Summary

Psychotherapy is a profession that attempts to ensure that we, as therapists, do well and do good. To do so, we have developed a set of ethical guidelines for therapists to follow and aspire to. Each field in psychotherapy might have their own ethical codes; however, by and large, they mainly overlap. It is important for you to have a good working understanding of the ethical codes of your profession. Working from these standards and expectations will be one way to help ensure you are practicing competently. However, ethics are not always crystal clear. There will be times when you find yourself in the gray areas of therapeutic practice. When these times come, you will need to make ethical decisions. This chapter presented several ethical decision-making models that can help you to choose a course of action that is most beneficial for your client while adhering to the field's expectations.

References

Alonzo, D., & Gearing, R. E. (2018). *Suicide assessment and treatment: Empirical and evidence-based practices* (2nd ed.). Springer.

American Association for Marriage and Family Therapy. (2015). *Code of ethics.* www.aamft.org/Legal_Ethics/Code_of_Ethics.aspx

American Counseling Association. (2014). *2014 ACA code of ethics.* www.counseling.org/resources/aca-code-of-ethics.pdf

American Mental Health Counselors Association. (2020). *AMHCA code of ethics.* www.amhca.org/events/publications/ethics

American Psychological Association. (2017). *Ethical principles of psychologists and code of conduct.* www.apa.org/ethics/code/ethics-code-2017.pdf

Bell, L. (2021). *Helping people overcome suicidal thoughts, urges and behaviour.* Routledge.

Bronfenbrenner, U. (1979). *The ecology of human development: Experiments by nature and design.* Harvard University Press.

Caldwell, B. E., & Stone, D. J. (2016). Using scaling to facilitate ethical decision-making in family therapy. *The American Journal of Family Therapy, 44*(4), 198–210. http://dx.doi.org/10.1080/0192 6187.2016.1150797

Centers for Disease Control and Prevention. (n.d.). *Suicide prevention.* www.cdc.gov/suicide/index.html

Corey, G., Corey, M. S., & Corey, C. (2023). *Issues & ethics in the helping professions* (11th ed.). Cengage.

Ferguson, S. (2023). Assessment writing. In M. D. Reiter (Ed.), *A therapist's guide to writing in psychotherapy.* Routledge.

Flemons, D., & Gralnik, L. M. (2013). *Relational suicide assessment: Risks, resources, and possibilities for safety.* Norton.

Katafiasz, H., Patton, R., Tefteller, D., & Takeda, M. (2020). Ethical decision-making in marriage and family therapy: An introduction of a new model. *Journal of Systemic Therapies, 39*(4), 40–55. https://doi.org/10.1521/jsyt.2020.39.4.40

Leaune, E., Durif-Bruckert, C., Noelle, H., Joubert, F., Ravella, N., Haesebaert, J., Poulet, E., Chauliac, N., & Cuvillier, B. (2021). Impact of exposure to severe suicidal behaviours in patients during psychiatric training: An online French survey. *Early Intervention in Psychiatry, 15*(1), 149–157. https://doi.org/10.1111/eip.12923

Lee, R. E., & Nelson, T. S. (2022). *The contemporary relational supervisor* (2nd ed.). Routledge.

Moffett, L. A., Becker, C.-L. J., & Patton, R. G. (2014). Fostering the ethical sensitivity of beginning clinicians. *Training and Education in Professional Psychology, 8*(4), 229–235. https://doi.org/10.1037/tep0000054

Montreuil, M., Séguin, M., Gros, C. P., & Racine, E. (2021). Everyday ethics of suicide care: Survey of mental health care providers' perspectives and support needs. *PLoS One, 16*(4), e0249048. https://doi.org/10.1371/journal.pone.0249048

National Association of Social Workers. (2021). *Code of ethics of the national association of social workers.* https://www.socialworkers.org/About/Ethics/Code-of-Ethics/Code-of-Ethics-English

Okiishi, J., Lambert, M. J., Nielsen, S. L., & Ogles, B. M. (2003). Waiting for supershrink: An empirical analysis of therapist effects. *Clinical Psychology & Psychotherapy, 10*(6), 361–373. https://doi.org/10.1002/cpp.383

Pope, K. S., Vasquez, M. J. T., Chavez-Dueñas, N., & Adames, H. Y. (2021). *Ethics in psychotherapy and counseling: A practical guide* (6th ed.). Wiley.

Chapter 9

Navigating Therapy-Based Dilemmas

Myth About the Field

"Clients come to therapy being open, honest, and ready to change."

Therapists oftentimes wish this were the truth. Unfortunately, not all clients who come to therapy actually want to be in therapy. Whether, for example, it be an individual who is coming in at the request of their partner or a teenager being forced into therapy by their parents, some clients are going to be less than thrilled to be sitting in front of you. Even if clients willingly come to therapy, they may think it is someone else who needs to change. These are some of the therapy-based dilemmas that we will address in this chapter.

When Clients Don't Want to Be in Therapy

As mentioned previously, clients not wanting to be in therapy—or willingly coming to therapy under the pretense that it is another who needs to change—is one therapy-based dilemma that you are likely to encounter at your site. You may hear this dilemma referred to as client **resistance** (Yaman, 2021). There are some therapists who accept this notion that clients can be resistant to therapy; other therapists don't like to label clients as resistant (de Shazer, 1984). Regardless, the reality of some cases will be that there are clients who don't want to be there or are not opening up in ways which you find important for therapy to be helpful.

So how do you navigate working with these clients? As you may expect, there is not one clear answer for everyone, as each client's context plays a role in the best approach. We have found that one thing you can do across most of these cases, however, is to start by validating the client. Until they feel like you understand why they don't want to be there or why they think someone else needs to change, they will likely not give in to any other tactic you employ to invite them to open up. For instance, Kayleigh primarily works with teenagers who are often placed in therapy against their own wishes and are at the mercy of their parents. Instead of trying to tell them that they are in therapy, so they have to talk, Kayleigh empathizes with them and says things like, "This has gotta be really frustrating for you that you have to be here just because mom and dad said so." The majority of the time, Kayleigh has found the clients start to feel more comfortable and can relate to what she is saying. Then, she will often say, "So listen, we both know that you have to be here for the time being. The good part, though, is that this is your space—so in the end, you really get

DOI: 10.4324/9781003433484-9

to use it however you want. Is there something that *you* want to talk about?" If you find that your client does not want to be in therapy, you might consider using many of the principles of motivational interviewing (Miller & Rollnick, 2023).

When Clients Lie

We would like to think that everything a client tells us is the truth, as we are there not to punish them but to help them. But for various reasons, clients will lie to us. About 89–93% of clients reported lying to their therapist (Blanchard & Farber, 2016; Curtis & Hart, 2020). They may feel embarrassed about what they did or thought and may want to avoid a perceived judgment from us. Depending on the setting, they may lie to avoid consequences. For instance, if you are doing your field placement in an in-patient facility, there are a lot of rules for the clients/patients to follow. If they are honest with you about breaking a rule, you may have to report this to the authority at the facility.

Trust is one of the core components of therapy. Kottler and Carlson (2011) explained that "the foundation of counseling and psychotherapy is based on trust—not just trust in the therapist, but just as critically, trust in the client" (p. 3). Part of trust is about truth and honesty, or, conversely, that the person doesn't lie to you. However, what is a lie? Are all lies the same? We might categorize **lies** in terms of falsities, obfuscations, partial disclosures, hidden reactions, secrets, and things left unsaid (Farber et al., 2019). Curtis and Hart (2020) categorized **deceptions** into those of omission, failed deception, half-truth, white lie, distortion, and blatant lie.

When you realize that a client has lied to you, we encourage you to take a second and think about what they were really trying to tell you. What was behind the lie? There was a reason for it. Perhaps it was because they were trying to gain your approval or protect themselves from embarrassment and shame (Kottler & Carlson, 2011). Blanchard and Farber (2016) surveyed clients about the topics of their lies. The results might be quite interesting for you. Here are the top ten topics of lies reported by clients (p. 98):

1.	How bad I really feel—I minimized	54%
2.	The severity of my symptoms—I minimized	39%
3.	My thoughts about suicide	31%
4.	My insecurities and doubts about myself	31%
5.	Pretending to like my therapist's comments or suggestions	29%
6.	My use of drugs or alcohol	29%
7.	Why I missed appointments or was late	29%
8.	Pretending to find therapy more effective than I do	29%
9.	Pretending to be more hopeful than I really am	27%
10.	Things I have done that I regret	26%

What Do You Think About These Reasons?

So why do clients lie? For therapy-related topics, they tend to lie to be polite, to not upset the therapist, or so their therapist doesn't disapprove of them (Blanchard & Farber, 2016). For non-therapy-related lies, it tends to be because the topic is uncomfortable, the client didn't want to look bad, the client wanted to avoid shame, or the client wasn't ready to discuss the topic.

So who lies? All clients lie. However, they may do so differently based on age. Younger clients tend to report lying about more topics than older clients (Blanchard & Farber, 2016).

So when do clients lie? They might lie anywhere along the therapeutic process; however, they tend to be more willing to lie in the first session the most (Curtis & Hart, 2020). This is because they have not yet developed a strong therapeutic alliance with the therapist. The greater the emotional connection between people, the less likely they are to lie to the other person. This dynamic should prompt you to figure out how to, as quickly as possible, develop a positive therapeutic connection with your client.

So what do you do when your client lies? It is important to be aware of your own reactions when you find out that a client has deceived you. Most therapists tend to hold negative attitudes toward clients who lie (Curtis & Hart, 2015). This can negatively impact the therapeutic alliance. We encourage you to engage in a **therapeutic confrontation**, in which you point out the discrepancy that is happening. "I'm confused. On the one hand you said that you didn't talk to your ex, and now on the other hand you are saying that the two of you spent the night together last night. Can you clarify that?"

Quick Tip: Remember, you are not alone as a therapist. There will always be therapy-based dilemmas for you to deal with. The longer you are in the field, the more comfortable you will be with making therapeutic decisions on your own. However, you are still new in the field. Engage in consultation and supervision. It is better to talk with someone about what your best courses of action are rather than flounder on your own.

When Clients Are Extremely Emotional

Some people think that therapy is effective when the client cries. Perhaps. But some people will cry at the drop of a hat, while other people will never shed a tear. You will have a client that will cry in your office at some point. What do you do when this happens?

To hand clients a tissue or to not hand clients a tissue? That is the question. Though perhaps a seemingly small issue, this is actually a meaningful dynamic to address before you go into the therapy room. We call this the **tissue dilemma**. And there is not a right answer to it. Still, we want to discuss the different approaches that you can take when you are faced with this decision.

On the one hand, people think that if you give a tissue to a client who is crying, it can be a signal to them to stop crying. You should think to yourself, "Why am I giving them a tissue?" Your first response will probably be about them—maybe to have them feel better or so that snot isn't running down their nose and face. But if you take a longer look, it might really be for you. Most people are not comfortable when someone else is in such emotional pain. They will try to get the person to stop being so emotional and crying not only to try to make the other person feel better but to get themselves to stop feeling uncomfortable. If this is the case, we recommend that you maybe refrain from taking this initiative and quickly passing over the tissue box.

On the other hand, people think that giving a tissue is a sign to the other person that it is okay for them to emote—that having the tissue is a sign that it is safe for them to cry. It also may convey that you are really attuned to the client's emotions and are responding appropriately.

Whichever choice you decide, make sure you have the tissue box near where the client might be seated so *they* can easily reach it if they decide they want it. We both tend to follow the latter approach, but we have both been in situations in which we forgot to put the tissue box near the client while they were crying (sometimes they get moved around in sessions). So we weren't handing the client a tissue, yet they could also not get the tissue for themselves. These are situations in which we got up and grabbed the box to give to the client. It's better to prevent this from happening altogether and just check the location of the tissue box before each session. (As a side note, make sure you have a trash bin in the therapy room. We have also been in situations in which there was no trash can and the client had to hold onto their soiled tissues throughout the session.)

Tales From the Field: Intern

My internship site was a community-based agency with a private dimension, catering to clients from the state and those with private insurance. In the midst of my responsibilities, I was assigned a client for case work based on the knowledge and experiences I have that aligned closely with the client's needs. However, what began as a seemingly straightforward case quickly spiraled into a complex situation. There were multiple providers involved, each with their unique contributions. However, from the outset, I sensed an unusual tension among some of them and a protective barrier forming around the client.

As I worked closely with the client, I observed a troubling shift—a marked increase in sadness, frustration, and anger and a noticeable decline in her overall mood. She made alarming statements that began to deeply concern me. In response to each concern, I promptly alerted the appropriate channels, seeking support for the changes I was witnessing. However, each of these care providers thought that the client was crying wolf.

Despite my best efforts, her deterioration accelerated, leading to a pivotal two-hour discussion between myself and the family case manager. During this conversation, I asked probing questions inquiring whether the client had ever been off her medications and what it looks like when she is off them. I asked whether there was any concrete evidence to challenge her narrative that she was severely distressed. I also offered alternative perspectives, suggesting that we should enter her world rather than insisting she conform to ours. After a series of meetings and concerning interactions among providers, I approached my supervisor and requested an in-person shadowing session. This allowed my supervisor to witness our interactions, observe the client's behavior, and gain insight into her concerns.

Tragically, the client's struggle persisted. She would regularly call and text, ensuring our sessions would take place so that she did not miss any. One day, she messaged me to cancel because she felt unwell. I offered my well wishes and promised to check on her later. It was not less than an hour after that I received a call informing me of her suicide. The aftermath left me hazed in a whirlwind of emotions. The overwhelming hurt and profound sadness intertwined with a seething anger. My anger wasn't just directed at the circumstances but also at the system that had seemed so preoccupied with ignoring her truth that they failed to recognize the depth of her pain.

As the news of her suicide swept throughout the team, condolences poured in accompanied by an acknowledgment of my close connection to her. It was this bond that led her grieving mother to reach out to me, her anguish manifesting as blame directed at me for her daughter's untimely death. In this tumultuous time, the family case manager—who had been a vital part of our support network—retreated into a disheartening silence. The weight of these accusations, coupled with the profound loss, heightened my emotions and made it hard to contain the anger that needed time to subside.

In recognition of my emotional turmoil, I decided I needed some time off. My anger was too raw to immediately address the situation, but with time, I began to process the ordeal. To the credit of the organization, I was offered the respite needed, which started with granting my leave and providing access to five counseling sessions through their Employee Assistance Program (EAP). Returning to work within the same system proved to be a challenge. I could not get past my feelings of hurt and pain in the time permitted. Each attempt to navigate the familiar environment would unravel me, leading to uncontrollable bouts of tears and heavy, labored breathing.

In the end, I made the difficult decision to extend my leave indefinitely, ultimately opting to sever my relationship with the organization before the leave period formally concluded. This painful chapter reinforced the critical importance of advocating for robust mental health support and highlighted the pressing need to address systemic shortcomings that had prevented the recognition and appropriate response to the profound suffering of an individual in distress.

Victoria Nichols, MS intern in Family Therapy, Capella University

When Clients Are Inappropriate With You

We know that therapy is a contractual relationship in which you are a business professional. However, we also know that it is an intimate endeavor in which we are engaging clients on levels they likely don't experience in most of their other relationships. This may lead them to develop an attraction to you beyond the scope of the therapist-client relationship. Your psychotherapy program has likely not introduced you to this topic.

Harris and Harriger (2009) surveyed therapists-in-training on what they might do if a client who was coming in for couples therapy expressed attraction to them. Fifty-three percent of the therapists-in-training said they would process the expressed attraction with the couple. Thirty-three percent were uncertain about discussing it. Seventy-six percent would not meet individually with the person who expressed the attraction, and 70% wouldn't meet with the non-attracted partner.

There can be several ways in which your client may specifically be inappropriate with you. One example is when Kayleigh was a student intern with Michael as supervisor during their graduate program's one-way-mirror practicum. Kayleigh and a co-therapist (another female who was in her mid-20s) were seeing a 78-year-old male client who had been in therapy for several semesters at the university's clinic. Kayleigh and her co-therapist had developed a good relationship with their client, who was a sentimental yet old-fashioned guy. However, the team of other student therapists thought that there were times when the client was flirting with both therapists. He would not be overt (e.g., "I want to take you out to dinner") but had made several innuendos and would use various terms when referring to them, such as "Sweetie" or "Honey." One day, he asked them if he could take a picture of them to show the people at his AA meeting. He explained that he was so happy with the therapy and the progress he was making that he wanted to promote the therapists who were helping him. Kayleigh and her co-therapist were not really comfortable with this request and declined it.

This is just one example. Another, perhaps more common example, is when clients want to hug you. Earlier, we asked, "To hand clients a tissue or to not hand clients a tissue?" Now, the question is, "To hug your client or to not hug your client?" There may be some moments when a hug can be a therapeutic intervention. For instance, in a case that Michael supervised (and Kayleigh watched behind the mirror), the student intern's client came into therapy because he was having issues with embracing his emotions and then expressing those emotions to others. In one session, Michael entered the therapy room and talked with the client about how he could express his emotions nonverbally, as the client was an older male who was struggling with his physically and psychologically ailing wife. Michael explained that he wanted to communicate his support for the client without saying anything and asked the client to stand up. Michael then hugged the client and held the hug, allowing both himself and the client to experience the sensation of being connected to another person and not having to do anything but feel the support. The client shared how powerful this was in feeling those emotions and allowing them to be shared with another.

In this situation, Michael initiated a therapeutic hug. In other cases, your clients may ask for or physically initiate a hug first. This is where you consider the ethics and appropriateness behind a hug, as a hug does include the element of physical touch. If you believe a hug is appropriate and therapeutic, then a hug should be okay. For example, Kayleigh was working with a couple in their 70s for almost a year during her practicum. At the end of their last session, after Kayleigh had walked them out to the clinic's lobby, the wife started to tear up, thanked Kayleigh for everything, and started to reach for a hug. Kayleigh returned the hug, and afterwards, the husband did the same. This is an example of when a hug initiated by a client was appropriate as it signified the growth and the positive end of a long and deep therapeutic relationship.

Now, if a client expresses their romantic interest in you after the end of a session and quickly goes in for a hug and starts rubbing your back a bit too intimately, that is obviously on the inappropriate side. When something like this happens with a hug, even if a hug seemed appropriate and therapeutic at first, you need to address it with your client. Michael was supervising a mid-20s female therapist who was working with a mid-30s male client. At the end of the fourth session, the client got up, walked over to the therapist who was sitting, and leaned in to kiss the therapist. She stopped him before he kissed her, explained that wasn't part of their relationship, and walked him to the front. In supervision, she explained that she was not comfortable working with him anymore and arranged for him to meet with a different therapist.

What Would You Do?: 9.1

You have a client that keeps making comments that you are perceiving to be subtle flirtations. They are not saying, "You are so attractive," but are making statements that are trying to shift the therapeutic conversation from them to you. They are asking you about things you like, such as types of food, television shows, and music. They are asking you about your personal life. You are getting the sense that, if not your client, they would be trying to date you. Each session they are increasing these types of comments but have never been overt about flirting. What would you do?

When You Are Inappropriate With Your Client

Just as clients have the potential of being attracted to you, you are likely to occasionally be attracted to one of your clients. It is actually normal for therapists to be sexually attracted to a client (Martin et al., 2011). About 70% of therapists find at least one of their clients sexually attractive, and 25% fantasize about having a romantic relationship with a client (Vesentini et al., 2022). If you think this is strange, how come? The client is first and foremost a human being who, if they weren't in your office, you would not only find physically attractive but also interpersonally attractive in which you might seek out a relationship with them. But because they are your client, you cannot. All ethical codes hold that you cannot have a sexual relationship with your client. For instance, NASW (2021, Standard 1.09) states, "Social workers should under no circumstances engage in sexual activities, inappropriate sexual communications through the use of technology or in person, or sexual contact with current clients, whether such contact is consensual or forced." They further stipulate that therapists not have sexual contact with a client's relatives or others closely connected with the client, former clients, or people they've had a past sexual relationship with.

Okay, so that is clear. Don't have sex with your client. But what happens when you are attracted to your client? What do you do? This is probably a difficult question for you to answer since many graduate programs provide little training on this topic (Harris, 2001). Ladany et al. (1997) found that only about 50% of therapists-in-training brought up their sexual attraction to their client with their supervisor. This is compounded because their supervisors were unlikely to initiate the conversation. When the topic is brought up, interns found it quite helpful when the supervisor normalized the attraction and provided a space for them to explore their feelings during the supervision session. However, it is very important to explore and talk about these feelings, especially with a supervisor or a more senior therapist (Vesentini et al., 2021). This can be difficult since many therapists believe it is taboo to have sexual feelings about a client. Further, younger and more inexperienced therapists may have a more difficult time talking about sexual feelings toward clients. So if you do find that you have strong sexual feelings toward a client, in which you think it is playing a role in how you are conceptualizing the case and what you are doing therapeutically in the room, please make sure that you consult with someone. This could be your supervisor or a more experienced therapist.

The person you should probably not talk with about these feelings is your client. Fisher (2004) argued that self-disclosing your sexual feelings to your client may run the risk of harming them and is potentially unethical. He discourages therapists from doing so since it puts the clients in a very awkward position in which what is being discussed is about you and not about them or their concerns that they brought into therapy. Rather, Fisher suggests utilizing supervision, personal therapy, and consultation to help therapists manage their sexual feelings so that they maintain their professional ethics.

There are various ways that you can be inappropriate with your client, with sexual boundary breaches being one of the most visual. Anytime you are inappropriate with your client, you open yourself up to possible ethical and legal consequences. Even if you are not licensed, you can come in disfavor with the licensing board of your state or area. Perhaps you are not sexually attracted to your client but are interpersonally attracted. You will likely have a client who, if conditions were different for your meeting (perhaps at a party or somewhere outside of therapy), you would want to be friends with. Almost 4% of therapists started a relationship with their client during therapy, and 13% did after therapy (Vesentini et al., 2022).

Now, all healthcare practitioners have complaints made against them. However, mental health practitioners had them at a rate double to physical health practitioners, such as doctors and chiropractors (Veness et al., 2019). Further, male and older practitioners were at increased risk of having a complaint lodged against them. While these rates are not only for sexual boundary breaches or interpersonal behavior (they also include issues of confidentiality, reporting, recording, and the mental health of the practitioner), they are higher than any of us would like them to be.

Tales From the Field: Supervisor

I have two tales that I would like to share with you, as they demonstrate that what may seem like a small thing can actually be a big thing and that, as a student intern, it is extremely important to think about the larger picture of the therapeutic context. First, John was a mental health counseling intern at an in-patient addiction treatment center and was being supervised by the site's clinical director. John had completed all of his course work, and this internship was the final requirement of the program before graduation.

During the addictions group he was co-leading, John had a bad headache. He took a pill bottle out of his pocket, popped a pill into his mouth, and then put the pill bottle back into his pocket. The group co-leader reported this activity to the site's clinical director, and John was asked to not come back to the internship site.

The issue was processed in group supervision. John initially had difficulty understanding how what he did could lead to his discharge from the site. However, other interns in the supervision group helped John see how such behavior could be a serious trigger for some of the group members. Additionally, I talked with John about being aware of how his actions, whether intentional or not, have an effect on clients. John was able to see how the context of his behavior was so important and that he needed to be mindful of the impact of his behavior on others. I encouraged John to become more self-aware of his behavior and the context in which he is counseling. John was referred to the school's Professional Standards Committee, which is required when an intern is let go from a site. The results of the committee were that this seemed like a rookie mistake. John was required to write an ethics paper on why this behavior was not acceptable, and he was permitted to find another site.

Second, Sondra was a White female mental health counseling intern at a community mental health center. She was being supervised by the clinical director. At the end of one work night, Sondra just finished a therapy session with a client. When they walked out of the office, they realized there was a severe thunderstorm. The client remarked that they would have to walk three blocks in the rain to catch a bus to be able to get home. Sondra, in wanting to maintain a therapeutic alliance, offered to drive the client to the client's home. The offer for a ride was overheard in the hallway on the way to the exit and reported to the clinical director. Sondra was asked to not come back to that internship site.

During our next group supervision, this issue was processed, and Sondra was unable to see how such behavior is crossing boundaries with the client, even though it was a very nice gesture. Like John, Sondra was referred to the school's Professional Standards Committee. It was uncovered that Sondra was being picked up by their spouse and that the client was introduced to the spouse as well as being given a ride to their home. The results of the committee were for Sondra to write an ethics paper about why this behavior was unacceptable from a counselor. Instead of writing this paper, she voluntarily withdrew from the program.

Dale V. Wayman, PhD, LCAC, LMHC, ACS, Mental Health Counseling program, Capella University

When You Do Not Like Your Client

You probably have a view that you should like all of your clients. We would like to disavow you of this belief. Clients are people, and you do not like all people (nor are you supposed to). However, we want to just tweak our language just a little bit. When we say the word "like," we are more so referring to not liking what our client thinks or does. But be guaranteed, you are going to have clients that, for one reason or another, you are not excited about when you see them on the schedule. This feeling is not problematic unless you do not do anything about it.

Carl Rogers, perhaps the most influential therapist of all time, held that one of the core conditions of psychotherapy was that the therapist was able to provide **unconditional positive regard** for their client (Rogers, 1961). He also talked about this in terms of therapeutic caring. What this means is that you accept and support the person without any judgments or expectations. It is a demonstration of the client's inherent worth. Now, you may work with some clients who have done very bad things, such as assault, rape, and murder. You shouldn't like that they did any of these acts. However, unconditional positive regard holds that if that person's context were different, they would move toward self-actualization, and their behaviors would be more positive.

So how do you deal with your negative reactions to clients? One way is to use them as a transformation device (Flemons, 2002). Instead of trying to take away your negative feeling, you can complement it with curiosity. This is a twofold curiosity: First about your own reactions and second about your client. You might ask yourself the following questions about yourself:

1. What is it about me that I'm having difficulty with the client?
2. How are my reactions a message from myself to myself?
3. What can I learn about me, based on this situation, that I didn't know before?

You might then ask yourself the following questions about your client:

1. What is it about the client that I haven't learned yet?
2. How does the client's behaviors or philosophies make sense, given the conditions the client grew up in and were living in?
3. What are some of the similarities that I have with the client?

The answers to these questions may provide you a bridge of connection to your client. The more that you hold the view of "I do not like this person" in your head, the more you will likely avoid them and have the potential of a self-fulfilling prophecy. It is important for you, as early as possible, to begin to open yourself to new experiences and perceptions of your client.

Exercise 9.1   Getting Curious About Someone

Think about someone in your life that you do not like too much. It might be a client, but perhaps it is better if it is not. Maybe it is a family member or coworker. This should be someone with whom you have some frequent contact. Perhaps someone whom you would like a better relationship with. Once you have decided on the person, answer the following questions based on the questions in the previous section:

1. What is it about me that I'm having difficulty with this person?
2. How are my reactions a message from myself to myself?
3. What can I learn about me, based on this situation, that I didn't know before?
4. What is it about the person that I haven't learned yet?
5. How does the person's behaviors or philosophies make sense, given the conditions they grew up in and were living in?
6. What are some of the similarities that I have with the person?

After answering these questions, how are your thoughts and feelings about the person different? How likely are you to try to know more about them now?

Another way that you can develop greater unconditional positive regard for your client is to adopt the perspective of "**not-knowing**" (Anderson & Goolishian, 1992). This is a therapeutic stance in which the therapist comes into an encounter with openness and curiosity. It is not that you do not know anything. You've taken a lot of courses, read tons of books and journal articles, and watched lots of therapy videos. You also know yourself. What you don't know is how the client makes meaning of their life. The more you have this not-knowing viewpoint, the less you will objectify the client as being only a certain way. You will be able to be curious about the client's way of understanding self, which should bring some type of humanity to them (at least in your eyes). While you will still not like some of the client's behaviors, you will hopefully appreciate that they are a human being, which is worthwhile in itself.

When Clients No-Show

We can guarantee that at some point during your practicum/internship, a client is going to no-show. For outpatient therapy, the no-show attendance rate might be as high as 30% (Muppavarapu et al., 2022). This means that they simply do not show up to the session at all and give no notice that they are not coming. If this happens with your client and it was truly just an accident that one time, then it is usually not a big deal, and you can move on with therapy like usual. Most sites reflect this approach, as they often have a one-time waive of any no-show fee as a courtesy because life happens.

Where you will have to intervene in some way is when no-showing for a client becomes a pattern. DeFife et al. (2010) discussed that consistent no shows can create problems in a variety of ways: administrative difficulties (e.g., billing), clinical issues (e.g., monthly documentation or the therapist-client relationship), and issues in therapeutic effectiveness (as a client who doesn't consistently come to therapy is likely not gaining as much from treatment). While this shouldn't affect you as a student intern, it is also important to note that—depending on your future therapy workplace—you may not be paid for a no-show session. While we need to consider the client's situation, no-showing can also affect us financially.

This is a therapy-based dilemma in which you will need to balance both your practicum/ internship site's policies and your own contextual understanding of the client and their situation. The first step in doing this is to make sure you know the parameters of your site's no-show policy. For example, at one site, a missed session or a session canceled within one hour of the appointment may be considered a no-show; another site may only consider missed sessions as a no-show. If a client asks you what constitutes a no-show, you should be able to accurately answer that question. Other parameters to consider include whether your site has a courtesy waive of the fee or waives the fee in emergency situations.

The second step is to try to prevent the no-shows from becoming a pattern. You should always find out why a client no-shows each time it happens. Typically, a site policy involves calling a client if they haven't shown up around 10–15 minutes into the session. If they don't answer, you should either leave a voicemail and/or send them an email or text (again, depending on your site's procedures). More often than not, a client will later reach out to you and let you know why they didn't show up. If you don't hear from them and then they do show up to the next session, you can ask them about missing the previous session. You usually want to do this in a non-blaming way: For example, "I wanted to check in and see if you had gotten my message about missing our session last week. Is everything okay?" Typically, they will say that they completely forgot to come or completely forgot to cancel. Again, when it's the first time for a reason that isn't a big deal, you can usually let it go.

Now, if this happens a second time and the client gives the same/similar reasons (e.g., they forgot, they have a lot going on right now, they couldn't get a ride and forgot to cancel, etc.), you need to have a therapeutic conversation with them about why it is important for them to attend therapy regularly. You can talk about how this space is for them and you want to make sure they are getting the most out of it. You can also gently remind them of your site's policies, as some sites will discharge a client after three consecutive no-shows, for instance. It may also be beneficial to proactively ask the client if the day and time of their appointment still works for them or if they need to switch to another session time. Sometimes clients' schedules change, and they don't want to be a burden and change their therapy time (even if they aren't showing up); initiating this conversation may be just what they need. Perhaps they are even appropriate for biweekly therapy and this is a better option for them to attend consistently instead of once a week.

So what do you do if none of this works and a client keeps no-showing? Well, on the one hand, you need to follow your site's policies to some degree. If you have had the aforementioned conversations with a client and they are still not showing up to sessions consecutively, then you may just need to move forward with the discharge process based on your site's policy. Kayleigh had a client who no-showed for three sessions, and each time would email Kayleigh back the day after the missed session stating she was so sorry and she just forgot (this client also sporadically no-showed throughout the course of therapy). Despite Kayleigh reiterating the no-show policy and giving the client an extra chance past this policy to attend the next session, the client did not show up to the fourth session, and Kayleigh had to discharge her. Not only was the client past the no-show policy, but she was also no longer benefiting from therapy. In these cases, it is important to email your client when you do need to officially discharge them and offer for them to reach back out if/when they want therapy and are able to attend consistently.

On the other hand, you also need to consider your client's context. For instance, Kayleigh had another client who attended therapy very regularly. The client never missed a session unless she had canceled it well in advance. About a year into therapy, the client did not show up to her weekly session three weeks in a row despite Kayleigh reaching out to her (and her emergency contact, since this was very odd for her client) each week through phone and email. Kayleigh wanted to wait another week to hear back from her instead of discharging after three sessions (as was her workplace's policy) since this was very out of character for her client. (Kayleigh consulted with her site supervisor about extending the policy based on the circumstance, and this is something that you should do as well.) Sure enough, the next week, Kayleigh's client showed up to her session, and Kayleigh had asked her if everything was okay and where she had been. The client had gone on vacation for a few weeks, did not check her emails or voicemails, and stated she had thought she had told Kayleigh about needing to cancel. This was a very rare occurrence for the client and was the first time anything like this had happened, so Kayleigh was happy that she did not simply discharge this client.

Overall, you will need to play it by ear with each no-show case. Part of this is going to involve using your therapeutic intuition on how to handle a client who no-shows. We recommend that you proactively communicate with your client about the no-shows. Additionally, don't just jump the gun and assume a client no-showed because they forgot. Wait to hear back from your clients after you reach out to them—for example, Kayleigh's client had once no-showed because she had to go to the emergency room and was physically unable to send an email. No-showing is a dilemma in which you should always consult with your supervisor as well.

Tips From a Supervisor

You've probably seen the car bumper sticker that says "Sh*t happens" or "Life happens." My main tip here is to accept this and be prepared that you are going to have experiences in the therapy room that are not ideal. You've probably read about how to do a technique and thought of how to do it well. Then when you try to implement it, it fails, and you fall on your face. We don't have pristine conditions when therapy happens. It is the real world with real clients and a real therapist.

This is where the science and art of therapy overlap. The science is what to do and why. The art is how to do it. Be prepared that there are going to be "issues" that come up in therapy. You will become frustrated, angry, concerned, and confused. When this happens, slow down, take a breath, and think about what is happening. The second tip here is to not keep the therapy-based dilemma to yourself. Remember that you have a lot of resources at your disposal. You have fellow classmates at school, other interns at the placement, your site supervisor, and your faculty supervisor. The more that you can consult with these various people, the more you can be thoughtful about what your next therapeutic step will be rather than be reactive.

When Clients Ask You Personal Questions

Therapy is frequently viewed as being predicated on the therapeutic relationship. Clients get invested not only in the therapy process but in their therapist. They want to know that they are making a human-to-human connection. When they do, they may ask you personal questions. If they do, will you answer? If so, for how long? If not, how will you respond in your non-answering?

Self-disclosure occurs when the therapist shares information about themselves to the client. Our recommendation is to be genuine while being therapeutic. Self-disclose appropriately while quickly shifting the focus in what you are saying from yourself to the client. For instance, Michael was working with a young adolescent who was having sibling rivalry with his brother. Michael said to the client, "My brother and I used to fight all the time. For a time, it was bad. However, we figured out how to be with one another that was more enjoyable. How might you and your brother start to change your relationship?" Here, the self-disclosure helps to normalize the client's situation and provide hope. It then ends on the client and their situation.

We think being genuine—a real human being—is so important that if you aren't genuine with your clients, you can harm the therapeutic relationship. Michael was a therapist and supervisor in a clinical psychology outpatient clinic and saw a consistency across the psychology interns. When they were asked any personal question by the client, regardless of the intensity of it, the interns had the same response: "How would it help you to know that about me?" Clearly, they were learning this response in class. We don't recommend this response, at least for most client inquiries. If a client is going into the woods for vacation and asks you whether you like hiking, "How would it help you to know that about me" is not a beneficial response. If a client asks if you watched the Super Bowl, it is not likely a beneficial response. But if they ask you about your favorite sexual position, then this response seems quite appropriate.

We understand that, based on your model, self-disclosing might have serious therapeutic implications. However, that was mainly classical psychoanalysis. When we appropriately self-disclose, we can strengthen the therapeutic relationship. This is beneficial since 30% of positive therapeutic change is based on a strong alliance between you and the client (Lambert, 1992). We cannot help but self-disclose to our clients. How you style your hair, your jewelry, your clothing, and your accent are all forms of self-disclosure. We cannot not self-disclose. So it is not a matter of "Do I self-disclose?" but "What do I self-disclose and why?"

Quick Tip: When thinking about whether you should self-disclose or not to the client, think to yourself: "Who am I self-disclosing for?" If the answer is for yourself, do not self-disclose.

Tips From an Intern

We've talked about a lot of different therapy-based dilemmas in this chapter—clients lying, giving hugs, clients no-showing, and more. As a student intern, it can be overwhelming to figure out how to respond to each of these situations since there is not a one-size-fits-all approach. However, I want to bring up something we mentioned in Chapter 8: beneficence. My tip is that beneficence should be your guiding principle when deciding how to navigate the therapy-based dilemmas we presented in this chapter (and any other related dilemmas that you come across).

Above all else, we need to practice beneficence and do good to and for our clients. When you are trying to navigate a therapy-based dilemma, always ask yourself what would be best for the client. Along with making decisions based on ethical, legal, and policy-related considerations, we also need to include beneficence when determining the most clinically appropriate decision. Remember the couple whom I gave hugs to after the closure of our last session? Imagine what it would have been like for the wife if I retracted from her when she went to give me a hug after thanking me for everything. In that situation, it was more clinically beneficial to give her and her husband a hug.

Summary

Therapy is not a straightforward or simple endeavor. Besides the case conceptualization that you have and the treatment plan you develop, there are many other potential events that can happen that can lead to a therapy-based dilemma. Clients may not want to come to session, no-show, lie, challenge you, be emotional, or be overly intimate. Each of these situations will happen to you to some degree at some point in your therapeutic career. That is a guarantee. The question is not will it happen, but rather, what will you do when it happens? This chapter has introduced you to some of the common therapy-based dilemmas that occur for all therapists so that you are one step closer to being able to handle them effectively.

References

Anderson, H., & Goolishian, H. (1992). The client is the expert: A not-knowing approach to therapy. In S. McNamee & K. J. Gergen (Eds.), *Therapy as social construction* (pp. 25–39). Sage.

Blanchard, M., & Farber, B. A. (2016). Lying in psychotherapy: Why and what clients don't tell their therapist about therapy and their relationship. *Counselling Psychology Quarterly, 29*(1), 90–112. https://doi.org/10.1080/09515070.2015.1085365

Curtis, D. A., & Hart, C. L. (2015). Pinocchio's nose in therapy: Therapists' beliefs and attitudes toward client deception. *International Journal for the Advancement of Counselling, 37*(3), 279–292. https://doi.org/10.1007/s10447-015-9243-6

Curtis, D. A., & Hart, C. L. (2020). Deception in psychotherapy: Frequency, typology and relationship. *Counselling & Psychotherapy Research, 20*(1), 106–115. https://doi.org/10.1002/capr.12263

de Shazer, S. (1984). The death of resistance. *Family Process, 23*(1), 11–17. https://doi.org/10.1111/j.1545-5300.1984.00011.x

DeFife, J. A., Conklin, C. Z., Smith, J. M., & Poole, J. (2010). Psychotherapy appointment no-shows: Rates and reasons. *Psychotherapy: Theory, Research, Practice, Training, 47*(3), 413–417. https://doi.org/10.1037/a0021168

Farber, B. A., Blanchard, M., & Love, M. (2019). *Secrets and lies in psychotherapy*. American Psychological Association.

Fisher, C. D. (2004). Ethical issues in therapy: Therapist self-disclosure of sexual feelings. *Ethics & Behavior, 14*(2), 105–121. https://doi.org/10.1207/s15327019eb1402_2

Flemons, D. (2002). *Of one mind*. Norton.

Harris, S. M. (2001). Teaching family therapists about sexual attraction in therapy. *Journal of Marital and Family Therapy, 27*(1), 123–128. https://doi.org/10.1111/j.1752-0606.2001.tb01145.x

Harris, S. M., & Harriger, D. J. (2009). Sexual attraction in conjoint therapy. *The American Journal of Family Therapy, 37*(3), 209–216. https://doi.org/10.1080/01926180802152032

Kottler, J., & Carlson, J. (2011). *Duped: Lies and deception in psychotherapy*. Routledge.

Ladany, N., O'Brien, K. M., Hill, C. E., Melincoff, D. S., Knox, S., & Petersen, D. A. (1997). Sexual attraction toward clients, use of supervision, and prior training: A qualitative study of predoctoral psychology interns. *Journal of Counseling Psychology, 44*(4), 413–424. https://doi.org/10.1037/0022-0167.44.4.413

Lambert, M. J. (1992). Psychotherapy outcome research: Implications for integrative and eclectic therapists. In J. C. Norcross & M. R. Goldfried (Eds.), *Handbook of psychotherapy integration* (pp. 94–129). Basic Books.

Martin, C., Godfrey, M., Meekums, B., & Madill, A. (2011). Managing boundaries under pressure: A qualitative study of therapists' experiences of sexual attraction in therapy. *Counselling and Psychotherapy Research, 11*(4), 248–256. https://doi.org/10.1080/14733145.2010.519045

Miller, W. M., & Rollnick, S. (2023). *Motivational interviewing: Helping people change and grow* (4th ed.). Guilford.

Muppavarapu, K., Saeed, S. A., Jones, K., Hurd, O., & Haley, V. (2022). Study of impact of telehealth use on clinic "no show" rates at an academic practice. *Psychiatric Quarterly, 93*(2), 689–699. https://doi.org/10.1007/s11126-022-09983-6

National Association of Social Workers. (2021). *Code of ethics of the National Association of Social Workers*. https://www.socialworkers.org/About/Ethics/Code-of-Ethics/Code-of-Ethics-English

Rogers, C. (1961). *On becoming a person: A therapist's view of psychotherapy*. Houghton Mifflin.

Veness, B. G., Tibble, H, Grenyer, B. F., Morris, J. M., Spittal, M. J., Nash, L., Studdert, D. M., & Bismark, M. M. (2019). Complaint risk among mental health practitioners compared with physical health practitioners: A retrospective cohort study of complaints to health regulators in Australia. *BMJ Open, 9*(12), e030525. https://doi.org/10.1136/bmjopen-2019-030525

Vesentini, L., Van Overmeire, R., Matthys, F., De Wachter, D., Van Puyenbroeck, H., & Bilsen, J. (2022). Intimacy in psychotherapy: An exploratory survey among therapists. *Archives of Sexual Behavior, 51*(1), 453–463. https://doi.org/10.1007/s10508-021-02190-7

Vesentini, L., Van Puyenbroeck, H., De Wachter, D., Matthys, F., & Bilsen, J. (2021). Sexual feelings toward clients in the psychotherapeutic relationship: The taboo revealed. *Qualitative Health Research, 31*(5), 999–1011. https://doi.org/10.1177/1049732321990654

Yaman, N. (2021). Working with resistance in therapy: A theoretical evaluation. *IBAD Journal of Social Sciences, 9*(9), 481–495. https://doi.org/10.21733/ibad.835243

Chapter 10

Navigating Site-Based Dilemmas

We hope that from the first contact you have with your site to the last, you have an amazing experience. For most of you, for the most part, you will. Many interns find their placement to be the highlight of their degree program experience. Even so, there will be hiccups or even earthquakes along the way. In this chapter, we'd like to talk with you about being aware of site-based dilemmas and possible routes that you can take when they occur.

Now, we know that the previous chapter was on ethical dilemmas. Some of the points from that chapter may apply to this chapter because some of the ethical dilemmas that we outlined are obviously going to happen at your site. However, there are other dilemmas that you will come across that may or may not be ethical in nature but are present solely because of how your site is operating (rather than being a general ethical dilemma that is not related to your site specifically). That is why we thought it was prudent to make two separate chapters.

Myths About the Field

"Once I'm at my site, things will go smoothly."

We wish this were true, but it's important for us to dispel this myth. If you have ever had a job before—even if not in the psychotherapy field—we are willing to bet that you have experienced hiccups due to your workplace. (If there is any workplace that is fully functional and efficient, then let us know because we'd love to work there.) This means that you will experience site-based dilemmas during your practicum/internship. Being prepared for this fact beforehand will help you to navigate these situations more easily rather than being caught off guard.

Addressing the Reality of the "Real World"

Perhaps the information we presented in the last chapter seemed a bit more expected and/or inevitable. Essentially, we think it is realistic to expect some of the ethical situations that we talked about, such as a suicidal client. What may seem less expected is for you to have to deal with ethical dilemmas as a result of your site specifically.

As an intern, you may have the mindset that you are the student who is going to receive valuable information and guidance from a fully functional therapy-based facility. This expectation makes sense, as that is exactly what a practicum/internship is supposed to be. As we

DOI: 10.4324/9781003433484-10

noted previously, for the most part, this is exactly what the case will be. However, we think it is unhelpful and unrealistic to pretend that every practicum/internship site will be perfect. This is unfortunately not how the world works even in other settings and fields.

This is why we want to prepare you for the potential that you may encounter dilemmas at your practicum/internship site. For some optimistic, bright-eyed interns, it is natural to think that things at your site run properly and smoothly; there may, however, be situations and challenges that you may face, and we don't want you to be caught off guard by them. These situations may range from ethical dilemmas, to issues with personnel, to a lack of internship hours being provided. We will go over some of these dilemmas that you are most likely to encounter later on in the chapter.

What Is Your Role?

As an intern, you are in a bit of a precarious position. The site is very important to you, your growth as a therapist, and to the completion of your academic program. However, you are likely not a paid employee and are only there temporarily. As such, the level of power that you have is probably quite low. Further, you'll probably not want to make waves or rock the boat, as you need the site to complete your hours and degree.

It is important for you to maintain your role. However, that does not mean that you have to be silent. As an intern, you are likely able to notice some things from a different vantage point. If you are seeing that something is happening that may be a site-based dilemma that isn't being addressed at your site, bring it up with your university's program supervisor first. Sometimes, you both may come to the conclusion that this is something you can leave be (if your supervisor has a different perspective on the ethical or functional nature of the situation). Other times, your supervisor may suggest that you talk with the appropriate parties at your site about your concerns if the issue is manageable enough for you to handle on your own. In more intense scenarios, your supervisor may need to handle the situation themselves. The main point here is to constantly consult with your program supervisor to brainstorm what the appropriate action would be for you to take.

One important thing to note here is that you should always stay true to yourself. Perhaps your parents and/or guardians told you this when you were a kid: You shouldn't do something (or not do something) just because someone else is doing it (or not doing it). If you see that other student interns or even paid therapists and employees at your site are mishandling a situation or are perpetuating a site-based dilemma, that does not mean that, as a student intern, you should just sit back and let the situation unfold. If you really believe that the dilemma is problematic and you do not feel comfortable participating in whatever it is, then let your supervisor know. Although you are not licensed yet, you never want to sacrifice your own future license and integrity because you are simply following what others are doing.

Tips From an Intern

My tip for Chapter 8 was about acknowledging that ethical dilemmas will happen and listening to your gut when it tells you that something is off. My tip for this chapter is similar but relates even more to a specific topic from this chapter, which is about your role as a student intern at a site. As we mentioned, you may feel like you are in an awkward position as a student intern if you experience dilemmas due to your site. This is natural, and it is okay.

I really want to emphasize, however, that your practicum/internship is about getting you to start thinking and practicing like a licensed therapist. So it is unhelpful for you to experience certain issues at your site (e.g., therapists not writing their notes properly) and take a back seat and say, "Well, that's not my problem. I'm just going to do what they do." It *is* your problem because, as you may hear a supervisor say in the future, "It's your license that's on the line." Even though you are not licensed yet, I recommend that you start thinking this way because one day your actions will reflect your license.

Even if you see, for example, a paid therapist at your site writing notes like "Client is sad" instead of "Client stated she is sad," that does not mean you have to do what they do. If you know there is a more ethical and/or appropriate way to handle something, you should do it that way, even if it is against the norm of your site. With the previous example, your site probably won't say anything because it will not be a big enough of a difference to them. Other times, they may talk to you about it. This is where you use the conversations with your supervisor beforehand to bring this up. This is the fine line that we had mentioned earlier—both in terms of if you make a decision that goes against the flow of your site and how you will need to address it with your site prior and/or after. As we have suggested throughout this book, you should usually consult with your faculty and/or supervisor about these things beforehand instead of just making decisions on your own.

What Dilemmas Might You Face?

Based on our own experiences and what we have seen from other student interns, there are some common overarching site-based dilemmas that we can go over. Because the nuances at each site are different, we won't be able to cover every single possible scenario. We did, however, want to give some general examples to give you as much of a heads up as we can if you find yourself experiencing one of these situations.

Hours-Based

We mentioned back in Chapter 3 that one thing you should do before starting your practicum/internship is calculate how many hours you need on average per week to get your program's total required hours. We also discussed how, based on this calculation, you need to pick a practicum/internship site that can offer you this number of hours or get a second site if necessary. So while this is not an ethical or legal issue, not getting the amount of hours that you were expecting to at your site could potentially be a site-based issue.

We have unfortunately seen this—though rarely—happen with other students. They discussed the weekly hours they will need with their site prior to accepting the internship, and their site assured these students that they would be able to attain those hours at that facility. Part of the way through the semester, however, these students began realizing that they were not getting enough hours. This may be for a variety of reasons—perhaps the site wound up hiring too many interns and had to split the hours evenly or maybe the practicum/internship is taking place during the summer when there are generally more cancellations.

Michael was recently supervising a student whose site assured her she would be able to meet the minimum semester clinical hours her program required. However, right when the student started, things changed at the site, and their clientele they were expecting didn't happen. The student was left in the lurch, as she needed the minimum hours to advance in the practicum sequence. Unfortunately, she did not achieve this number and had to repeat her first practicum. This is where you will need to be your own advocate. Make sure you have a clear and open conversation with the site about your expected hours. If you are not on pace to achieve that, then you will need to talk with them again to see what they can do to fulfill the clinical hours. If nothing changes, reach out to someone from your department at the university to either reach out to the site, see about adding an additional site, or change sites.

Ethical

In your program, hopefully, you have spent a lot of time focusing on the ethical component of psychotherapy. You took the ethics course, which is usually mandatory before you can engage in practicum/internship, and perhaps were threatened to some degree that if you didn't behave in an ethical manner, then you would have severe consequences within the program, your site, or with the licensing body. However, you don't need these warnings, as you plan to act with the utmost adherence to ethical principles and standards. Yet not everyone does. Further, ethics are not a black-and-white process. There is a lot of gray.

Staff at some sites have found that things are easier and quicker when some paths are taken rather than others. Thus, there will be times when you may question the ethicality of someone's actions at the site. You will then have to decide what to do. You might consult your discipline's ethical codes. For instance, American Psychological Association (2017, Standard 1.03) Conflicts Between Ethics and Organizational Demands states:

> If the demands of an organization with which psychologists are affiliated or for whom they are working are in conflict with this Ethics Code, psychologists clarify the nature of the conflict, make known their commitment to the Ethics Code, and take reasonable steps to resolve the conflict consistent with the General Principles and Ethical Standards of the Ethics Code. Under no circumstances may this standard be used to justify or defend violating human rights.

American Counseling Association (2014, Section D.1.d.) explains that counselors working in a team setting (in an organization) first attempt to resolve an ethical dilemma within the team. If there is not a satisfactory outcome, then they should pursue avenues outside of the team while keeping in mind the well-being of the client. Thus, turning a blind eye is not an expectation from any ethical body. However, doing something about the situation is easier said than done.

Our tip here is to not think that you are alone. It is important for you to maintain your integrity. However, we understand that you are likely to feel you have little power at the site. This may be the case, which is why you should consult with someone in a higher position than you. This may be your site supervisor, the agency director, your faculty supervisor, or the field placement coordinator.

Michael supervised a practicum student who was working at a site where the site supervisor told her that she could put down four direct clinical hours each time she came. However, the intern was only there for three hours a day. Thus, there would be an extra hour being documented that the student did not work. The student expressed this concern during the faculty supervision she had with Michael. Michael agreed with the student that this was not ethically correct for her to document the four hours. Given that the student therapist was in a lower power position than the site supervisor, Michael reached out himself to inquire about the communication about documentation of hours. After some conversation, the site supervisor changed how they communicated about the hours. The student only listed the three direct client contact hours in which they saw clients.

What Would You Do?: 10.1

Put yourself into the shoes of one of Michael's supervisees. They were interning at a substance abuse facility that was a semi-inpatient program. The facility did not have living arrangements on its campus; however, there were several group homes closely located that were owned and run by one of the staff therapists. Getting into the home and maintaining the housing was a prized event because it ensured the person would be able to stay in the substance abuse program. However, this put the staff therapist and client into a dual relationship. The client goes to the therapist for substance abuse therapy but also pays them rent for housing. Further, the therapist knows more information about them than they normally would because of often going over to the group home and making decisions as to who will be the group home client manager. During a session, one of the clients complains to you about the setup but thinks that there is nothing they can do because this is just "the way things are." What do you do?

Practice-Based

Okay. We just talked about some ethical dilemmas that might occur at your site. These are a little easier, as you should always maintain your ethical position and follow your discipline's ethical codes to the best of your ability. However, there may be times when your site supervisor will ask you to do something you are not comfortable with. At these times, it will be important for you to follow your gut. If there is something within you that says, "Hold on a second. This doesn't feel right," it is probably best to take a second and examine why you feel this way.

You can also become more curious as to the reason your site supervisor wants you to do what they are asking. They likely have a good reason for it. They have more experience, know their clientele better, and know their site better. That doesn't mean that they aren't fallible. As we will discuss in Chapter 11, we all make mistakes. Your site supervisor will as well. Maybe they aren't making a mistake and are asking you to do sound clinical work, but you might not have the conceptualization of that yet. This is why it will be important for you to talk with them about it. However, at the end of that conversation, if you still do not feel comfortable doing something, err on the side of not doing it. But don't just refuse. Have a continuing conversation with the supervisor. If something more comes of it, bring in your program administrator.

What Would You Do?: 10.2

It is Friday afternoon. You are interning at an outpatient agency but only come in Mondays to Thursdays. Your supervisor calls you up to let you know that the two therapists who normally do the groups on Saturday are both ill and won't be able to come in. The supervisor says that they really need you to come in. You have plans to meet a friend for lunch. It is not imperative like if you were going out of town or had a wedding to go to. However, you've never run a group by yourself and don't know these clients. You don't quite feel comfortable but also don't want to let the site down. You know your supervisor is really hoping, and maybe even expecting, you to say yes. What do you do?

Personnel-Based

In Chapter 9, we discussed the situation of when either you or your client may be attracted to the other. It is clear in these situations that no romantic or sexual relationship should occur. But what happens when there are flirtations, inquiries, or more serious attempts at connection outside of the proper roles at the agency? Let's take a moment to talk about sexual harassment and what you might do if this occurs.

Sexual harassment is when there are unwanted or inappropriate sexual advances from one person to another. It can be overt, with one person stating what they want to do sexually with the other person, or more covert, such as the way one person looks at or how close they get in proximity to another. Being sexually harassed in the workplace (the field placement for you) can have serious negative consequences for people, including depression (Diez-Canseco et al., 2022). Women are sexually harassed at a much greater rate than men, usually by someone in a higher position. Unfortunately, it is prevalent at such rates that people have come to view it as a normal part of women's workplace experiences (Spiliopoulou & Witcomb, 2023).

There are several subsets of sexual harassment; each of which is problematic. We will briefly talk about each of them here in hopes that, if they do start to happen at your site, you can quickly recognize them and determine how to handle them. Perhaps you watched *Silence of the Lambs* and remember the scene between Hannibal Lecter and Clarice Starling in which Clarice wants Lecter's help to track down a serial killer. Lecter tells her he will but only if she agrees to a quid pro quo—that is, she provides self-disclosure from her childhood to appease his analytic mind. In work settings, a **quid pro quo** happens when a person in power demands sexual favors in exchange for some other type of benefit, such as a raise, promotion, or keeping of one's job.

There is also verbal and physical harassment. **Verbal harassment** occurs when there are unwanted sexual jokes, comments, innuendos, or remarks. This might also be when the person consistently asks to go out on dates or to have sexual relations. **Physical harassment** happens when one person engages in unwanted touching of the other person. This physical touching may be patting the person somewhere, touching their hair, groping them in sexual places, or trying to hug and/or kiss them.

A **hostile environment** is the accumulation of verbal and/or physical harassment and occurs when there are repetitive and pervasive unwelcome activities occurring at the site.

This may be repeated sexual jokes, innuendoes, comments, or explicit materials (such as sexual pictures on the walls or in emails). When this happens over time, the person usually experiences a lot of stress and anxiety being in the site, let alone thinking about going to the site.

What Would You Do?: 10.3

You are interning at a therapy agency where one of the staff therapists has tried to mentor you since you first started. Over time, they slowly begin to shift conversations from the site's policies, procedures, and therapy to your personal life. They ask about your dating history and tell you that they are single. You are not interested in dating them, but they haven't yet been overt about asking you out for you to tell them no. They now have started to ask you if you want to talk about the work over lunch outside of the agency. What do you do?

Will sexual harassment happen to you? We hope not; however, we know that it does occur. Seventy-three percent of female and 22% of male internal medicine residents reported they were sexually harassed during medical school or residency (Komaromy et al., 1993). Only 1% reported this experience to an authority. While these are striking numbers, this was a small sample at one university. However, people tend not to report sexual harassment for a variety of reasons, including not thinking that the event was significant, not thinking that the report will be believed, or believing that nothing will come out of the report (Kirkner et al., 2022).

As with all site-based dilemmas, it will be important for you to make sure that you maintain your ethical and personal integrity. You should not be placed in a situation that makes you uncomfortable or violates your personhood. If this does happen, then it is your right to seek intervention to make the environment safer for you and/or the clients and other staff members. If a dilemma does arise, please reach out to the appropriate professional to help navigate you through it. You might also consider legal options; however, your legal rights might depend on whether you are considered a paid or unpaid intern of the organization. Also, depending on the country that you live in, there is likely to be different sexual harassment policies or no policy at all. For 22% of high-income, 26% of middle-income, and 34% of low-income countries, sexual harassment in the workplace is still legal (Heymann et al., 2023).

There are a variety of options for you to take based upon the structure of the organization, your academic program, and the severity of the offense. We will briefly discuss talking with your supervisor or your program administrator.

Talking With Your Supervisor

There will be events that happen at your site, perhaps with clients, colleagues, staff, or administrators, that leave you feeling confused, angry, embarrassed, or ashamed. What many people would likely do is keep these feelings inside. This will only lead to these feelings festering. It is important in these moments to talk with your site supervisor. They are there to not only help you develop as a therapist and grow while you are in the therapy room but to also help you navigate aspects of the site. They can't do this if they don't know what you are experiencing.

Michael was supervising a couple of student therapists who were doing their internship at the same agency. One day, they came into supervision saying that they were highly disturbed by something that happened at their site. These were two young female therapists, and they explained that their site had just hired a male in his late 30s. With one of the student interns, he was doing co-therapy with her and treating her in a way that was uncomfortable, such as treating her as his personal assistant rather than co-therapist. For the other student intern, she was a co-therapist with him in a group of teen girls. She stated that he had told them not to trust any men, as all men will eventually cheat on them. There were other concerns as well, such as him saying inappropriate sexual things about a female faculty member that they knew. The student interns were unsure of what to do. They didn't feel comfortable working with him and were concerned about the quality of his therapy with the clientele. Michael encouraged them to talk with the site supervisor, as she needed to know what was happening not only for the student interns but also for the clients. They did so, which led to the site supervisor having a discussion with the therapist and coming up with an action plan for his continued employment.

Tales From the Field: Intern

Before my doctoral internship began, I had assumed that people in the mental health field had it all figured out. I assumed that they had done the work to improve their emotional intelligence to avoid reactions and respond to situations compassionately. Throughout my internship year, I quickly realized this was not always the case. I encountered individuals who reacted emotionally and often escalated situations. This was a big source of the dilemmas I encountered at my internship site.

For example, I received an email from a supervisor inquiring about the gap between the finalization of a psychological testing report and the feedback session with the client's primary therapist. The supervisor stated, "Even taking into account therapist being on vacation for a week, this lengthy time frame for providing testing results to the therapist doesn't make sense." To me, this seemed passive-aggressive and accusatory. Initially, the therapist had not responded to my emails and seemed to be out on vacation for two weeks. It had been a month since the finalization of the psychological testing report. Finally, the therapist responded and apologized for the delay in getting back to me. The feedback session happened, and the same supervisor was part of the feedback session with the therapist, who had not notified me of the therapist's presence. Thankfully, my individual supervisor informed me of this the day before, which allowed me not to be surprised by the therapist's presence during this meeting.

At the end of the feedback session, the therapist shared negative feedback about me to the supervisor. She, per the supervisor's report, shared that I was condescending and did not collaborate well with her. The therapist also shared that she purposefully did not reply to my emails because she was frustrated with me and my lack of availability to meet with her. I had provided two dates and times because it was what I had available. She appeared to perceive this as a lack of collaboration on my part.

This feedback was provided to my primary individual supervisor. I didn't quite understand where the therapist was coming from until I processed this feedback with my individual supervisor, which was extremely helpful. We realized the therapist wanted to confirm a certain diagnosis that testing did not support. The therapist also appeared to be under the assumption that one had to assign a trauma-related diagnosis to a client to engage the client in trauma-focused cognitive behavioral therapy, which is not the case. Had I been informed of what was happening with this therapist behind the scenes, this issue would have likely been resolved during the feedback session and the therapist would have probably left feeling more supported instead of emotionally reactive. I wish all of us had been on the same page to help the therapist receive the feedback and help her process her reactions to the feedback. However, processing this with my individual supervisor significantly helped me make sense of the situation and respond accordingly.

I understand that we are all human and at times will react. We have the right to feel our emotions. However, there needs to be a balance between validating our own experience and taking accountability for our actions instead of pointing fingers.

Goldie Barajas, PsyD program, California School of Professional Psychology, Alliant International University

Tips From a Supervisor

I have had hundreds of supervisees who have had thousands of site-based dilemmas. Some are quite minor, in which my involvement is not necessary, such as minor scheduling issues or small miscommunications. However, there have been plenty that were important for me to know so that I could either help the student therapist to process or actually contact someone at the site to see how the issue might get resolved.

My main tip when you have a site-based dilemma is to not hold off but rather contact your supervisor about it sooner rather than later. If you have both a site-based supervisor and a faculty supervisor, then I would triage the dilemma, seeing how serious it is. For many of these dilemmas, your site supervisor will be the first person that you go to. They know the site better than your faculty supervisor and can perhaps problem solve with you in ways your faculty supervisor could not. However, if the situation at the site is more severe, is with your site supervisor, or doesn't get resolved after talking with your site supervisor, talk with your faculty supervisor.

I've had a few supervisees who were having quite problematic experiences at their site that I didn't know about because they either tried to ignore it or were anxious about bringing it up in supervision (thinking perhaps that doing so would negatively impact their field placement). There have been a few times when the outcome of the conversation between me and the supervisee is them leaving the site. However, for the most part, the resolution of the dilemma comes about through open conversation (either between myself and the supervisee or with the inclusion of one or more people at the site). Yet the resolution would likely not occur if not brought up. So the primary tip here is to talk with someone. Get guidance on who the most appropriate person is to talk to and talk with them with the mindset of resolution.

Talking With Your Program Administrator

There are going to be some site-based dilemmas that you will decide to let go as they come to some resolution. After you consult with your supervisor, you will come to the decision that it is a small enough issue to look past and move on from. There may be some other site-based dilemmas, however, that are too concerning to ignore. We hope that this is not the case for you. But in case it is, we obviously want to provide some sort of preparation for these more difficult situations.

Your site and your university program are not separate. Rather, they are connected in that they are both there to try to help you in your training to become a therapist. It is important that there is an open line of communication between the two. Sometimes, this communication will happen outside of you. For instance, many programs will automatically send the site supervisor access to fill out your midterm and/or end-of-term evaluation. While this may happen without you needing to be involved, you should always talk with your site supervisor about your evaluation so that you can take that feedback and apply it the next time you enter the therapy room (see Chapter 14).

Although there is a connection between site and school, there is also a disconnection. Unless your site is run through your program, the people at your school likely do not know what is happening at the site and whether it is an appropriate situation for you to be in. This is where it is important for you to maintain open communication with administrators in both contexts. When a situation cannot get resolved at your site, it is important to talk with someone from your university to see if they can help expedite a favorable resolution for you. This person might be the clinical coordinator, university faculty supervisor, or the program director for your program. Based on the situation, you will have to figure out who is most appropriate to get involved.

Many student interns that we know were hesitant to involve school personnel in site-based issues because they didn't want to upset the people at the site by "getting them in trouble." We don't think that this is a useful way of looking at things. Yes, there might be some nerves and concerns that you have about bringing the dilemma outside of the placement, but there are times when this is imperative.

Quick Tip: Things done now are usually better than things put off. While you might not talk with your supervisor or program administrator at the first inkling of a dilemma (unless it is something quite significant), the longer you don't, the bigger the dilemma is likely to become. They are there to help you navigate any issues that come up. Utilize them.

Tales From the Field: Supervisor

Paul was a senior bachelor of social work student who was passionate about the basic human right for housing for all individuals and families. He was happy to obtain a coveted internship at a homeless shelter. As a seasoned student who had some work experience in the helping professions, he felt prepared and easily adjusted to the challenging situations he encountered in his early weeks at the internship. He jumped right into counseling individuals at the facility, working on employment and housing goals with individuals, and negotiating disagreements that occasionally arose between the residents at the facility. What Paul did not anticipate was an outbreak of bed bugs at the facility.

The outbreak triggered Paul, who had witnessed the challenges of eliminating a bed bug outbreak firsthand when he was a child. Paul was also worried about exposing his wife and children to possible risk. However, Paul felt obligated to his clients and to the agency and did not tell his internship instructor or his internship supervisor that he was uncomfortable going to the internship site. He felt that bringing up his discomfort would be selfish and would take away from the dignity and respect he felt for his clients.

Paul finally mentioned his discomfort to me, the field director, who also served as the instructor of the internship seminar. I validated that it was okay for Paul to worry about health and safety. I notified the site that Paul would not be attending his internship for a few days and requested a meeting with the agency-based supervisor. During the meeting with the field placement site, Paul and I learned about the precautions that the agency had taken to safeguard interns, employees, and clients. Paul was assured that his clients and their wing of the building had not been exposed and that the areas of exposure had been mitigated. Paul felt more comfortable and expressed that he wished he had asked for support and explanations earlier. The agency-based supervisor and I encouraged him to bring up concerns early, as soon as something might make him uncomfortable, so that they could collaborate to work through problems together.

Janice Nuss, DSW, LCSW, Social Work program, Gwynedd-Mercy University

Summary

Not only will there be dilemmas that happen in the therapy room that you will have to navigate, but there will occasionally be site-based dilemmas as well. Regardless of how well organized and functional an agency is, there will likely be some type of issue that will present itself. These dilemmas might be in the ethical, practice-based, personnel-based, or hours-based realm. Throughout, you will need to keep your role in mind and balance that you are an intern at the site while maintaining your integrity. Our recommendation is that whenever a site-based dilemma occurs, you talk with your site supervisor, faculty supervisor, and/or your program administrator.

References

American Counseling Association. (2014). *2014 ACA code of ethics*. www.counseling.org/resources/aca-code-of-ethics.pdf

American Psychological Association. (2017). *Ethical principles of psychologists and code of conduct*. www.apa.org/ethics/code/ethics-code-2017.pdf

Diez-Canseco, F., Toyama, M., Hidalgo-Padilla, L., & Bird, V. J. (2022). Systematic review of policies and interventions to prevent sexual harassment in the workplace in order to prevent depression. *International Journal of Environmental Research and Public Health, 19*(20), Article 13278. https://doi.org/10.3390/ijerph192013278

Heymann, J., Moreno, G., Raub, A., & Sprague, A. (2023). Progress towards ending sexual harassment at work? A comparison of sexual harassment policy in 192 countries. *Journal of Comparative Policy Analysis, 25*(2), 172–193. https://doi.org/10.1080/13876988.2022.2100698

Kirkner, A. C., Lorenz, K., & Mazar, L. (2022). Faculty and staff reporting & disclosure of sexual harassment in higher education. *Gender and Education, 34*(2), 199–215. https://doi.org/10.1080/09540253.2020.1763923

Komaromy, M., Bindman, A. B., Haber, R. J., & Sande, M. A. (1993). Sexual harassment in medical training. *The New England Journal of Medicine, 328*(5), 322–326. https://doi.org/10.1056/NEJM199302043280507

Spiliopoulou, A., & Witcomb, G. L. (2023). An exploratory investigation into women's experience of sexual harassment in the workplace. *Violence Against Women, 29*(9), 1853–1873. https://doi.org/10.1177/10778012221114921

Chapter 11

Honoring Diversity and Inclusion

You have probably already taken at least one whole course focused on the notion of honoring diversity. Your program might call it differently, such as Culture and Wellness, Multicultural Counseling, or Diversity and Cultural Issues. Whatever the title, the course was developed to introduce you to the impact that diversity has on you and your clients. In this chapter, we want to highlight some of the main concepts that you learned about in that course (and hopefully a lot of other courses and other areas) as well and talk about how they might be present during your placement.

Myth About the Field

"I can overcome any differences between me and the client since we are both human beings."

This is not what honoring diversity and inclusion is about. Honoring these factors means knowing when beneficence is compromised because of differences that create a space that is no longer trusting or therapeutic. It is similar to the concept of being **color blind**: pretending that race does not exist in an effort to see everyone as equal human beings. This ignores the fact that there are differences between us that change the context of our experiences. These factors need to be acknowledged and understood because they provide meaning to our lived experiences and interactions with one another.

Diversity

We can define **diversity** as the differences between people. Usually when we think about diversity, we think about race. This has been the primary way that psychotherapists have explored diversity—how people from different races are similar and different. Most of psychotherapy's history was written by White individuals. The way that they understood the world was from a White perspective. Fortunately, clinicians realized that there might be differences in viewing self, other, and the therapeutic process when you are non-White. This led to looking at the difference between those who were White and Black, which eventually expanded to include Asian, Hispanic, American Indian/Alaska Native, and Native Hawaiian/Pacific Islander as well as other groups.

Being aware that there is diversity within people and between people is significant, as people's experiences are multivarious based on these differences. You have undoubtedly taken a course that primarily focused on diversity, which may have included terms such as diversity,

DOI: 10.4324/9781003433484-11

multiculturalism, or cross-culturalism. One of the reasons you have taken this course (and covered notions of diversity in aspects of most courses) is because working with diverse clientele is perhaps the most challenging issue for psychotherapists (Lee & Park, 2013).

However, diversity is much more than race. We said that psychotherapy's history was mainly written by White individuals. We can look more deeply to understand that these people were mostly males. And mostly in the middle or upper class. And mostly heterosexual. And mostly able-bodied. And mostly middle-aged. And so on. To some degree, this has informed us about psychotherapy practices. In each of these areas, there is not a bifurcation but rather a continuum in which people can be viewed across a range of positions. This has led to a better appreciation of intersectionality. And in all transparency, this book is written by two White, heterosexual, cisgender, middle-class, able-bodied individuals. We understand that there will likely be aspects of the book that may not fully fit for you based on your own social location factors. We have tried to incorporate different voices throughout the book in the Tales From the Field section to account for this. When reading this chapter, please consider it within the context of your individual situation and larger context.

Intersectionality

The term **intersectionality** was first used by Kimberlé Crenshaw in 1989, who, as a law student, was interested in critical theory. The Oxford dictionary defines intersectionality as "the interconnected nature of social categorizations such as race, class, and gender as they apply to a given individual or group, regarded as creating overlapping and interdependent systems of discrimination or disadvantage."

Each of us is housed in our own intersectionality (see Figure 11.1). Based on the combination of many of these aspects of personhood, some people have gained privilege while others have been oppressed. Thus, in each society, power practices occur based on peoples' demographics. It is important for you to consider this, both for yourself and your clientele.

Roper-Hall and Burnham developed a mnemonic for thinking about the notion of power and social location, which was originally called the social **GRACES** and then was shifted to **GGRRAAAACCEEESSS** (Burnham, 2012). The mnemonic refers to gender, geography, race, religion, age, ability, appearance, class, culture, ethnicity, education, employment, sexuality, sexual orientation, and spirituality. Any one of these contexts has a significant impact on a person's identity and living situation. By holding the mnemonic in mind, you will be better able to keep consideration of how the client you are working with is a multifaceted individual that cuts across multiple contextual systems.

Social Location

Your specific combination of these various categories is your **social location**. Mock (2008) explained, "An individual's social location means the groups that he or she belongs to because of his or her position in society and history. It also refers to the relative standing between the groups" (p. 426).

Each person has their own social location. Two people from the same family will have a lot of overlap but will not have the same social location. Their geography, race, class, culture, and ethnicity will likely be the same. However, there may be significant differences based on ability, appearance, or sexual orientation, for example. While just one difference out of all these categories may seem minor, it can have a huge impact on how the person views themselves and how others view them.

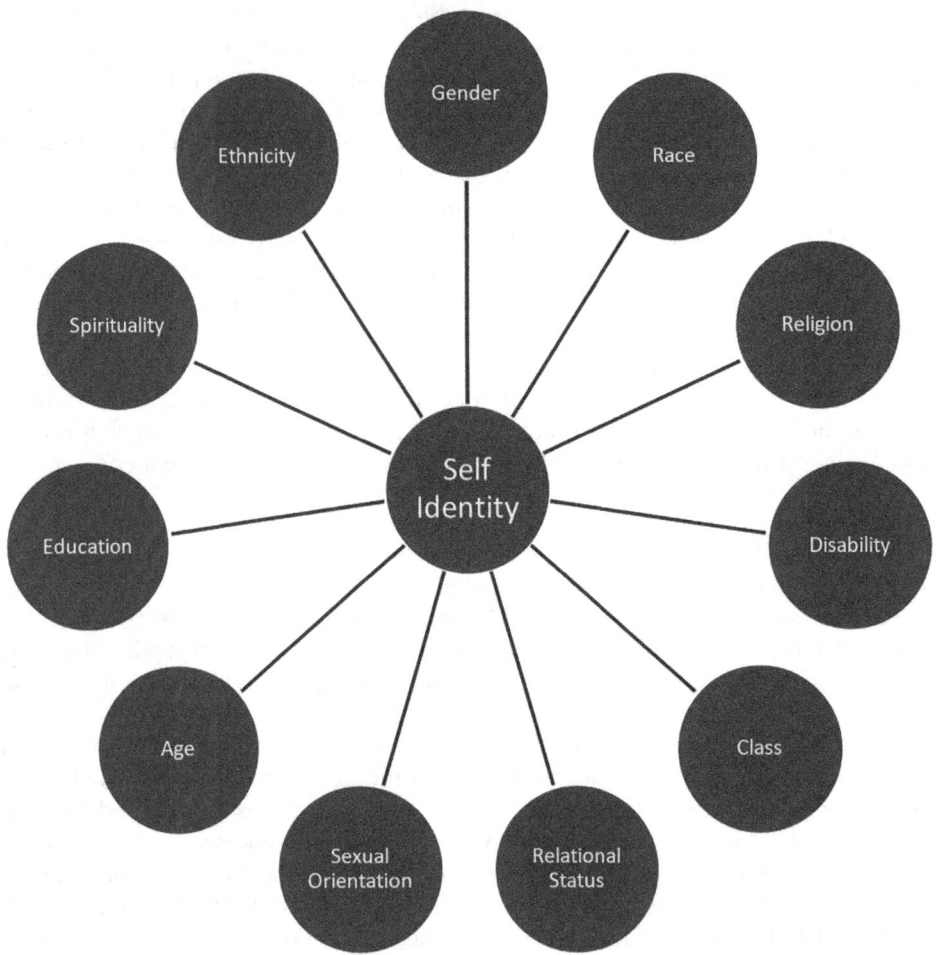

Figure 11.1 Intersectionality is the combination of the various aspects of self and how they privilege or oppress us.

Exercise 11.1   Your Social Location

Take a second to think about your own social location. Fill in each of the following areas.

- Gender:
- Geography:
- Race:
- Religion:
- Age:

- Ability:
- Appearance:
- Class:
- Culture:
- Ethnicity:
- Education:
- Employment:
- Sexuality:
- Sexual Orientation:
- Spirituality:

When you take all of these aspects in combination, what does that tell you about yourself? How have you experienced privilege based on one or more of these categories? How have you experienced oppression? What areas of power have you had? What areas of lack of power have been present for you?

The more that you become aware of the various identities, systems, and ideas that inform who you are, the more likely you are to become curious to how clients' identities have been informed. One way to explore your cultural experience is to create a **cultural genogram** (Hardy & Laszloffy, 1995). The cultural genogram has all of the information that a typical genogram has along with your national origin, ethnicity, racial identity, religion, socioeconomic status, migration history, and other cultural variables.

Now, expand your imagination and think about what happens when you come in contact with someone else. You are connected with someone that comes from their own social location. How do these two social locations interact? We're sure you can imagine certain categories in which connection will be easier and other areas in which it might be more difficult. So let's explore that just a bit more.

Exercise 11.2   Interactions of Social Locations

Go back to the list of your social location and think about a client whose social location might make it easier to connect with you and one whose social location might make it more difficult to join with. We present again each of the social location areas. This time, fill in the two columns. Write in a social location of a client that you think it would be easier for you to connect with and harder to connect with.

	Easier social location	Harder social location

- Gender:
- Geography:
- Race:
- Religion:

- Age:
- Ability:
- Appearance:
- Class:
- Culture:
- Ethnicity:
- Education:
- Employment:
- Sexuality:
- Sexual Orientation:
- Spirituality:

What did you learn about yourself from doing this exercise? What are ways that you think you can work on yourself to make it easier to work with people from different social locations? Was there one or two categories that you find are more triggering for you? How come?

Ethics That Honor Diversity

Regardless of your discipline, the ethical codes associated with each mental health field pay a keen interest to diversity and cultural competence. This is because you will, regardless of where you are practicing, come into contact with diverse clientele. Remember, diversity is more than race. So what are some of the ethical aspects of diversity for you to consider and honor? We will present just a few codes from a variety of ethical bodies here to start that conversation.

The American Psychological Association (2017, Standard 3.01) Unfair Discrimination states the following:

> In their work-related activities, psychologists do not engage in unfair discrimination based on age, gender, gender identity, race, ethnicity, culture, national origin, religion, sexual orientation, disability, socioeconomic status, or any basis proscribed by law.

The American Counseling Association (2014, Section C.5) states the same thing. They also have subcodes for various aspects of therapy, such as informed consent (A.2.c. Developmental and Cultural Sensitivity):

> Counselors communicate information in ways that are both developmentally and culturally appropriate. Counselors use clear and understandable language when discussing issues related to informed consent. When clients have difficulty understanding the language that counselors use, counselors provide necessary services (e.g., arranging for a qualified interpreter or translator) to ensure comprehension by clients. In collaboration with clients, counselors consider cultural implications of informed consent procedures and, where possible, counselors adjust their practices accordingly.

The NASW (2021) Standard 1.05 is all on cultural competence:

a. Social workers should demonstrate understanding of culture and its function in human behavior and society, recognizing the strengths that exist in all cultures.
b. Social workers should demonstrate knowledge that guides practice with clients of various cultures and be able to demonstrate skills in the provision of culturally informed services that empower marginalized individuals and groups. Social workers must take action against oppression, racism, discrimination, and inequities, and acknowledge personal privilege.
c. Social workers should demonstrate awareness and cultural humility by engaging in critical self-reflection (understanding their own bias and engaging in self-correction), recognizing clients as experts of their own culture, committing to lifelong learning, and holding institutions accountable for advancing cultural humility.
d. Social workers should obtain education and demonstrate understanding of the nature of social diversity and oppression with respect to race, ethnicity, national origin, color, sex, sexual orientation, gender identity or expression, age, marital status, political belief, religion, immigration status, and mental or physical ability.
e. Social workers who provide electronic social work services should be aware of cultural and socioeconomic differences among clients' use of and access to electronic technology and seek to prevent such potential barriers. Social workers should assess cultural, environmental, economic, mental or physical ability, linguistic, and other issues that may affect the delivery or use of these services.

As you can see, an ethical focus is much more than nondiscrimination. That is the easiest part of our work with clients, that we will work with almost any client (you should not work with a client if the problems they are dealing with are outside of your scope of competence).

Tales From the Field: Intern

It was August, and I felt eager and terrified to begin my doctoral internship. At that time, I did not admit to myself that I was experiencing imposter syndrome. I simply noticed the thoughts and allowed them to pass. I told myself, "You belong here, and you have earned your spot." As a bilingual, first-generation everything (as I describe it), it is difficult to feel as though I belong. I sat amongst other doctoral interns from a different ethnic background than me. I was the only Mexican American. The internship program director was a White, middle-aged, cisgender woman. I immediately noticed she approached me differently, and I could not quite pinpoint why. I allowed time to pass, telling myself, "Maybe you are thinking too much into this, Goldie. Let it unfold." Months passed, and after "letting it unfold," I provided her with feedback on my reactions to some of the statements she made. She did not take ownership of her statements and did not acknowledge a possible implicit bias. More months passed: This time, I could not move past the fact that she had, in front of other interns, stopped me and said, "Doesn't she sound harsh?" as I was expressing why healthy boundaries are important to me, given that I was a parentified child. I noticed myself internally frowning in confusion.

I consulted with my individual supervisors to gain clarity about how to navigate the situation. I consulted with one of my dissertation committee members of the same ethnic background as me, and she said, "As a minority and woman of color, you are perceived as passive if you do not share enough and as aggressive if you do." I reflected on this internally while I was not sure if it was safe to bring up the issue with the internship program director. I made the decision to confide in my fellow doctoral interns during a Friday group supervision and share about my experiences with this individual. I thought everyone was supportive and had made the decision to bring up these issues with the internship program director the following week. On Monday, when I returned to work, I came back to an email from my school asking to meet to discuss ethical concerns shared by the internship program director about me. Two of the interns violated my confidentiality and texted the internship program director after our discussion letting her know I was, for lack of better words, "bad-mouthing her." I met with my school's program director and the director of training to discuss the matter. They provided me with encouragement and support; they also facilitated a meeting between me and the internship program director.

During this meeting, the internship program director did not apologize, did not take ownership for the microaggressions she had engaged in, gaslighted me, and placed the responsibility on me—a student with systemically less power than her—to fix the issue. Considering my internship evaluation was pending, I decided to take the "high road" and agreed that moving forward I would bring any issues I may have with her and directly address them with her and/or the director of DEI at my internship site. I was disillusioned with how poorly this conversation went and how much of the responsibility to resolve the issue was placed on me. I went home and cried. I questioned whether I should have spoken up about such crucial issues. I thought, "Goldie, you do not have the power yet, why did you do that?" I started questioning my own reality and had to engage in a tremendous amount of self-validation and grounding. The next week, I had a meeting with the program and training director at my school. To my relief, they had the same thoughts as me and were supportive of how skillfully I navigated the situation. My individual supervisor also offered emotional support, shared that my efforts and self-advocacy were not in vain, and stated that this individual was now on their "radar" and that it would probably take a significant amount of challenging to increase her multicultural competence. I felt empowered and proud.

Goldie Barajas, PsyD program, California School of Professional Psychology, Alliant International University

Stereotypes

Do you stereotype people? Don't be so quick in answering. Stereotyping is a common means that human beings use to quickly categorize information. **Stereotyping** is holding a general belief about a particular category of people. All of us stereotype people. We cannot help but do so. We think, "Well, they are a teenager, so they probably X," or "They are married, so they probably Y," or "They are a biker with tons of tattoos, so they probably Z." These quick conceptualizations help us to quickly navigate a situation. The problem comes when we hold these initial thoughts about a person based on a group they are associated with and don't adjust our understanding based on that person's uniqueness.

When it comes to stereotyping, we have both implicit and explicit stereotypes. **Implicit stereotypes** happen unconsciously, when they are out of our awareness, and we have little control over them. **Explicit stereotypes** are conscious, when we are aware we hold this belief.

As we discussed when we talked about your values in Chapter 5, it is important to become aware of what stereotypes you may be holding and using when engaging with your clients. The more aware you are of them, the better able you will be to not allow them to impact your conceptualization and interactions with your client. Once you recognize how you utilize stereotypes, you can then question your assumptions. Challenge yourself to go beyond what you originally thought. This may come in the form of educating yourself; challenging the influence of media, friends, culture, and enculturation; and exposing yourself to a variety of aspects of diversity that you hadn't before. Talk with people who are quite different than you. Watch movies from other countries. Stay on top of current events since what is going on in the world and your community can affect your clients.

Perhaps our biggest tip here is to give yourself some leeway. Don't expect yourself to be perfect. Rather, appreciate that you are in a constant state of growth and learning. You are learning psychotherapy. But perhaps even more importantly, you are learning about yourself and growing as a therapist and a person.

What Would You Do?: 11.1

You get assigned a family case that includes a father, mother, and a 12-year-old son. The father and mother are both fairly recent immigrants, and their English is not very good. They can communicate very basically but not in-depth enough to have the session. The 12-year-old is bilingual. The family is coming in because they are concerned about the boy's behavior at school. He has been getting detentions because he has been disrespectful to teachers and has gotten into a few fights with other students. During the first session, when you realize that the parents were not really understanding you, you find yourself turning to the 12-year-old to help you translate to the parents and vice versa. However, your preference is for the son not to be in the translator role. What do you do?

Tips From an Intern

As we have discussed throughout this chapter, there are a range of considerations to make when we talk about diversity, as they involve a complex interplay between multiple factors of life. These things can be overwhelming and complicated to navigate—you may often feel like you don't know if you are honoring diversity and inclusion in the "right" way. This makes sense, though, because even different professionals in the field have different opinions and approaches on how diversity and inclusion "should" be honored.

I want to qualify that the tip I am going to give is just another one of those approaches based on my time at my practicum/internship sites and the classroom learning of my graduate programs. I believe that honoring diversity and inclusion requires a balance between meeting the client where they are at and being able to be aware of and appropriately incorporate larger systemic considerations that may be at play.

To provide some clarity on what I am saying, I'll give a quick example: I had a client who was navigating his South American culture (where his family was from) and his American culture (where he was born and primarily raised). He came into therapy stating that he felt inauthentic from giving too much to others (which is more so what his family expected) yet wanted to focus on himself sometimes, too. This was something that was important to him, so this is what we focused on in therapy (e.g., through him engaging in more hobbies and career goals of his own). At the same time, we talked about the larger systemic factor of the acculturation between a more individualistic American culture and, from what he stated, a more collectivistic South American culture.

In the end, my client obtained great benefit from being able to give himself some of the love and attention he was giving others. He also found value in having those conversations about the difficulty of navigating between two different cultures. Although he was wanting to focus on himself more, which may be seen as a more individualistic value, he was able to do so without guilt from the recognition that he was able to experience both cultures in different ways.

Your job as a therapist, then, is to listen to what the client is stating they need and then also look at the larger context and see how that may be playing a part in what the client is saying they need in the first place. You can both work from where the client is currently at and also invite them to take a look at these larger societal discourses that often influence how we feel and what we want. Honoring diversity and inclusion can thus be about providing a therapeutic space to incorporate all these elements of a client's experience and of life in general.

Barriers to Cultural Competency

Our field is set up to help you continue to move forward toward **cultural competency**. The more diverse clientele you work with, the greater understanding you have about the differences between groups. You aren't supposed to be fully culturally competent—in some ways, it is similar to self-actualization in that it is an ideal to move toward but never fully attained. What is important is that you are making movement in that direction and away from being culturally incompetent.

Cultural incompetence happens when we have a lack of knowledge, understanding, and sensitivity toward those who are from a different culture than us. What usually happens is when someone experiences this, they try to avoid contact with people who are different from them, which only perpetuates their difficulty in working with diverse individuals. Cultural incompetence can be seen when someone incorporates stereotypes and prejudice in their understanding of others, functions from a position of ethnocentrism (thinking that their culture is better than other cultures), isn't able to be flexible and adapt, and has a lack of knowledge of other cultures.

Cultural incompetency also happens when the person believes that White ethnic groups and ethnic minority groups are similar in terms of their acculturation and assimilation patterns (Sanchez et al., 2010). This can lead to **cultural tunnel vision**, in which the therapist is unaware that they are having difficulties working with someone from a different cultural background (Corey & Corey, 2020). This occurs when we are ethnocentric, thinking that our culture's beliefs and practices are correct and other cultures' practices are wrong. Cultural tunnel vision leads us to not honor the client's culture and attempt to impose our own.

Cultural competency can be seen in macro and micro practices and is housed within cultural assumptions that you have. Corey and Corey (2020) explained that there are many assumptions of our culture that we are aware and unaware of which impact our perceptions. In the therapy room, this comes out when we think about self-disclosure, nonverbal behavior, relationships, self-actualization, and directness. People from different cultures will tend to think and behave differently in each of these areas. When we are assessing and working clinically with clients, we need to account for these types of cultural factors to prevent us from pathologizing a person's behavior that is culturally rooted.

This seems like a very daunting task. We said that you are going to work with a variety of diverse clientele. How can you know about all these different cultures? The good news is that you are not expected to be an expert on all cultures and ethnicities. However, your openness to talk about them is what is key in therapy. You should be able to ask your client how their way of thinking and acting is based upon their culture(s). They may or may not have thought about that before, but either way, it becomes a foundation for opening up space in the therapeutic conversation to do so.

Exercise 11.3   Enhancing Cultural Experiences

Part of becoming more culturally competent is having exposure to people, practices, and ideas from a variety of cultures. This allows you to appreciate the differences. For this exercise, we encourage you to engage in each of the following activities, some of which you will be able to achieve today, while others may take some time. That is fine because cultural competence isn't an end goal but a continual process.

- Eat at an ethnic restaurant where you have never tried that cuisine.
- Read a book by an author from a different country than you.
- Watch a movie in a different language than yours (that has subtitles so you can follow the plot).
- Have a conversation with a person who is quite diverse from you in some aspect(s), focusing on how they view the world.
- Travel to a country that you have never been to, preferably one that doesn't speak the same language as you.

Broaching

No matter what site you are at, you will almost be guaranteed that you will work with one or more clients who are racially and/or culturally different than you are. This trend will continue as our world continues to become more multicultural. Thus, you will find yourself in a therapeutic relationship with a client who is of a different race and/or ethnicity than you. These differences may become significant for the therapeutic relationship, in which both client and therapist find that they are not understanding the other person or are having difficulty in connecting with the other.

How do you bring racial and cultural issues into the therapeutic discourse? You do this through a process called **broaching**. Day-Vines et al. (2007) defined broaching as "the counselor's ability to consider the relationship of ethnic factors into the client's presenting problems and inviting the client to explore these factors in treatment using an ongoing attitude of openness and genuine commitment" (p. 404).

Tales From the Field: Supervisor

Alison accepted a position as an in-home therapist. The in-home counseling agency served the local diverse, marginalized, and underserved communities through federal and state funding. Alison was passionate about helping others and working with children and families, although she was not quite prepared for what in-home therapy entailed.

Alison shadowed another therapist for about four weeks before she was assigned her own geographical area in which she would provide services. The population and neighborhoods in her assigned area were very different than what she had become accustomed to. As Alison drove through the neighborhoods and entered the homes of her clients, she became uncomfortable and worried about her safety. She found herself struggling to focus throughout client sessions, which she connected to anxiety and discomfort. Alison was upset with herself for having this reaction and was embarrassed to bring it up during group supervision because she was afraid of how others would perceive her.

While speaking to a close colleague, Alison admitted she was having difficulties with certain aspects of the placement. The supervisor worked with Alison to process her discomfort, biases, and safety concerns. Alison discussed how her lifestyle framed her perspective of what a home should look like and ways she could begin to appreciate how other people lived. Alison and her supervisor also focused on specific things she had control over to enhance her safety, such as how she dressed, what jewelry she chose to wear, and the hours she worked. Over time, Alison became more comfortable working with clients in their homes and was able to appreciate different cultures and family systems while being able to identify when a bias may be clouding her perspective.

Natalie Rothman, PhD, Director, Brief Therapy Institute, Nova Southeastern University

---

More recently, broaching has been focused on to discuss racial and/or cultural issues happening in the therapeutic connection between therapist and client. Lee et al. (2022a) explained that "broaching inevitably means addressing both similarities and differences in cross-cultural dyads" (p. 325). It is not a confrontation or conflict. Rather, it consists of having a conversation about each person's social location, position, and worldview and how there is overlap and non-overlap between the two of you. This will hopefully allow both of you to work more cohesively together, understanding that you are two distinct people that have different perceptions, experiences, and pressures.

Sometimes, having this conversation seems a bit too much to do and could be quite scary. You might ask yourself, "Do I have to?" Lee et al. (2022a) argued that broaching is not just an option for therapists but is an integral part of therapy. Many times, it is better to address the unsaid than to let it fester. The more that you can get things out in the open, the greater opportunity that you can use the topic as a platform for growth—both for you and the client. Broaching is one way to strengthen the therapeutic alliance.

How might you engage in broaching with your clients? There are three main microskills that you could utilize (Lee et al., 2022b). First, you can engage in self-disclosure. Second, you can pay attention to **cultural immediacy**—how the here-and-now moments in therapy between you and the client that are racially and/or culturally based are impacting the therapy process. Third, you can incorporate the use of reflective listening, especially complex reflections in which you make an inference and/or reframe the information present in the conversation so that a deeper exploration is attained.

Not only do therapists sometimes have hesitation in broaching racial issues with minority clients, but minority clients tend to refrain from bringing up racial and cultural concerns with their therapists (Chang & Yoon, 2011). However, these clients tend to find that the racial differences between them and their therapists are not that significant when they find that their therapist is accepting, compassionate, and comfortable in talking about racial issues. Hopefully, this research finding encourages you to be more open and overt when navigating racial differences.

Quick Tip: Take a chance, get out of your comfort zone, choose one client (to start with), and engage in broaching about the ethnic, racial, or gender differences between you. Make sure that you feel confident doing so, as your willingness to talk about these dynamics will likely lead to your client feeling more confident about them as well.

Power

One thing that you will need to accept as a therapist is that you have inherent power based upon this role. Murphy and Hecker (2017) explained, "Power exists in relationship between at least two people, as it suggests differences between two (or more) people in some way" (p. 100). You will have **expert power** as a therapist, which comes from having knowledge and expertise. You may have clients come to you calling you "Doctor" and looking to you for the right answer on how to fix their situation or lives. This can sometimes seem overwhelming, especially when you are at the beginning stage of your training as a therapist.

For any Marvel Comics fans, particularly those of Spider-Man, you know the phrase, "With great power comes great responsibility." You have great power as a therapist. Clients will come to you in some of the most severe points of distress in their lives and will look to you to help them through it. It is your responsibility to take this position seriously and to do good with it. It is okay to accept that you have power in the therapeutic realm. Having power is not problematic. Using it in ways that are antithetical to proper therapy are.

Tips From a Supervisor

The focus on diversity may be one of the most emotionally intense experiences my supervisees have, particularly within the classroom. In the therapy room, clients seem to be more accepting than what happens in the classroom, as teachers and students are charged when talking about these ideas. Therapists have become much more attuned to issues of power, privilege, and social justice than the lay individual.

My main tip here is to not expect anyone to "have it" and "know it" or be perfect when it comes to aspects surrounding diversity and therapy. This includes yourself. All of us have blind spots, which is why it is easier for us to see the bad predicament our friend has put themselves into rather than them seeing it. And we have to remember that we are still learning. As a society, our understanding of acceptability is extremely different today than it was 1 year ago, 5 years ago, or 20 years ago.

Unfortunately, I have seen student therapists argue and have a very bad experience with one another when they are discussing issues of diversity. This happens when both people are trying to be accepting, inclusive, and socially just. My tip is to step first with connection and acceptance rather than showing the other person where they are at fault. Understand that they are probably trying but might not do so in the most currently acceptable way. Perhaps they use a term that has fallen out of favor, or they haven't thought of an issue that is impacting their client that is based on different cultural aspects. To enact my tip, I recommend reaching out to the other not with a slap but with an embrace (psychologically rather than physically). Lead with your appreciation of their effort and then talk about how they might think, speak, or behave differently. This is what my mentor, Salvador Minuchin, talked about when he recommended the use of a stroke/kick (Minuchin et al., 2021): Challenge comes from connection. Connect with the person first and acknowledge their positive intentions to honor diversity and inclusion. Then it will be easier to talk about how they might do so differently and more effectively.

Summary

Every interaction you have with someone includes some type of diversity. This may be based on gender, culture, age, religion, socioeconomic status, and so on. This is because each person comes from a social location that has many components. This intersectionality occurs for you and for your client. When you engage in therapy, these two unique people come together. This chapter provided a foundation for understanding diversity so that you can honor your own social location as well as that of your client.

References

American Counseling Association. (2014). *2014 ACA code of ethics.* www.counseling.org/resources/aca-code-of-ethics.pdf
American Psychological Association. (2017). *Ethical principles of psychologists and code of conduct.* www.apa.org/ethics/code/ethics-code-2017.pdf
Burnham, J. (2012). Developments in social GRRRAAACCEEESSS: Visible-invisible and voiced-unvoices. In I.-B. Krause (Ed.), *Culture and reflexivity in systemic psychotherapy: Multiple perspectives* (pp. 139–160). Routledge.

Chang, D. F., & Yoon, P. (2011). Ethnic minority clients' perceptions of the significance of race in cross-racial therapy relationships. *Psychotherapy Research, 21*(5), 567–582. https://doi.org/10.1080/105 03307.2011.592549

Corey, M. S., & Corey, G. (2020). *Becoming a helper* (8th ed.). Cengage.

Day-Vines, N. L., Wood, S. M., Grothaus, T., Craigen, L., Holman, A., Dotson-Blake, K., & Douglas, M. F. (2007). Broaching the subjects of race, ethnicity, and culture during the counseling process. *Journal of Counseling & Development, 85*(4), 401–409. https://doi.org/10.1002/j.1556-6678.2007. tb00608.x

Hardy, K. V., & Laszloffy, T. A. (1995). The cultural genogram: Key to training culturally competent family therapists. *Journal of Marital and Family Therapy, 21*(3), 227–237. https://doi.org/10.1111/ j.1752-0606.1995.tb00158.x

Lee, C. C., & Park, D. (2013). A conceptual framework for counseling across cultures. In C. C. Lee (Ed.), *Multicultural issues in counseling: New approaches to diversity* (4th ed., pp. 3–12). American Counseling Association.

Lee, E., Greenblatt, A., Hu, R., Johnstone, M., & Kourgiantakis, T. (2022a). Developing a model of broaching and bridging in cross-cultural psychotherapy: Toward fostering epistemic and social justice. *American Journal of Orthopsychiatry, 92*(3), 322–333. https://doi.org/10.1037/ort0000611

Lee, E., Greenblatt, A., Hu, R., Johnstone, M., & Kourgiantakis, T. (2022b). Microskills of broaching and bridging in cross-cultural psychotherapy: Locating therapy skills in the epistemic domain toward fostering epistemic justice. *American Journal of Orthopsychiatry, 92*(3), 310–321. https:// doi.org/10.1037/ort0000610

Minuchin, S., Reiter, M. D., & Borda, C. (2021). *The craft of family therapy: Challenging certainties* (2nd ed.). Routledge.

Mock, M. R. (2008). Visioning social justice: Narratives of diversity, social location, and personal compassion. In M. McGoldrick & K. V. Hardy (Eds.), *Re-visioning family therapy: Race, culture, and gender in clinical practice* (2nd ed., pp. 425–441). Guilford.

Murphy, M. J., & Hecker, L. (2017). *Ethics and professional issues in couple and family therapy* (2nd ed.). Routledge.

National Association of Social Workers. (2021). *Code of ethics of the National Association of Social Workers*. https://www.socialworkers.org/About/Ethics/Code-of-Ethics/Code-of-Ethics-English

Sanchez, D., del Prado, A., & Davis, C. III. (2010). Broaching ethnicity competently in therapy. In J. A. E. Cornish, B. A. Schreier, L. I. Nadkarni, L. H. Metzger, & E. R. Rodolfa (Eds.), *Handbook of multicultural counseling competencies* (pp. 93–116). Wiley.

Chapter 12

Learning From Mistakes

We have good and bad news for you. First, the bad news: During your practicum/internship, you are going to make a mistake. Actually, you are going to make a *lot* of mistakes. Every single time you meet with a client, you will make not only one but plenty of mistakes. Michael has been practicing as a therapist for over 30 years and makes mistakes each and every session. He also makes mistakes during each supervision session.

Now, the good news: These mistakes aren't usually debilitating. Most of them are extremely small, such as asking a closed rather than an open question or forgetting a client's dog's name. Some other good news: As a beginning therapist, you will not be alone. All of your colleagues will be making therapeutic mistakes, but so will more experienced therapists. Even master therapists make mistakes, fail, and engage in bad therapy (Kottler & Carlson, 2003).

Further, there is actually a benefit to making mistakes. We understand this may sound a little strange, that it might be good to have made a mistake. We believe this is the case when you learn from your mistake. Maybe this is intuitive to some of you already. You might be thinking, "Well, of course I'm going to make a mistake and I'm going to learn from it. That's what my practicum/internship is all about." If this is your mindset going into your field placement, that's great. We want to stress the importance of this anyway (and take an entire chapter to talk about it) because, as it turns out, thinking about making a mistake and learning from it in your mind tends to be quite different than actually being in the moment and making a mistake at your site. As Dennett (1995) stated, "Making mistakes is the key to making progress" (p. 137).

Myths From the Field

"I need to be an excellent therapist to pass my practicum/internship."

You wouldn't really need to be in a practicum/internship if you were already an excellent therapist. You are a beginner, and your site knows that. You are there to learn how to provide therapy, likely for the first time ever, so being an excellent therapist even at the end of a practicum/internship is a silly expectation. Rather than seeking perfection, your site is more so wanting to see your willingness to put forth effort, learn, and grow. It is more about being an excellent student intern than being an excellent therapist.

DOI: 10.4324/9781003433484-12

What Is a Mistake?

As a student, you probably try hard not to make a mistake. One reason is that you've learned that each mistake you make means a deduction of points on an assignment. You make a mistake on a test question, and you go down from a 100 to a 97. Several mistakes on one test or assignment leads to you achieving a B instead of that A you wanted. You've also learned that there are differences in severity of mistakes. If you put a comma in the wrong place, maybe the instructor will actually see it, maybe they will point it out, and likely they will *not* take off any points for it (unless it is done in conjunction with multiple other punctuation issues). But if you make the mistake of plagiarizing (which we encourage you never to do), you might receive a zero on the assignment and could get on probation, suspension, or dismissal from your program. So there could be a lot on the line if and when you make a mistake.

But things change in the therapy room. While you will be graded (your site supervisor and your university supervisor will both be filling out evaluations for you), the mistakes you make in therapy are fodder for growth. Wenzel (2002) stated, "Making mistakes and learning from them are natural components of human existence" (p. 439A). We all make mistakes, which is why there is the saying (attributed to the Enlightenment poet, Alexander Pope), "To err is human" (the end of the saying is "to forgive is divine"). In this chapter, we are going to encourage you to do both—make a mistake and forgive yourself for making it. But better yet, we will also help you to not only forgive yourself but learn from the mistake.

So what is a mistake? Crigger (2005) defined **mistakes** "as unintentional acts that may or may not result in harm that can be judged to be erroneous by practical and reasonable standards" (p. 13). Crigger explained that mistakes can be categorized as either omission or commission. **Omission** occurs when we fail to act on something. In therapy, this may be when you do not conduct a suicide assessment with a client who states, "I've never felt this low before." Or you can engage in a mistake of omission when you do not do a case note or call a client back when they've left a message. Mistakes of **commission** occur when we do something incorrectly. Here, perhaps you say something that does not fit for the client and actually offends them.

Our perspective is that we learn both from what we do well (right) and what we didn't do well (mistakes). Usually, it is better to make therapeutic mistakes when practicing in class. Michael teaches a therapy skills class and prefaces the course by saying that he wants the students to make mistakes so that they can discuss them as a class, learn from them, and then not make those mistakes with clients. In this way, the mistake becomes useful not only for you but for your client as well. The mistake actually becomes something that is desirable. As Roberts (2001) boldly exclaimed, "Guard your mistakes like they are your most valued possessions" (p. 13).

Exercise 12.1   Identifying Past Mistakes

We have all made thousands upon thousands of mistakes in our lives (depending on how we define a mistake). For this exercise, identify some of the mistakes you have made that have been at varying intensities. These mistakes do not need to be therapy related.

Minor Mistake

What was it?:
How did you know it was a mistake?:
How did it impact you?:

Moderate Mistake

What was it?:
How did you know it was a mistake?:
How did it impact you?:

Major Mistake

What was it?:
How did you know it was a mistake?:
How did it impact you?:

Accidental Versus Intentional Mistakes

As we just explained, as a student, you try hard not to make mistakes. And you do the same as a therapist. You think that if you make a mistake, it might negatively impact the client. However, some therapists will make tactical mistakes. Mazzetti (2012) made a distinction between strategic mistakes and tactical mistakes. **Strategic mistakes** happen when the therapist engages in a significant misunderstanding which impacts the diagnosis or treatment plan of the client. If not addressed and corrected, they can have a serious negative impact on the therapy. **Tactical mistakes** intentionally engage in inappropriate moves that have adverse effects. They are more likely to be useful to the therapeutic relationship as the therapist has to learn how to engage in repair behavior.

This is one of the important things to know as a budding psychotherapist—there are always choices to be made as a therapist. You can never know exactly what will happen. Improvisation plays a significant role in the therapeutic process, which means that, in the moment, we might not always make the correct or best choice. What we do is become intentional and hypothesize how our actions will impact our client, the therapeutic relationship, and the therapeutic process. Hopefully, we are correct more often than we are not:

> While it is advisable to predict to some extent how a client might react to an intervention, we have to remember that there is always a level of projection involved in developing empathy. So it is important not to berate ourselves or feel humiliated when an intervention backfires.
>
> (Alschuler, 2014, p. 45)

Therapists tend to feel embarrassment and/or shame from making a mistake. The most frequent of these being making a scheduling mistake, forgetting and/or incorrectly stating client information, being visibly tired, and being late to a session (Klinger et al., 2012). From our own experiences as therapists and being around a lot of therapists, you will do every one of these things. We don't encourage you to do them intentionally but to be aware that it happens. Traffic, confusion, sickness, academic demands, interpersonal demands, and more will present themselves in your life. We call this life! Prepare to try to avoid them but accept them when they happen. Be prepared to apologize to your client or site supervisor and see if you need to change your preparation to try to avoid them in the future.

What Would You Do?: 12.1

Let's give you a scenario that happened to one of Michael's supervisees during a live supervision session. Put yourself into the therapist's position. You are working with a woman who is in her early 30s. She is coming in because she is having difficulties with her husband who is still too connected (at least in your client's eyes) to his ex-wife. Your client feels quite inferior to the ex, thinking that she is smarter and prettier and that the husband probably cares about the ex more than your client. It was very hurtful to the client, that once during sex the husband called her by the ex-wife's name. This caused serious conflict in their relationship and was the final impetus for her entering into therapy. During the course of the session, you try to be personal, so you call the client by name; however, you use the wrong name. You call her by the ex-wife's name. You then realize that you made this mistake. What do you do?

Microskills Mistakes

In Chapter 7, we presented a review of some of the primary microskills that all therapists utilize. Here, we want to present some common microskills mistakes that many therapists do but that we encourage you to avoid. These microskills mistakes include "why" questions, "don't you"/"do you think" questions, "I understand," "basically," "how does that make you feel," "so," and using jargon (Reiter, 2022). Let's quickly go over each so you minimize the possibility of making these mistakes.

"Why" questions are potentially problematic because clients usually don't know the answer to the question and are led to perhaps become defensive. Put yourself in the place of the following client:

Therapist: Why did you decide to confront her?
Client: I don't know. I guess I got fed up.
Therapist: Why is this so important for you?
Client: Because I had enough.
Therapist: Why are you keeping at it?

What are you experiencing when reading this? For us, we can imagine moving backwards rather than wanting to move forward to connect. This pathway will likely lead to client frustration and disconnection from you.

"Don't you think"/"do you think" questions are usually not designed to get the client's opinion into the forefront of the conversation but rather the therapist's. These are really covert ways for the therapist to tell the client what they are thinking without taking ownership for it. Here are a few examples:

- Don't you think that you ought to be nicer to your mother?
- Do you think that this is the best way for you to try to win her back?
- Don't you think that you should be more sensitive to him?

In each of these questions is an implied message from the therapist to the client: They should be nicer to their mother. They should try to win back the person in a different way. They should be more sensitive to the other person.

We would think that one of our primary statements to clients would be "I understand." Isn't that a big part of a therapist's job? To understand the client? Isn't that what empathy and active listening are about? Yes. However, when you try to tell the client this overtly, they will have to let you know that you do not. While people want to be understood, they don't want to be so easily understood. Check out this scenario:

Client: So this has been really difficult for me.
Therapist: I understand.
Client: No, no, no. But you see, it's more than that. I've put everything into this relationship, and I'm not getting what I want out.
Therapist: I understand.
Client: No, no. You see, it's . . .

So what do you do instead since we do want our clients to feel understood? You do so by using all of the microskills that we talked about in Chapter 7. When you do so accurately, the client will respond with "Yes" rather than "No" and will know you understand them without you ever having to say it overtly.

When you start a sentence with "Basically," you are diminishing the client's experience. They have just told you a very important aspect of your life. "Basically" wraps up the complexity of their experience and shrinks it to a simple phenomenon.

Client: My mother is aging and having difficulties. I'm trying to take care of her, but that takes a lot of time and is having a negative impact on my marriage. My husband is not happy with how much I am there and not at home.
Therapist: Basically, this has been a tough situation.

While the therapist may be accurate, the client probably doesn't feel fully appreciated in their situation.

This next microskills mistake might be the one that is most used by therapists, which is one of the reasons that it is a mistake. Watch almost any session by a novice therapist, and we can almost guarantee you that you will hear, at least once (but probably much more than that), "How does that make you feel?" While the intent of the question isn't problematic, the wording is. This is because this sentence has become trite. It is expected. Have you ever seen *Freaky Friday* where Lindsay Lohan swapped places with her mom—who is a therapist—and keeps saying, "And how does that make you feel?" to her mom's clients because she doesn't know what else to say?

Take a second and do an activity that Michael has his therapy students do during class. He has them text someone who is not in the therapy field and ask them, "What are two things that a therapist is likely to say to a client?" The responses are usually in the realm of, "What brings you in?" and "What was your relationship like with your mother?" However, almost every single student will say that the person they asked gave one response, and that was, "How does that make you feel?" Clients expect this, and when you deliver this line, you will likely be perceived to be in therapist mode. You can go after the same information but just phrase it differently:

• What is that like for you?
• How is that for you?
• When that happened, what happened for you?

These variations mine the same depths without the expected response from you.

So what is wrong with "so"? Nothing. As long as we don't use it too often. However, most of us have a few vocalisms that we use to fill space: for example, "Um," "uh," and "hmm." The word "so" is also one that we tend to put at the beginning of our questions or sentences. When used too much, it can seem like we are being inquisitorial. Further, its overuse (and this refers to any word/phrase we overuse) tends to become focused on by the client. When they start to notice and think to themselves, "Is my therapist going to say 'so' again?" they tend not to pay as much attention to what you are actually saying. Here is a brief transcript of this:

Therapist: So what are you hoping to do?
Client: Well, I think it is time for a change.
Therapist: So what change are you thinking about?
Client: Maybe a change of careers. Or even locale.
Therapist: So how are you going to make that decision?

As you can see, there is a pacing that happens that can become troublesome. There is an easy solution to this problem: Stop saying "so." But we know that this is easier said than done. So you will have to figure out how not to say it (whoops, we just did it, and it is not a deadly mistake but is a subtle way to negatively impact the therapeutic alliance).

The last common microskills mistake we want to talk about is the use of jargon. Jargon is words or expressions that are used by a certain profession that others outside of that profession might not know. The first issue is that the clients will likely not understand what you are talking about. A second issue is that the use of this technical language may lead the client to feel stupid because they aren't understanding what you are saying.

Client: We have been going on this merry-go-round with each other, doing the same damn thing every time.
Therapist: You're actually experiencing a competitive symmetrical relationship with one another.
Client: What's that?

We recommend that you try, as much as possible, to use the client's language when you talk with them. The more that you do, the more likely they are to understand you.

We've presented some of the common microskills mistakes. They are all avoidable. However, it will take active effort on your part. Our biggest tip for you here is to record every session that you can (as long as the client has signed a consent to be video recorded). Watching yourself, you will be better able to take a step back and observe what you are doing. The more that you are aware of doing any of these (or other) microskills mistakes, the more likely you will be in avoiding them in future sessions.

Perfectionism

Do you think that you need to be perfect? That you can't make any errors? When you do make an error (or don't get a 100% on a paper or test), do you chastise yourself for it? Over and over? If so, you likely have a tendency for perfectionism. **Perfectionism** happens when we strive to be flawless and have extremely high standards for ourselves.

People tend to think of perfectionism in a negative way and is associated with narcissism (Juwono et al., 2022). That is, the person is very self-focused. It can lead to anxiety and depressive disorders, low self-worth and self-esteem, high stress, and even suicidality. A striving for perfectionism also decreases one's ability for creative thinking (Goulet-Pelletier et al., 2022). Instead of striving for perfectionism, you can strive for **excellencism**, which is pursuing excellence while also allowing yourself to make mistakes and learn throughout the process (Gaudreau et al., 2022).

For those with a tendency for perfectionism, there are a few things that you can do. To start, set more realistic goals. Appreciate that you are beginning to learn and are not a seasoned or master therapist that you've seen in videos such as Carl Rogers or Salvador Minuchin. You can borrow from cognitive behavioral therapy and challenge some of your cognitive errors, such as all-or-nothing thinking or comparing yourself to others. Another strategy to avoid perfectionism is to focus on the process rather than the outcome. Rather than what happened, you can think about what you are learning along the way. You might also practice self-compassion. Provide yourself with a little grace and understand that you are early in your therapy career and are not expected to be perfect, now or ever!

Tips From an Intern

Oh boy, does this topic resonate with me heavily. We just talked about perfectionism and how it can sometimes get in the way of accepting your inevitable mistakes and embracing the lessons you can learn from these mistakes. For any of my friends who may read this, they are likely chuckling right now because I may or may not be known as a perfectionist. While that can be a helpful trait for me to have in certain situations (e.g., like when I am editing the grammar for this book), I knew before going into my practicums and internships that I had to leave perfectionism at the door.

If you feel like you need to be perfect at your practicum/internship, I am here to tell you that you aren't supposed to be, nor should you. It will prevent you from growing as a therapist, plain and simple. If I had gone into my sites with my normal perfectionistic mindset, I would have likely not explored certain things with my clients in fear of them not working, not brought up my mistakes with my supervisors, and not have been open to feedback. My guess is that similar effects would happen to you as well. However, letting my perfectionism go and embracing my mistakes freed me to feel open and confident. That is my advice for you as well. (Oh, and as a note, I will likely miss some grammar edits in this book. And that is okay, too.)

Quick Tip: Intentionally make a mistake! We know this one will be a hard one, especially if you have a tendency to want to be perfect. But when you intentionally make a mistake, you might give yourself more grace. (Just make sure it is not a serious mistake, just a minor one.)

Models of Mistake Making

There are two main models of making mistakes for healthcare providers (Crigger, 2005). The first is the **perfectibility model,** which holds the healthcare provider responsible for functioning in a way that they do not make mistakes. Thus, if a mistake happens, it is because the therapist is at fault since they did not do their job correctly. One of the negative outcomes of using this model is that the health care provider will be much less likely to divulge to someone when they have made a mistake because they would potentially be perceived as incompetent.

The second model is the **faulty systems model** (Crigger, 2005). Here, mistakes can occur from the individual or the system. The errors that people make are expected and anticipated, and there are safety measures built into the system to account for them. When we look at ethics in psychotherapy, we can see this model at work. Not everything is black and white. While there are certain areas that are clear (e.g., don't ever have any sexual relations with a current client), there are many gray areas (which is why we have ethical decision-making models).

Tips From a Supervisor

As I've mentioned a few times throughout this book, I have been a teacher for almost 25 years now and a supervisor for about the same. One of my favorite courses to teach is the counseling skills class in which we would do a lot of role-plays. One of the things I encouraged was for the students who came to the front of the class to be the therapist was to feel comfortable making mistakes. I told them I would stop them when they do make a mistake so we could talk about it. Hopefully, once they understood the mistake, they would not make it with an actual client.

Perhaps your counseling skills instructor did the same for you. But now, you are in your placement and working with actual clients. One tip is to think back to your skills class and remember all of the things your instructor taught you. What were the errors and mistakes they pointed out that you or one of your classmates made? Think about them because the more aware you are of them, the less chance you have of making them.

The next tip that I have for you is to embrace the notion that you are not going to be perfect. I make mistakes every time I enter the therapy room. I hope that most of them are minimal. Hopefully, your mistakes will be as well. Go into your sessions knowing that you will do well *and* will make mistakes. Try to record your sessions so you can watch them with your supervisor and pay attention to what you did well and what you could have done differently.

Learning From Mistakes

Mistakes can be viewed as the only opportunity that we have to really learn something new (Dennett, 1995). The next time you try something similar, you will not be in the same position, as you'll have the experience of the first attempt to help guide your second attempt. Take a second and think about if you had to throw a ball 50 feet through a four-foot opening. Your first throw goes left. You then tell yourself, "Okay. That wasn't correct. I have to adjust and aim more toward the right." Your next throw goes too far right. You then take that learning into consideration and aim more for the center. You then come up ten feet short, and for your next throw, you put more power into it. With each throw, you are learning from the previous ones and making successive approximations. Eventually, you throw the ball through the opening, not because of luck, but because you learned from your mistakes.

Clinical mistakes often lead to useful information that therapists can utilize with their clients (Gilhooley, 2011). Gilhooley explained that a mistake can be seen as a mis-take, where the therapist didn't quite see the client's position. Thus, making these mis-takes provides an opportunity to refocus and better bring forth aspects of the client that one or both parties had not previously seen as clearly (see Figure 12.1). You have made many of these mis-takes, and many of them have been made about you.

Take a second to think about the last time each of these has happened for you. How have you made an attribution of understanding of someone only to find out sometime later that how you viewed the person was not quite accurate? Perhaps you didn't initially like the person but are now good friends with them, or maybe they are even your romantic partner. Or conversely, you initially thought someone was great and now think they are poop.

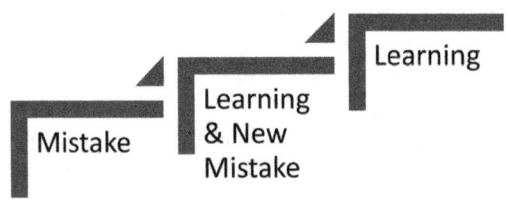

Figure 12.1 Mistakes are opportunities for us to be able to gain a better understanding of ourselves and the situation, learn, and to improve for the next time.

People have done the same with you. What has been a recent conversation during which someone tried to put their understanding of you out there and you disagreed with them? What was that conversation like? How did that conversation lead to a bettering of the relationship between the two of you?

Roberts (2001) promoted the notion that your role should be as a human first and a therapist second. As he explained, "A person makes mistakes honestly and, hopefully, learns from them" (Roberts, 2001, p. 13). Clients can and usually will forgive mistakes that you make when they see that you are invested in their active growth.

Exercise 12.2   Learning From Our Mistakes

In Exercise 12.1, you identified several mistakes that you had made in your life. For this exercise, consider what you learned from making those mistakes and how they have been useful for you.

Minor Mistake

What did you learn from making that mistake?:
What did you learn about yourself from making that mistake?:
How was making that mistake useful to you?:

Moderate Mistake

What did you learn from making that mistake?:
What did you learn about yourself from making that mistake?:
How was making that mistake useful to you?:

Major Mistake

What did you learn from making that mistake?:
What did you learn about yourself from making that mistake?:
How was making that mistake useful to you?:

Appreciating Our Resources

Throughout this chapter, we've discussed the inevitability that you will make mistakes. It will happen. We've emphasized that these are not failures but opportunities to learn. But we don't want to end this chapter on that note. We are both strength-based therapists. We recognize that while there are times you don't engage in therapy in the most efficacious manner, there are many more times that you do. You should also be on the lookout for these occurrences, as we believe in the motto, "Once you know what works, do more of it" (Berg, 1994).

Take a moment and think about your best and most effective therapeutic skills. How have you engaged at your site in a way that has assisted in your learning? How have these skills been present in this process? In what ways are your competent therapeutic skills a product of your learning—that they have built off of past mistakes? What are some of the ways that you conceptualize cases and engage in therapeutic skills that you are most proud of?

Sharing Your Mistakes

You probably don't look forward to telling friends or family members that you made a mistake. Perhaps you will, but it likely depends on the severity of the mistake. On the basketball court, you throw a bad pass and will say, "My bad." No worries, it was just a pickup game, and the bad pass doesn't really mean much in the grand scheme of things. But if you cheat on your partner, you probably won't say, "My bad." Small mistakes can be funny: "You'll never believe what I did. I called Sylvia by the wrong name," "I went to Burger King, and when I ordered their chicken nuggets, I called them McNuggets," or "I gave Bill the soda to drink but didn't realize that when I was walking from the fridge to him, my hand was moving up and down. When he opened the bottle, it sprayed all over him."

When you view your mistakes through a lens of humility, you have an opportunity to grow. While they share the same etymological root, there are big differences between humility and humiliation (Alschuler, 2014). Humiliation is an internal experience of not thinking that you are good enough and may include aspects of shame. Humility, in contrast, promotes an idea that there is more for you to learn. Sharing your mistakes with others provides the space for you to appreciate yourself as a human being and explore areas of how you can improve.

Tales From the Field: Intern

Going into my practicum as a doctoral-level student, I knew I wanted to put my best foot forward and present professionally and competently. I have been a professional counselor for ten years, and I am confident in my therapeutic skills. However, I was not as confident being at the doctoral level. There was some level of imposter syndrome: Did I belong here? Was I good enough? How could I be smart enough for this?

The agency I was completing my practicum with had never taken on a doctoral-level student before, so I knew there may be a learning curve for both me and the agency. I pride myself in being an authentic practitioner, which I believe helps clients feel comfortable and facilitates a positive rapport. But I was nervous about being the first doctoral student, and there were many thoughts running through my head. For example, if I were "too" professional, would I not come across as authentic? And if I were "too" authentic, would my clinical supervisor think I was not professional enough? Needless to say, I put a lot of pressure on myself.

My duties at the site were mainly in psychological testing; this was by design because this is an area in which I wanted to learn and gain experience. The first time I conducted a psychological assessment—independent of my supervisor's observation—I was assessing a 17-year-old male for an attentional disorder. I prepared the battery of tests the clinical supervisor typically used. I felt comfortable with how the administration went, and after the three-hour testing session, I told myself, "Dang girl, you nailed it!" I was certain my clinical supervisor was going to feel the same way. I saw the client out and went to my office to begin scoring the tests, and there it was: the mistake. I had given the WISC-V (for children ages 6–16) and not the WAIS-IV (for adults ages 17–90). A wave of anxiety came over me. How could I have made such a huge mistake? I was worried about what my supervisor would say, and all the catastrophic thoughts came to my head. I thought, "Of course I am going to be let go from the practicum, because why wouldn't I be?" Then I thought of the client: He had spent all of this time in testing, and his results were not valid because he was over the age limit of the WISC. I was terrified to bring this to the attention of my clinical supervisor, but I knew I must.

I reluctantly went to my supervisor and informed him of my grave mistake. I was waiting for the look of disappointment that would be crushing to my ego. However, to my surprise, my clinical supervisor smiled and said, "I made the same mistake during my training." Wait . . . what? Did I hear that right? Mistakes happen when you are in training? My supervisor asked to review the client file, which included his date of birth, previous testing from three years prior, and his school records. Turns out, the supervisor felt the results could be considered valid, as the client had scored in the very low range for his FSIQ and was on an IEP. The supervisor explained that the client may not have been able to complete the WAIS because it would have been too challenging for him. In fact, he said it was better to repeat the WISC in order to compare results and to identify any changes in index scores, which then could allow for more confidence in results.

What I learned from this experience is that mistakes happen, and as a student, you are bound to make them—they make room for growth and learning. Experiencing anxiety at this stage is completely normal. I also learned that being authentic yet professional when reporting mistakes is important, and being open to feedback and constructive criticism is an absolute necessity if you want to succeed at your site.

Shauna Putzy, PhD in Clinical Psychology program, Capella University

Apologizing

Some mistakes you make will not impact anyone else and are just for you to learn from. However, other mistakes may have negative implications for others. When they do, consider offering an apology. Apologies are beneficial, as they allow us an opportunity to take ownership of our actions, lead to us thinking about our actions (or inactions) and learning from the situation, repair a relationship, resolve a situation, and lead to emotional healing for both parties.

There are a variety of ways that you can apologize to someone, depending on the context. If you make a mistake with a client, it is perfectly fine to apologize to them. While there is an inherent power imbalance between therapist and client, an apology helps to humanize you and can enhance the therapeutic alliance.

Apologies tend to consist of the following components. You might add or delete components based on the severity of the mistake and the type of relationship you have with the other person.

- Let the other person know you would like to apologize to them.
- Be specific about what it is you are apologizing for.
- Take ownership of your actions.
- Say "I'm sorry" or "I apologize."
- Be remorseful about the actions and empathetic about how those actions impacted the other person.
- Explain your position (without trying to justify it) if the other person wants to know why you did what you did.
- Accept that there may be consequences to the mistake.

However you do the apology, make sure that you are doing so from a place of genuineness and sincerity. If it comes across that you are giving lip service, this might exacerbate the situation.

Tales From the Field: Supervisor

Allana was midway through her master of family therapy program, and she was excited to begin her internship at her first practicum site. Her site of choice was a private practice that worked with individuals, couples, and families. She attended my online university supervision class before she began her internship. During class, we discussed the transition from academic case conceptualization to in-person application of what she had learned over the previous year and a half. Like many of her peers, Allana reported feeling nervous about seeing clients for the first time. She was also anxious about the school requirement to record video of her work with clients to show our class.

Luckily, Allana's very first clients—a heterosexual couple in their 50s—agreed to be recorded to fulfill Allana's school requirement. In the middle of the session, the husband cursed, stood up, and walked out the door, leaving his wife annoyed and Allana stunned. Not knowing what to do, Allana continued speaking with the wife alone for the remainder of the session.

When Allana told her site supervisor about what happened, her supervisor normalized her experience, saying, "Great, you got that over with!" They discussed how this session was a good learning opportunity for Allana and contained a lesson that sessions may not go the way you envision them. They continued to process Allana's feelings of embarrassment and doubt.

We also watched the recording and discussed Allana's case in online supervision to provide additional feedback. I asked Allana if she knew why the husband had left. Allana shared her realization that the husband walked out because she was aligning with his wife and not providing enough space for him to speak, sometimes even interrupting him. She needed to balance the session more, giving each person time to speak and feel heard.

I also asked about her choice to see the wife alone for the second half. She said it was not a choice so much as her not realizing her own authority to end the session early. Allana explained how she had not considered that it would be okay for her to end the session early since they had paid for a full session. Allana and her peers considered ways to get therapy back on track if the clients came back.

The couple returned the next week, and Allana opened the session with an apology. She disclosed that she reviewed the session with two supervisors since their last meeting. Allana shared she could see herself interrupting him on the video and understood why he left. She also apologized for continuing to speak with his wife after he left, and she guessed that made him feel like even more of an outsider. Her client was appreciative of her admission and that she had worked to review the case in such detail between their sessions. They kept Allana on as their therapist. She later reported they had developed excellent rapport and were making progress toward the client's goals. Allana continued to check in regularly to make sure both individuals felt heard, and she said she was grateful for the learning experience.

Kelsey Railsback, PhD, LMFT, Family Therapy program, Touro University

Accepting Feedback

Many people say that they want feedback so that they can improve. The question is, do they really want this feedback? What about you? We tend not to want to hear what we are doing wrong. Instead of receiving this information as feedback, we take it as criticism. Your supervisor is trying to provide you with constructive criticism that will help you to become a better therapist. **Constructive criticism** occurs when you receive feedback that is intended to improve your skills while being respectful and supportive.

Perhaps you've watched a lot of competitive cooking shows hosted by Gordon Ramsay in which he yells at the chefs and sometimes even throws food at them. This will be rare for you to experience in the therapy world. On the other end of the spectrum, we have seen supervisors only give compliments as feedback—that is, they only comment on what you are doing well and omit anything you could work on for future sessions. It is our belief that this approach only provides you with half of the opportunity to improve as a therapist. To us, it is equally important to know what you could refine and vice versa.

Hopefully, whoever is supervising you will provide feedback in an appropriate manner. Whether they do or don't, you are able to engage with them in a way that you can better use the feedback so that you can learn from your mistakes and improve your therapy. Here are some general tips on accepting feedback:

- Maintain an open mindset
- Listen actively
- Seek clarification if you need to
- Stay calm and manage your emotions
- Avoid personalizing the feedback
- Ask for specific examples
- Reflect before you respond
- Express gratitude
- Take ownership and set goals
- Seek support and follow up

It is your supervisor's responsibility to provide you with useful feedback (including constructive criticism) to help you become a better therapist. However, it is your responsibility to get yourself in the right mental frame to receive that feedback and then to implement it.

Summary

No one wants to make mistakes, but we all do. This chapter has attempted to normalize this notion so that you don't chastise yourself for making a mistake but, more importantly, that you will learn from your mistake. Psychotherapy is about growth, and your practicum/internship experience is about your growth. Another way of viewing growth is as learning. We encourage you to accept that you make mistakes; apologize when appropriate; share your mistakes with relevant people (such as colleagues and supervisors); seek out and accept feedback; and appreciate that not only did you make a mistake, but you also did a lot of things that were useful. Each mistake you make can be used as a stepping stone to become a better psychotherapist.

References

Alschuler, M. L. (2014). Learning from and with humility. *Reflections: Narratives of Professional Helping*, *20*(2), 42–46.

Berg, I. K. (1994). *Family based services: A solution-focused approach*. Norton.

Crigger, N. (2005). Two models of mistake-making in professional practice: Moving out of the closet. *Nursing Philosophy*, *6*(1), 11–18. https://doi.org/10.1111/j.1466-769X.2004.00203.x

Dennett, D. C. (1995). How to make mistakes. In J. Brockman & K. Matson (Eds.), *How things are* (pp. 137–144). William Morrow.

Gaudreau, P., Schellenberg, B. J. I., Gareau, A., Kljajic, K., & Manoni-Millar, S. (2022). Because excellencism is more than good enough: On the need to distinguish the pursuit of excellence from the pursuit of perfection. *Journal of Personality and Social Psychology*, *122*(6), 1117–1145. https://doi.org/10.1037/pspp0000411

Gilhooley, D. (2011). Mistakes. *Psychoanalytic Psychology*, *28*(2), 311–333. https://doi.org/10.1037/a0023080

Goulet-Pelletier, J.-C., Gaudreau, P., & Cousineau, D. (2022). Is perfectionism a killer of creative thinking? A test of the model of excellencism and perfectionism. *British Journal of Psychology*, *113*(1), 176–207. https://doi.org/10.1111/bjop.12530

Juwono, I. D., Kun, B., Demetrovics, Z., & Urbán, R. (2022). Healthy and unhealthy dimensions of perfectionism: Perfectionism and mental health in Hungarian adults. *International Journal of Mental Health and Addiction*. https://doi.org/10.1007/s11469-022-00771-8

Klinger, R. S., Ladany, N., & Kulp, L. E. (2012). It's too late to apologize: Therapist embarrassment and shame. *The Counseling Psychologist*, *40*(4), 554–574. https://doi.org/10.1177/001000011416372

Kottler, J. A., & Carlson, J. (2003). *Bad therapy: Master therapists share their worst failures*. Routledge.

Mazzetti, M. (2012). Teaching trainees to make mistakes. *Transactional Analysis Journal*, *42*(1), 43–52. https://doi.org/10.1177/036215371204200106

Reiter, M. D. (2022). *Therapeutic interviewing: Essential skills and contexts of counseling* (2nd ed.). Routledge.

Roberts, T. W. (2001). Therapeutic use of the unpredictable: When mistakes lead to therapeutic change. *Reflections: Narratives of Professional Helping*, *7*(1), 13–20.

Wenzel, T. J. (2002). Using mistakes as learning opportunities. *Analytical Chemistry*, *74*(15), 439A–440A. https://doi.org/10.1021/ac022078z

Chapter 13

Navigating a Work/Life Balance

Many students need to work while going to school to not only pay for school (or the impending student loans they are accruing) but for living expenses as well. During your practicum/internship, you may also be taking other courses to complete your degree. Then you have the actual hours that you are putting in at your site. Depending on your personal situation, you may have a family that you need to take care of. This amount of responsibilities can be overwhelming for a lot of people. In this chapter, we want to talk about these potentially competing responsibilities and provide ideas for you to think about while you navigate them to attempt to develop a work/life balance.

As we discussed in Chapter 2, it is important to talk with your site, before you both agree on that placement, about what their expectations are in terms of the number of hours they want you to be at the site. However, we recognize that while you likely agreed to the amount of time at the site, many times our eyes are bigger than our stomachs. That is, you probably told yourself that you would be able to put in the 20 hours (or however many was discussed) while also completing all your other responsibilities. After weeks or months, you may now realize that being at your site, being with your family, having a paying job, engaging in schoolwork, and just having time for yourself to chill doesn't provide you with the opportunity to do all of them. The optimistic hopefulness of beginning the practicum/internship may now be overrun by the overwhelming stress of juggling too many balls. And these balls may now seem like running chainsaws!

Myth About the Field

"I cannot have a life while I'm doing my practicum/internship."

This is not only false but something that we recommend you do the opposite of. It is important to not have therapy be all-consuming of your life. Your practicum/internship is an important part of your life, but it is not your entire life. It is necessary for you as a human being to engage in your own interests and hobbies as well as give time to your loved ones. While each person's balance of these important elements of life will look different, it is necessary that each person has some sort of balance.

DOI: 10.4324/9781003433484-13

Stress

While at your site, you will experience some level of stress, as you must work with clients, navigate paperwork, deal with ethical and site-based dilemmas, engage in schoolwork, and have a life. **Stress** happens when you experience emotional and/or physical tension. It can be both acute and/or chronic. **Acute stress** is time-limited. When you have a test coming up, you have a paper due, or you have to give a public speech, you will experience acute stress. Once the situation is finished, the stress goes away. **Chronic stress** lasts longer, sometimes weeks, months, or even years. Being in a miserable relationship, dealing with a serious illness, or working at a place that you hate are all situations that cause chronic stress.

At any one time, you have both acute and chronic stress factors impacting you. The longer you maintain stress, the higher potential there is for physical and mental difficulties. When experiencing acute stress, you might find that you are more tired than normal; have an upset stomach, diarrhea, headaches, lack of energy, focus, and appetite; and will likely have difficulty sleeping. Chronic stress may result in high blood pressure, depression, anxiety, eating issues, and a plethora of other ailments. It is important for you to stay in contact with yourself to assess your stress and determine if you need to do anything about it. Providing therapeutic services to others is not an easy endeavor. Given its demanding, draining, and exhausting aspects, being a psychotherapist is quite stressful (Rokach & Boulazreg, 2022). Many therapists experience physical isolation, emotional isolation, stress from negative interactions with clients, and a heightening of whatever personal situations are already occurring for them.

Tales From the Field: Supervisor

Marissa was a clinical psychology intern at a busy outpatient clinic at a dual-diagnosis treatment facility, and she was approaching the end of her graduate program. As the director of clinical training of her academic program, I reviewed her progress toward her training goals and received evaluative feedback from her site supervisor at several points of the training experience. Marissa demonstrated sound clinical skills and managed well with the many responsibilities she had as an intern. She was well-liked by other clinicians, staff, interns, and clients. Marissa consistently came prepared for weekly supervision, and client feedback showed high satisfaction rates. Marissa's description of supervision was overwhelmingly positive and supportive; her supervisor ended every supervision session asking Marissa how he could help. According to her supervisor, Marissa was far ahead of her three other peers in terms of clinical knowledge, therapeutic counseling skills, and time management. Although he didn't tell her yet, her supervisor was prepared to offer her an employment position once she completed her internship placement. About midway through her internship, Marissa shared with her classmates and me that she was excited to progress as the primary therapist of a therapy group. She explained that her supervisor would co-lead the group sessions, but Marissa was expected to lead the group. The first group session went well, and the supervisor was pleased with Marissa's growth during the internship experience thus far. The following week was a different story.

Marissa arrived late to the session, she neglected to bring the worksheets needed to complete the planned group activity, and she yawned numerous times while clients were sharing. Her supervisor invited her to an unscheduled supervision session following the conclusion of the group to check in. Marissa apologized for not being at her best. She added that she was up all night taking care of her sick daughter who was now at home with the flu. She shared that she was worried about her and had a lot on her mind during the group. Although she considered calling out, Marissa was concerned that her supervisor may view that as a sign she was not committed to the clinic. She felt torn between her commitment toward her family and toward her clients and the clinic.

Marissa's supervisor reassured her that her responsibility toward her family and to her own health were important. He reminded her that she is human and that "life happens." He explained that the important thing to keep in mind is to communicate her needs to ensure the outcome is best for everyone. He normalized the concept of self-care and emphasized the importance of prioritizing her basic needs, which include adequate sleep. He also reviewed the clinic's policies related to calling out, which ensured clinical coverage of her clients scheduled for the day. Marissa felt better after talking to her supervisor about this, but she also felt embarrassed that she made mistakes that day. With the support of her supervisor, she planned to take the following day off so she could get caught up with rest, spend quality time with her daughter, and return to the clinic ready to resume clinical services. Marissa shared this experience with me and her classmates during her seminar class the following week, reminding her peers to take care to balance work and life, as she had learned. I was proud of Marissa for her personal growth that day, which eventually led to being offered full-time employment after graduation.

Kristi L. Mueller, PsyD, LP, Clinical Psychology program Capella University

Wellness

While we talk about stress and the potential negative impacts it may have in your life, we are strength-based therapists and also want to focus on what you are striving for: **Wellness**. Wellness is not only your physical health. It focuses on your overall health, which includes the mental, emotional, social, spiritual, intellectual, and environmental aspects of your life (see Figure 13.1). The more of these areas that you feel happy with, the better your overall wellness. We would argue that this would lead to you being better able to be in the right mindset to do good therapy and be able to learn at your site.

You cannot separate the you of your daily life with the you of your professional life. The personal bleeds into the professional, and the professional bleeds into the personal. This is why it is extremely important for you to take care and monitor yourself in both realms so that you are well and are effective for yourself and your clients.

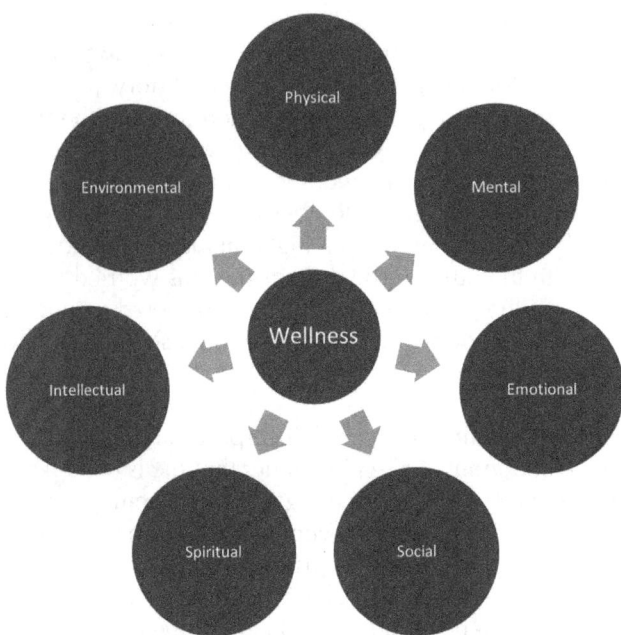

Figure 13.1 Wellness includes physical, mental, emotional, social, spiritual, intellectual, and environmental factors.

Exercise 13.1   Assessing Your Levels of Wellness

For the following areas of wellness, circle where you currently are on a scale of 1 to 10, with 1 being the lowest and 10 being the highest. Then, put a square around the number where you want to be in that area.

Physical	1	2	3	4	5	6	7	8	9	10
Mental	1	2	3	4	5	6	7	8	9	10
Emotional	1	2	3	4	5	6	7	8	9	10
Social	1	2	3	4	5	6	7	8	9	10
Spiritual	1	2	3	4	5	6	7	8	9	10
Intellectual	1	2	3	4	5	6	7	8	9	10
Environmental	1	2	3	4	5	6	7	8	9	10

Take a look at your scores. In which areas did you score the highest? Which is the lowest? How far off are you from where you want to be? Now, write down one very small thing that you can do this week in each of these wellness areas. Once you write them down, choose a different one each day for the next week and actually do it. This is you prioritizing your self-care.

Self-Care

Hopefully, you have heard a lot about self-care in your clinical program. Maybe it was refer-ring to clients, for you to talk with them about how they take care of themselves. There are many different ways of doing that which we won't talk about here. Rather, we are going to talk about *your* self-care. This is important since many training institutes and universities lack efficient and effective promotion of a self-care culture for their trainees and students (Vally, 2019). It is imperative that therapists ensure that they are functioning well so that they can help clients to function well. Why is this? You've heard this explained a different way when you're on a plane and the flight attendants are describing what happens if there is a loss of cabin pressure. Oxygen masks will drop down if this occurs. The flight attendant then tells you that you should put your own mask on first before you help those around you. This is because you need to be in a stable place before you can focus on helping the other person.

Self-care can be defined as "the deliberate and self-initiated attempt to take care of one-self" (Rokach & Boulazreg, 2022, p. 5660). It occurs when you try to engage in wellness practices and activities. It is respecting yourself and understanding that your physical, men-tal, and emotional energy is not everlasting. You need to put active effort into taking care of yourself.

Not only is self-care a useful thing (and potentially fun), but it is also an ethical impera-tive (Vally, 2019). The American Psychological Association (2017, Standard 2.06) Personal Problems and Conflicts states:

a. Psychologists refrain from initiating an activity when they know or should know that there is a substantial likelihood that their personal problems will prevent them from performing their work-related activities in a competent manner.
b. When psychologists become aware of personal problems that may interfere with their performing work-related duties adequately, they take appropriate measures, such as obtaining professional consultation or assistance, and determine whether they should limit, suspend, or terminate their work-related duties.

As you can see, being well physically, mentally, and emotionally is extremely important as a therapist, especially since we sometimes go and hang out in dark spaces with clients. Further, the more you engage in self-care, the more you learn and know about yourself.

Barnett and Cooper (2009) held that it is a therapist's responsibility in the development of their professional identity to have an active focus on self-care.

We have all heard about self-care but might not have the same understanding of what it is and the foundation upon which it rests. Suppes (2019) held that there are three assump-tions in self-care. First, it is proactive and intentional. Second, depending on the therapist, some may more naturally veer toward self-care activities while others will need to be more intentional about it. Third, when a therapist engages in self-care, they are demonstrating self-compassion.

An important thing to note about self-care is that it becomes much more beneficial if you engage in it proactively instead of just reactively. You are much more likely to burn out and produce less consistent work if you wait until the end of the semester to take a vacation, for example. In this circumstance, you are allowing the stresses of life to come crashing down at once, and you only do something after it has become too overwhelming.

While we understand that you can't just take a vacation whenever you'd like during the semester, there are smaller things you can do throughout your day-to-day life that are proactive acts of self-care. For example, we know students who take weekly yoga classes; others take baths a few nights a week. The beauty about self-care is that there are endless ways to engage in it. It is all about doing things that resonate the most with you and that allow you to take that break from your responsibilities and recharge.

If you don't have a proactive self-care routine going before you start your practicum/internship, now is the perfect time to start experimenting with what will work best for you. If you do have a proactive self-care routine, you may realize that you need to tweak this routine to fit your new practicum/internship schedule and responsibilities (e.g., maybe your days at your site conflict with your usual yoga class).

Examples of Self-Care

There are many different activities you can do for self-care. While we will talk about just a few of these, we want to take a broader view. Suppes (2019) characterized self-care into four types: cognitive, physical, emotional, and spiritual (see Figure 13.2). **Cognitive self-care** allows your mind to move away from therapy and think about something else or perhaps think about nothing at all. Activities you can do here include watching television, meditating, reading a fun book (other than this one), or other such practices. **Physical self-care** refers to your body. This includes ensuring that you are eating and drinking well, having nutritious meals and a lot of water. Exercise is also another excellent example of physical self-care. You might go to the gym, ride your bike, take a walk in a park, or engage in yoga practices. Don't

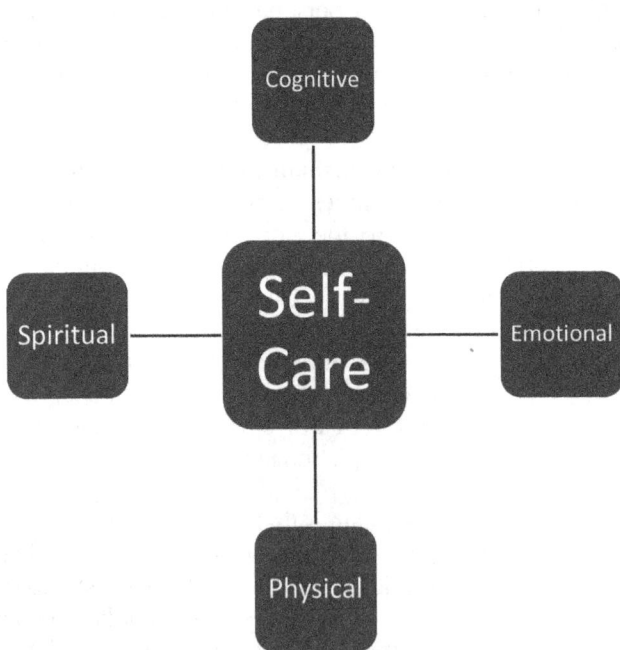

Figure 13.2 Self-care can be categorized into four types.

forget about ensuring that you are getting a good night's sleep. **Emotional self-care** includes you positively engaging with other people (who are not teachers, supervisors, or clients). This includes spending time with family and friends where you are enjoying each other's company. For instance, when was the last time you got together with someone and had a good laugh? The less you laugh, the more that potential burnout can enter the equation. **Spiritual self-care** refers to your connection to something larger than yourself. This might be your connection to nature, religion, or other entities.

Exercise 13.2   Being Aware of Your Self-Care

For this exercise, identify what you have already done in terms of self-care and what you'd like to further incorporate into your self-care routine.

	Cognitive	Physical	Emotional	Spiritual
What you are already doing				
1.				
2.				
3.				
What you would like to do that you are not				
1.				
2.				
3.				

As with exercise 13.1, it is important not only to become aware of where you are at and what you want to do but to actually do some or all of those activities. We challenge you to implement one or more of your answers this week—both continuing what you have done for self-care and introducing what you would like to do.

Bush (2015) promoted the idea that instead of going for big and seldom, it is often better to go for small and frequent. Bush calls this **micro self-care**, in which the person engages in small and quick replenishing practices during a day. Bush argued that this fits within the field of self-directed neuroplasticity where the brain can reorganize its neural networks from short and repetitive experiences. Micro self-care helps to promote repetition. What does this mean for you? While it might be quite useful to take that camping trip to get away from everything, that only may occur for 5 to 10 days a year. What about the other 360 or so days? Instead of thinking about the end of the day, end of the week, end of the month, or end of the year to engage in self-care, how can you think of doing so at least three or four times a day?

There are many ways to engage in these targeted micro self-care practices, which may help to prevent burnout, compassion fatigue, and secondary traumatization (Bush, 2015). You can do progressive muscle relaxation, stretching, positive self-talk, mindfulness practices, meditation, or other grounding practices. You don't need hours to do any of these. For instance, before you walk to the waiting room to get your client, you can close your eyes and think about how you are now part of a tribe of professionals who people come to for a more enjoyable life. By feeling connected to all other therapists, you can reacquaint yourself with the purpose that you have in being a psychotherapist. Or you can do as a therapist we know, who would do a five-minute meditation before each session.

Tips From an Intern

My tip for a good work/life balance relates to self-care. Self-care is spending time with your cat when it doesn't need a cone. Allow me to explain: Prior to writing this book, my cat had some medical issues that required her to be in the cone of shame most of the time before her medication kicked in (this was almost a year-long timeframe). In order to give her a break from the cone, I would take the cone off every day for around 30 minutes to an hour; however, I had to follow her every move to make sure she did not lick/bite herself and cause cuts and lesions on her skin. This was exhausting because—for those of you who don't have cats—cats are fast. I had to chase her around the apartment constantly during her "cone off time" to prevent her from hurting herself. This was all happening during my doctoral program.

I originally considered playing with my cat every day during her "cone off time" to be a part of my self-care. I love her very much, and it makes me happy to have fun with her. It also gave me a break from doing homework or working on progress notes for clients. However, I realized how drained I was after playing with her—it not only required a physical effort but a mental and emotional one as well. While the playing part was fun, the amount of energy it took me to play with her given the circumstances wound up taking more out of me than I thought. I have seen many colleagues do similar acts of self-care, which don't really wind up being self-care in the end (for example, answering work texts and emails while "relaxing" at the beach).

The moral of this story is that self-care is not self-care if you half-ass it. This logic applies to any type of self-care activity you choose: You have to make sure it is *really* self-care. You need to be able to (a) take a break from school/life responsibilities and (b) recharge. So I will repeat it again: Self-care is spending time with your cat when it *doesn't* need a cone. Now that my cat thankfully does not need a cone, the stress of "cone off time" has transformed into pure fun and enjoyment when playing with her. My tip is to revisit some of your self-care activities and really scrutinize them to see if they are providing the break that a self-care act should.

Mindfulness

Mindfulness is a practice that has become increasingly incorporated in the mental health field (e.g., Brody et al., 2018; Frostadottir & Dorjee, 2019; Hoffman & Gómez, 2017). It essentially consists of two components: (a) nonjudgmental (b) awareness (Stefan & David, 2020). It's a practice in which you are able to be aware of your present experience (e.g., thoughts, feelings, physical sensations) without getting frustrated at that experience. Mindfulness allows you to be in touch with yourself without becoming annoyed at what you are getting in touch with—for example, "Okay, I am noticing that I feel upset right now that I didn't get that internship placement like I thought I would." Usually, feeling this way produces a slew of emotions (e.g., frustration, anger, guilt, disappointment). Perhaps you are angry that you feel disappointed in the first place because you don't want the interviewer to have power over you. Mindfulness, however, allows for the recognition of our feelings and thoughts in a calm way. It gives us the ability to sit in our experience and simply reflect on and accept this experience without it becoming overwhelming.

Mindfulness is more frequently present in the therapy room, as therapists are utilizing mindfulness practices with their clients in a variety of ways for a variety of reasons (Kabat-Zinn et al., 1992; Stefan & David, 2020). We are able to not only use mindfulness with our clients but with ourselves as well. It is a practice that seamlessly ties into our discussion of a work/life balance because you can use mindfulness both in your professional life and in your personal life (and as a conduit to balance both).

A great example of the professional application of mindfulness is using it to help you process your biases. In Chapter 5, we talked about how you will inevitably have biases as a therapist. We also talked about how it is imperative that you acknowledge rather than ignore these biases. One way to do that is through mindfulness. We have both seen the reactivity that many student interns have had when a supervisor kindly yet constructively brings up an area of bias that a student may have based on their actions and words in the therapy room. This is hard feedback to take even if it is meant to be helpful, and it is understandable to feel upset, challenged, or defensive. Though understandable, these are not helpful responses to have when you are trying to grow as a therapist. Mindfulness can help you sit in those feelings and reflections without them overcoming you. It then frees you up to hear what your supervisor is saying with more open ears.

In your personal life, mindfulness can also be used to be in tune with your self-care practices. First, you can use mindfulness to determine whether or not you are engaging in self-care to the necessary degree or not. By being nonjudgmentally aware of your inner experience, you can truly sit with yourself and be able to recognize, "Whoa, I am not feeling my best. I need to look at this further" without this realization overtaking you. Second, you can use mindfulness to check in and determine whether the self-care activities you are engaging in are truly helping you (as mentioned in Kayleigh's tip previously).

There are many different ways to practice mindfulness. Mindfulness meditations are meditations that involve being present, paying attention to your experience moment by moment to understand it better, and also being able to let this experience go rather than ruminate over it. Journaling can also be a form of mindfulness. Breathwork, walking your dog, coloring, and more can all be mindfulness practices. Again, what makes it mindfulness is when the activity is done to bring about awareness while leaving the judgment at the door.

Let's take mindfulness out for a spin. We mentioned that one way to practice mindfulness is through journaling, so we want you to take a moment and try it out here. Take the next five or ten minutes (or longer, if you feel the mindful juices flowing) to simply journal about what you are experiencing right now—any thought, feeling, physical sensation, you name it, let the writing flow from there. Remember, it's not just about venting on the page and getting it all out. It is about *nonjudgmentally* being *aware* of your experience (it can be harder to do that when we are just furiously writing).

Instead, every time you write out a sentence or two, pause and reread what you wrote. Then, go ahead and keep writing, keeping your focus on the present moment. For example, "I am feeling really anxious about this big test on Friday. I honestly feel unprepared. [pauses and reads] Actually, I think the best way to describe the feeling is more like nervous than anxious. I'm even noticing that my mind is racing just bringing it up. [pauses and reads] That is actually something I do during my tests as well—my mind races like it's doing now. [pauses and reads] Oh wait, I'm thinking about the test . . . I got distracted, let me bring it back to what I'm feeling now . . . "

Some people like to journal on their computer or phone because they find it easier to type than write and more readily accessible. If you can, though, we'd like to recommend that you do this on a piece of paper with a pen or pencil. There is some literature to suggest that physically writing things out rather than typing them can produce a greater likelihood that you will retain and process the information you are writing (Ihara et al., 2021). In this case, it may also allow for a slower, more reflective writing process.

Boundaries

We all have people, organizations, and systems that impinge on us. This doesn't mean that they are wrong for wanting to connect with us. Even the relationships that we really want take a certain amount of energy to maintain. The more different people and organizations you are connected to, the more expectations there are that you will give some of your energy to them. When doing fieldwork, you have to give energy to your site, school, family, friends, and work. What is missing from that list? You! As humans, we have a limited amount of energy. If you give all of yourself to all these various entities, what is left for you? How much energy do you have at the end of the day?

To ensure that you are not completely depleted, you will need to ensure that you are clear with your boundaries. **Boundaries**, in this context, refers to the guidelines or limits we use to let other people know what we are and are not comfortable with. There are a variety of boundaries that we have with others. One of these is around proximity. If someone invades your physical space, you will do things to reestablish the distance that is comfortable for you, such as backing up or asking the other person to back up. We also have boundaries of what we are comfortable talking about. Sometimes people may ask us questions that we feel are too personal for the level of relationship we have. For instance, if a work colleague starts asking you about your dating history, you might not answer or let them know that you prefer not to talk about that topic. With your site, perhaps the most important boundary is about your time. Staff at the site may want or expect you to work more hours or different hours than you had agreed upon.

It will be important for you to preventatively set up boundaries not only with other people but with yourself as well. One reason is so you don't bring things that happen at your site home with you. Here, we are talking about bringing home the stress of what happens during a therapy session or while completing paperwork, for example. While it is hard to do, we recommend that, as best as possible, you leave your field placement at the site. Once you get into your car to leave, try to leave the stress behind. What you will want to take with you is what you learned. This will be important for you to talk about with your faculty supervisor. Boundaries can additionally manifest as changes in your lifestyle. For example, you may need to set a boundary with yourself that you won't take on a second practicum/internship site because you aren't spending the time that you'd like with your family.

Tales From the Field: Intern

When I applied to my doctoral program, I was already the parent of a teenage daughter. I was working and had just started a second master's degree in psychology at an Italian university. Despite being good at scheduling and managing several personal and family-related commitments, when I received the acceptance letter from Our Lady of the Lake University, I was not ready for what was about to come. No one provided me with a warning letter or instructions on how to manage life when starting a PsyD program.

At first, I thought I could manage everything. I told myself that I could keep the work I had because of the Rome time zone, continuing with both programs because my master's degree in Italy was already paid for. I could continue commuting 60 miles when going to practicum or university, doing my household chores, and making sure my daughter had the same attention she used to have. It did not take long to hit the low battery level even though my strong willpower kept me going. I knew I had to do something about it because I was totally out of balance. The first change I made was about my job—I needed to have more time because I was in the United States time zone. I kept studying for both programs, working a few hours, and more, but I started to make a few adjustments because I did not want to give up anything else in my life or risk potential burnout. So I took a second step and added items like breaks, meals, and physical exercise to recharge my batteries to my schedule.

Yet life is not always predictable, and things change not only each semester but even within semesters. For example, a few semesters ago, I ended up having not only several assignments due the same day but was told that one of my exams for the master's degree was anticipated to be on the same date I had those other deadlines. What I wanted to do was to cry, run away, and hide. What I did instead after taking a few long, deep breaths was prioritize things once again based on the progress on each course assignment. Another thing I did was to reach out to my professors and see if there was a chance of extending the deadline. Luckily, some faculty members in the psychology department were understanding and provided me with two extra days. However, the world and life do not stop when starting a doctoral degree, and even though a lot of time is spent studying, training, and working to become a psychologist, there is more out there. You may receive an invitation for a wedding or holiday season, illness could show up at the door, you may experience fatigue, there could be a neighborhood blackout, and much more.

There are some moments when it seems hard to balance life and work and others when it seems impossible. What I found useful is to engage in some mindfulness and breathing techniques and make time in my schedule for some social activities. I have realized it is a matter of quality and not quantity—that way, it does not feel like I have given up life or my doctoral degree. The key is to find what works and do more of it.

Grazia Raineri Acosta, PsyD Counseling Psychology Program, Our Lady of the Lake University

---

What Would You Do?: 13.1

You have been at your field placement for three months, and things seem to be going okay. Yes, there are times when you find that you are overwhelmed. For the most part, the staff and supervisor are friendly enough. However, there is one staff therapist that seems to have taken an interest in you above what you expect. You don't believe that they are coming on to you. They have never been inappropriate with you, asked you out, or anything of that manner. Rather, it is as if they are trying to be your best friend. Each Monday, they ask you questions about what you did over the weekend, specifically about your personal life. You are feeling uncomfortable with the in-depthness of the various inquiries. What do you do?

Burnout

At this point in your field placement, you have spent a lot of time and energy trying to succeed in your actual work with clients, such as through navigating the paperwork or thinking about whatever ethical and site-based dilemmas that may have arisen. If you haven't learned to establish strong and clear boundaries, all of these pressures, stresses, and situations may overwhelm you. This may have led you to feel exhausted, a condition that we call **burnout**. Suppes (2019) explained, "Therapeutic burnout is an emotional state of indifference or overt dread that results from stress and compassion fatigue" (p. 30). Burnout affects a large number of therapists, with a potentially large range somewhere between 20% and 70% (Miller & Hubble, 2015).

Compassion fatigue happens when people who are helpers take on their clients'/patients' pain and suffering. Burnout and compassion fatigue can lead to a severe impairment of your work in which you experience less empathy for your clients, feel overwhelmed, are emotionally disconnected, feel helpless, and have a loss of interest in what you are doing.

A related experience for therapists is known as **healing involvement**, which is when therapists feel deeply connected to their clients (Miller & Hubble, 2015). Master therapists rate healing involvement as less important to their work and identity than less experienced or effective therapists. They also experience less burnout. Miller et al. explained that instead of trying to focus on self-care when you are feeling burned out, you should instead focus on how to be effective and improve your clinical work.

A related phenomenon is **vicarious traumatization**, which occurs when therapists begin to take on the client's trauma-related behaviors. Vicarious trauma can lead to the therapist experiencing behavioral, physiological, emotional, and/or cognitive symptoms, which are usually related to the therapist's change in their views of self, other, and the world after being repeatedly exposed to client trauma (McNeillie & Rose, 2021). We highly encourage you to reach out to your supervisor, often, to talk about how being exposed to your clients' stories may be impacting you. It is okay to be impacted by our clients. That is normal. It happens because you are a caring human being. However, letting it have negative consequences on you and your therapeutic work is problematic. The more that you can get ahead of it and think about yourself and your relationship to the traumas that are being discussed, the more you can minimize their influence.

A good example to further differentiate between being an effective therapist who is connected to their clients without being overcome by your clients' experiences is from *Guardians of the Galaxy Vol 2*. In this popular Marvel movie, a character named Mantis is introduced who refers to herself as an empath (she literally feels other people's feelings when she touches them). As therapists, one of the big things we do no matter what specific field we are in or what model we practice from is demonstrate empathy to our clients. Empathy lets our clients know that we are there with them understanding their experience. However, there is a difference between being an empath and being empathic. As an empath, like Mantis, we would start crying when one of our clients is sad and crying. If we were to do this with all our clients' emotions, we probably wouldn't be very effective therapists. Being empathic, in contrast, involves being able to really see and sit in our clients' experiences to the point where we understand them but not to the point where we take that experience on ourselves. This might be a helpful comparison as you check in with yourself and your empathy throughout your field placement.

Quick Tip: Take a break. Actually, take lots of breaks every day. When you are doing schoolwork or at your site, stand up, stretch, take a quick walk, meditate, or do something to relax your mind.

Tips From a Supervisor

What's interesting for me is how quickly a student therapist's enthusiasm for beginning to provide therapy—what they've waited for and anticipated from the moment they first applied to their therapy program—wanes, and life overwhelms them. This has happened for most of the supervisees that I have had in the various programs I have been a supervisor. This is because life doesn't stop for them to be able to focus solely on the practicum/internship. They still might have classes to take (and books to read, papers to write, and tests to take), a paying job, and a family. The first few weeks of their experience are usually okay as they transition into it and are excited by what they are doing. Then everything catches up to them, and the novelty wears off.

Will this happen to you? It likely will if you are like most of my supervisees. My main tip is not to get discouraged about yourself. Most every one of your classmates (and most every student therapist in every program around the world) is going through something very similar. Talk with them. See how they are handling it. While their specific situation might be different from yours (perhaps they don't have a family or don't have to do the field placement while also holding down a full-time job), they can be both a support and a resource. They likely understand, for the most part, what you are experiencing. They also might have some tools that they are using to stay afloat that might also be useful for you.

I think when you can accept that while you are doing good (both for your clients and as a student therapist), the process of practicum/internship can be anxiety producing, stressful, and perhaps overwhelming. Know that going in so that you can, from the very beginning, try to figure out how to put into place frequent practices to cope with all of the demands that you will experience during your placement. Give yourself some grace and prioritize yourself as a person. It is okay to be frustrated and sometimes not know how to handle things. Don't keep it inside. Talk to people. Your colleagues. Your supervisor(s). Hopefully, you will incorporate into your therapy practice but also your life my number one rule of therapy: Have fun. Figure out how to be creative in the various parts of your life so that you never feel like you are on autopilot. I think the best therapy and the best way of figuring out how to have work/life balance comes from being creative. So that will be my main tip: Be creative.

Summary

This chapter explored how you might create a work/life balance. For most students, the internship experience is quite overwhelming as they have to negotiate schoolwork, the field placement, their paid job, and their personal life. For many, this can be quite a difficult challenge. The more that interns allow work to take over their lives, the greater the possibility that stress and potential burnout may occur. Here, at the beginning of your career, developing a self-care routine with a focus on wellness is key to being able to succeed in your practicum/internship and in your personal life.

References

American Psychological Association. (2017). *Ethical principles of psychologists and code of conduct.* www.apa.org/ethics/code/ethics-code-2017.pdf

Barnett, J. E., & Cooper, N. (2009). Creating a culture of self-care. *Clinical Psychology: Science and Practice, 16*(1), 16–20. https://doi.org/10.1111/j.1468-2850.2009.01138.x

Brody, J. L., Scherer, D. G., Turner, C. W., Annett, R. D., & Dalen, J. (2018). A conceptual model and clinical framework for integrating mindfulness into family therapy with adolescents. *Family Process, 57*(2), 510–524. https://doi.org/10.1111/famp.12298

Bush, A. D., (2015, May–June). Little and often. *Psychotherapy Networker, 39*(3), 24–27.

Frostadottir, A. D., & Dorjee, D. (2019). Effects of mindfulness based cognitive therapy (MBCT) and compassion focused therapy (CFT) on symptom change, mindfulness, self-compassion, and rumination in clients with depression, anxiety, and stress. *Frontiers in Psychology, 10,* Article 1099. https://doi.org/10.3389/fpsyg.2019.01099

Hoffman, S. G., & Gómez, A. F. (2017). Mindfulness-based interventions for anxiety and depression. *Psychiatric Clinics of North America, 40*(4), 739–749. https://doi.org/10.1016/j.psc.2017.08.008

Ihara, A. S., Nakajima, K., Kake, A., Ishimaru, K., Osugi, K., & Naruse, Y. (2021). Advantage of handwriting over typing on learning words: Evidence from an N400 event-related potential index. *Frontiers in Human Neuroscience, 15,* 67919. https://doi.org/10.3389/fnhum.2021.679191

Kabat-Zinn, J., Massion, A. O., Kristeller, J., Peterson, L. G., Fletcher, K. E., Pbert, L., Lenderking, W. R., & Santorelli, S. F. (1992). Effectiveness of a meditation-based stress reduction program in the treatment of anxiety disorders. *American Journal of Psychiatry, 149*(7), 936–943. https://doi.org/10.1176/ajp.149.7.936

McNeillie, N., & Rose, J. (2021). Vicarious trauma in therapists: A meta-ethnographic review. *Behavioural and Cognitive Psychotherapy, 49*(4), 426–440. https://doi.org/10.1017/S1352465820000776

Miller, S., & Hubble, M. (2015, May–June). Burnout reconsidered: What supershrinks can teach us. *Psychotherapy Networker, 39*(3), 18–23.

Rokach, A., & Boulazreg, S. (2022). The COVID-19 era: How therapists can diminish burnout symptoms through self-care. *Current Psychology, 41,* 5660–5677. https://doi.org/10.1007/s12144-020-01149-6

Stefan, S., & David, D. (2020). Mindfulness in therapy: A critical analysis. *International Journal of Clinical and Experimental Hypnosis, 68*(2), 167–182. https://doi.org/10.1080/00207144.2020.1720514

Suppes, B. (2019). Self-care of the therapist. In L. Metcalf (Ed.), *Marriage and family therapy: A practice-oriented approach* (pp. 25–39). Springer.

Vally, Z. (2019). Do doctoral training programmes actively promote a culture of self-care among clinical and counselling psychology trainees? *British Journal of Guidance & Counselling, 47*(5), 635–644. https://doi.org/10.1080/03069885.2018.1461195

Chapter 14

Benefitting From Supervision

Supervision is an integral element of your practicum/internship experience. If, as a budding therapist, you simply went to your site all willy-nilly, did some therapy, and then left it at that, there would probably be little learning or growing involved. This is the same for your regular courses: You have a professor with whom you consult, whom you learn and receive feedback from. You aren't simply given the readings and assignments and told, "Have fun." Rather, learning is the process of guided understanding in which a more experienced person with the material helps you to access and consider your engagement with it.

The process of discussing your practicum/internship experience with your supervisor is what allows you to grow as a therapist. You are able to reflect on what you are doing well, learn from any mistakes, and get into a groove of conceptualizing cases. Now, as with your other academic courses, you simply can't go into supervision and expect the benefits of the process to unfold on their own. You have to put in the work and do *your* part in making the most out of supervision. That is what this chapter is all about—providing a guide to the steps you can take to fully benefit from supervision.

Myth About the Field

"I have to do everything my supervisor tells me to do."

Nope. This is definitely not true. You do not have to do everything that another professional tells you to do, which we alluded to in Chapters 5 and 10 when talking about knowing yourself and site-based dilemmas, respectively. In every field, not every single professional is going to be correct 100% of the time. Even if they make a suggestion that may work for *their* therapeutic approach, it may not work for *your* therapeutic approach. And that is okay.

Defining Supervision

Supervision is the process of having a more experienced professional oversee your work. Given their advanced training and experience, they have a wider lens from which to understand the case as well as your development. We can break the word supervision down to *super* and *vision*. Their vision is more enhanced than your own. Storm and Todd (2014) explained as follows:

> Supervision is where one professional (who we call "supervisee") hoping for guidance enters into a learning relationship with another professional (who we call "supervisor")

DOI: 10.4324/9781003433484-14

with a mutual goal of advancing the supervisee's clinical and professional competencies while ensuring quality services to clients.

(pp. 1–2)

Your supervisor is there to provide you with guidance, support, and oversight. There are a couple of different formats of supervision. We will briefly talk about live and dead supervision. **Live supervision** occurs when the supervisor watches you while you are working with your client. In some programs, this may happen by the supervisor being behind a one-way mirror, through video, or on a videoconferencing platform. Live supervision is quite rare and usually occurs primarily in university settings. However, with the advent of videoconferencing platform use in psychotherapy, your supervisor may be on the video call (but perhaps with their camera turned off). They might direct message you throughout the session, providing you with suggestions for what you might do right then and there.

Dead supervision is what most people think about when envisioning supervision. Here, you see clients outside the scope of your supervisor seeing and/or listening to the session while it is happening. Rather, depending on your site and the agreement of your clients, you may bring in audio or video recordings for you and your supervisor to go over and discuss. However, getting recordings can be difficult. When you don't have them, dead supervision still occurs by you explaining to the supervisor about details of the case.

The Supervision Setup

The way your supervision is set up may differ depending on how your program structures practicums/internships. You may even have a different supervision setup for each type of practicum/internship you take within the same program. For example, Kayleigh's practicums were internal to her university's on-site family therapy clinic, while her two internships included an assessment-based counseling internship in a school and an internship at a nonprofit facility that provided group, individual, couple, and family therapy. For her practicums, the clinic consisted of therapy rooms that were next to a consultation room; these were connected by a one-way mirror. Her supervisor (which was Michael for some practicums) and fellow students were able to watch her therapy sessions live. About three-quarters of the way through the session, she'd take a break, go to the consultation room, and receive feedback from the supervisor and her colleagues before she wrapped up the session. The supervisor and students would also discuss cases during breaks in between sessions.

The supervision structure for her two internship sites were in some ways similar to and in some ways different from one another. For any internship in general, her program required that students had a supervisor for the entire semester of the internship (a professor in the program who was a qualified supervisor). The students would have weekly meetings with this supervisor to check in and discuss anything relevant to the internship experience. At Kayleigh's school-based site, there was a supervisor who would walk around the room in which interns did student assessments in case the interns needed help, so they also received supervision indirectly in that way. At her nonprofit site, they also required that interns meet weekly with the site's clinical director to discuss relevant supervision topics (as this person was in charge of the interns). Interns also received feedback from therapists whose sessions interns sat in on (which provided a bit of informal supervision).

This may sound like a lot of supervision. Thankfully, it is! Supervision is a necessary accompaniment to your practicum/internship experience, so you generally want to take advantage of getting feedback when you can. Again, your program—and your specific practicum/

internship sites—may have supervision organized differently. We are going to review the basics of benefitting from supervision that can apply across the board.

Selecting a Supervisor

Before you can even begin supervision, you have to select a supervisor. Once again, the ability for you to select a supervisor will likely depend on the structure of your program. In some programs, students are given a few supervisor options for both practicums and internships. Supervisors are often professors in the program (whether they are full-time faculty or even adjunct professors) who are also approved supervisors. It is essentially the same process as selecting a regular course—you usually have a few options to choose from.

Sometimes, you may have to select the practicum/internship option that best fits your schedule. However, if you are able to be flexible, we recommend that you really put some thought into who you'd like your supervisor to be. This philosophy applies to therapy as well: You may be an excellent therapist, but you are not the right therapist for everyone. Similarly, each supervisor will have a different way of providing supervision. For example, perhaps one supervisor values the use of constructive criticism and is more likely to give you feedback on what you can improve on, while another supervisor may believe that primarily highlighting what you are doing well is most helpful. This is where the fine line between being open to new experiences and knowing yourself and what works for you comes into play.

Tips From an Intern

I've had the privilege of having around ten different supervisors thus far in my therapeutic career. Some were for school, some for licensure, and some for work. Through these various supervisors, I have learned what type of supervisor I like and what type of supervisor I don't like. I've consequently learned how important it is to have a supervisor you like if you are wanting to get the most out of your supervision experience.

We talked about the process involved in selecting a supervisor, and we noted that sometimes you will not necessarily have a choice of your supervisor while you are in your psychotherapy program. However, I want to further highlight how vital it can be to pick the right supervisor when you do have a choice. I believe this may apply even more to your licensure supervision (which we will discuss more in Chapter 17).

You will likely pay for your licensure supervision if your work does not include it. While I know licensure supervision is not a part of your graduate program supervision, it is relevant to this chapter for a significant reason—you can use your experiences with your graduate program supervisors to help inform whom you choose for your licensure supervision after graduation. These supervisors may be professors in your program or perhaps your practicum/internship on-site supervisors. Regardless, my tip is that you create mental notes (or actual notes if you prefer writing things down) about the pros and cons of each type of supervision process/supervisor.

Such notes may include information about your preferred formatting of supervision (e.g., one meeting a week for one hour or one meeting every other week for two hours), the structure of supervision (e.g., each supervision meeting being structured versus the supervisees bringing up what is most important), and even the traits of the supervisor themselves (e.g., the supervisor providing primarily positive feedback versus including constructive criticism as well). You want to utilize your graduate program supervision experiences wisely to make your licensure supervision worthwhile.

What to Bring to Each Meeting

Supervisors spend a lot of time and training to become good at providing supervision for a variety of people. They may take courses, read articles, read books, go to workshops and trainings, and consult with other supervisors to become better at providing supervision. They take on a lot of responsibility for the supervisee's growth as well as legal responsibility for the supervisee's cases. Yet they are not the only one in the supervisory relationship that has responsibilities.

As a supervisee, *you* have responsibilities as well. You have to come to the context with motivation, initiative, and clear communication (Port, 2019). Just like your clients, whom you cannot change but can provide a context in which change is possible, the same is true for supervision. Your supervisor cannot make you a better therapist. They can set the stage for that possibility, but it will be up to you to take from the conversations and implement that into the therapy session.

There are a few main things that we recommend you take responsibility for and bring to your supervision meetings. First, bring questions. This may seem obvious, but this is something that you can easily forget to do. There is so much value in having a list of specific questions for you to ask at each meeting. While working at your practicum/supervision site, you will constantly experience situations that will produce a plethora of questions, even if they are small questions that tie up little odds and ends and any curiosities that you have. Writing these questions down throughout the week while you are at your site will prevent you from forgetting them. This way, you can bring a comprehensive list to your supervision meeting.

Second, bring cases that you want to conceptualize further with your supervisor. There will be some cases that you find a nice groove with, and there will be others where you will feel completely stuck at times. Bringing these cases up to your supervisor gets the creative juices flowing and allows for a new perspective on your understanding of and approach to these cases. If you are going to bring cases that you want to talk about, you should also bring a critical, thoughtful mindset. You aren't really doing your part if you just dump the case on your supervisor and expect them to do all the work. As the student intern, it is your job to think reflexively about these cases during supervision as well.

Third, bring an open mind to the feedback you will receive from your supervisor. Supervision is not going to be that helpful if you disregard everything your supervisor says. There are going to be moments in which your supervisor may make a suggestion about a case—whether it be a way to conceptualize it or an intervention to use—that you don't necessarily believe is the best move (we will talk about this more later on). This is okay. However, you have to at least be open to hearing what your supervisor says. If you approach supervision with skepticism or from a defensive position, you have already put up a wall that will prevent you from learning as much as you could.

Fourth, bring something with which you can write everything down. We have frequently seen students go to supervision, get some amazing insight on a case that they might not see until later in the week, and then forget everything that they discussed in supervision. Whether you write it down on a piece of paper or type it up on your computer, find the way that is best for you to write notes during your supervision meetings. These meetings will become much more useful if you are able to go back and reflect on what you talked about further instead of having to worry about remembering it all. As a note: Make sure any notes you take are confidential (i.e., there is no identifying information present in your notes). For example, use client initials or a pseudonym instead of a first or last name.

We want to bring up the difference between handwritten and typed notes. While we both love handwritten notes (as they prevent us from being in front of a screen more than we need to be), we have also seen many students handwrite their notes on paper and then (a) lose them or (b) not be able to sort through the information when they go back through their notes. This makes your notes much less helpful to you if you cannot locate where they are or cannot locate the relevant information within them.

Using technology helps keep track of these things more easily. For example, if you know you wrote about dialectical behavioral therapy for a client during a supervision meeting and want to see those notes, you could simply use the search function to type in a keyword (e.g., "dialectical") and then see all the places in your notes where you wrote about it. If you really prefer writing handwritten notes and yet are concerned about being able to navigate through them, you can always handwrite them first and then type them on your computer later (this might even really help you soak in the information from your supervision meeting). We just wanted to throw this out there preemptively as a consideration for you to make to see what is best for you.

Tales From the Field: Supervisor

In my position as a clinical supervisor, my job was to not only have a caseload of clients that I would meet with but to also provide guidance, education, and support to the clinicians working with me. The facility was primarily family therapy focused, but clinicians would also see children, adolescents, and adults individually. Supervision was done monthly with each clinician where they would discuss the cases they had and any challenges they had been facing. One such experience was with a registered intern in the MFT program who was working with a male adolescent struggling with depression.

The clinician described the client as having a depressive mood and affect, isolating himself from others, and having few positive connections with family and friends. The client was also struggling in school and had low motivation to make positive changes. The clinician had done well to build rapport and trust with the client, but the client still struggled to engage in interventions and different coping strategies. The clinician would describe the client as feeling stuck and becoming more resistant to change. Initial supervision sessions followed up on relational progress and any positive changes the client was making, but the client would struggle to recognize these positive changes in his life as valuable and would dismiss those successes.

Taking in all this information, what stood out to me as the supervisor was the client's continued hopeless perspective despite reported positive changes in grades and relational interactions. In the next supervision session, I explored the clinician's perspective on the goals and expectations of the work they were doing with the client. The clinician was able to explain the general goals and expectations, but they did not know the client's thought processes that were informing his expectations of success. I educated the clinician on the importance of understanding a client's perspective on success, failure, and change in order to meet the client where they are at. By understanding the client's thought processes, the clinician would be able to support, challenge, or even reframe those goals and expectations as well as be able to educate the client on realistic and unrealistic expectations. Supervision was also used to explore what the clinician understood about depression and how it can perpetuate poor motivation, internal failure narratives, and self-hatred.

As the supervisor, it was evident that the clinician gained a better understanding of meeting the client where they were at while also factoring in how the client's depression could perpetuate the internal narrative of failure by not reaching those unrealistic expectations. I made a plan with the clinician to have them explore these concepts with the client, not only to increase the clinician's understanding of the client, but also the client's understanding of their own expectations. The client could also then be educated on the perpetuation of negative narratives and the resulting impact on his experience with depression.

In the following supervision session, the clinician reported that the client responded well to the intervention and was looking at the pressure and expectations he had put on himself. The clinician proudly shared that the client became more open to making new short- and medium-term goals which were more realistic to his current experience. The clinician also expressed that the supervision sessions used to discuss this client created a new perspective of this case and allowed them to enhance their work with this client. This change would not have been possible without the diligent work done by the clinician to not only build a positive and supportive relationship with their client but to also be open to learning new skills and hearing new perspectives through supervision.

Christopher Valls, MS, LMHC, Private Practice

Exercise 14.1: Preparing for Supervision

As we've discussed, being a supervisee is an interactive process that requires you to be active. While your supervisor may have a view of what will be useful for your continued professional growth, you should as well. For this exercise, we want you to think about how you want to utilize supervision. Answer these questions and then use your answers to inform your engagement for your next supervision meeting.

1. What knowledge area would you like to explore this week in supervision?
2. What new skill would you like to incorporate into your therapy? How can you talk with your supervisor about its proper use?
3. Which client do you have the most questions about? What are the three primary questions that you have about that case?
4. What area of professional development would you like to know more about?
5. What mistake did you make this week that you would like feedback on?

Being Honest With Your Supervisor

As you begin to work with clients during your practicum/internship, you may come across situations in which your clients lie to you or keep something from you. Once your clients tell you the truth about something and you both talk about it, you and they may realize what a difference it made for the therapeutic process. The same goes for supervision—withholding information from your supervisor (or straight up lying to them about something) is more likely to hinder the supervision process than enhance it. Not wanting to disclose something that happened in your session—or for you as a therapist—is not new, as many supervisees experience the same thing (Hess et al., 2008).

Nondisclosure in supervision takes two paths: an unintentional withholding and intentional withholding (Hess et al., 2008). **Unintentional withholding** happens when you don't disclose something because you are not sure whether it is appropriate to talk about it in general or in supervision. Conversely, **intentional withholding** happens when there is a conscious choice to distort or not disclose some important piece of information. The latter is more problematic than the former since purposely not telling your supervisor something demonstrates that there is likely a rift either in the supervisory relationship or in your view of your own work. We highly encourage you, pretty much regardless of what it is about, to not withhold or lie to your supervisor. Whether it is to hide your embarrassment, to deal with anxiety, or most other reasons, the withholding will likely only further the current difficulty.

What Would You Do?: 14.1

You come to supervision discussing a case you are having some trouble with. It is a couple who are having a lot of conflict with one another where there is screaming and yelling between them. You are unsure of why they are together because in the three sessions that you've had with them, you haven't seen an instance where you would classify it as caring or love. While explaining the couple's dynamic and your uncertainty of what to do with them, your supervisor tells you that you need to tell them that they are making each other's lives miserable and that they should separate since they are no good together as a couple. This doesn't feel right for you, and you express that to the supervisor. They tell you that they've worked with thousands of couples and this one should not be together, and they want you to tell them that. What would you do?

Little Moments of Supervision

When your program refers to your supervision experience, they are likely talking about the regular meetings that you and your supervisor will have throughout your practicum/internship. This is the bulk of your supervision. However, your supervision does not just start and stop when you come for those one or two hours of scheduled supervision per week.

At the site, there are more than just these formal meetings. You might pass by your supervisor in the hallway, breakroom, or parking lot and ask a quick question. It is important to utilize these little moments of supervision (while still respecting your supervisor's boundaries and time) so that you have more immediate feedback or suggestions. If you wait until your next supervision session, there is a high likelihood that you will forget what it is you had a question about. That doesn't mean that if you forget about something it was not that important in the first place. All of us have forgotten about important things. What usually happens is that what we forgot about will come back and bite us in the ass.

Our recommendation is for you to think of supervision in this way: Whatever is agreed upon (usually the one hour of supervision a week) is the minimum contact between you and your supervisor. It is not the maximum. You are in your placement to learn (and to get your hours). Unfortunately, too many supervisees have a tendency to think of themselves as a burden on their supervisor and try not to be an imposition or take extra time. If this is your mindset, then you will need to adopt a different mindset. Your supervisor has agreed to work with you. They are there for you. And they are there for your clients. When you do not take that moment that you have to ask your supervisor a question, you are missing out on your own professional growth.

Quick Tip: Every day, write down one question that you have for your supervisor. Keep this in a journal (either on paper, your phone, or your computer). Review this list right before your next supervision session and ensure that you ask at least three of these questions during the supervision time.

Listening to Your Gut

One of the roles of the supervisor is to challenge the intern to move beyond their comfort zone. Therapists quickly become specialists, where you feel secure in what you are doing but in a very limited way. You might start to tell yourself, "I do well with adolescents but not older adults," "My area of competence is with substance abuse but not marital issues," or "I work best when things are calm."

When you do this, you begin to solidify a limiting identity. This will prevent you from being able to work with the widest range of cases you will encounter. Just like in therapy, one of the goals of supervision is to help the person shift from a limiting identity to a resourceful identity (Reiter et al., 2020). Your supervisor will likely push and challenge you to be richer than you think you are. When this happens, you will probably feel anxious, disoriented, and scared. And this is okay. Some of the times of biggest growth are when we feel discomfort.

Our suggestion to you is to go with the flow and see what happens when you follow the supervisor's challenges. But one major caveat here: Don't ever do anything that feels completely wrong to you. As we've said, your supervisor will push to get you out of your comfort zone. When you do this, you will expand and develop a greater array of therapeutic skills and alternative conceptualizations. However, you shouldn't do anything that someone suggests that goes against your core values or is possibly unethical. Take time to listen to your gut. If it is nervousness of doing something new, take the step and risk it. This is beneficial for both you and your clients, as you, as a therapist, are doing the same thing for them— challenging them to take a risk of living differently. If your gut tells you that something is not right, pause for a minute. Go back to your supervisor and discuss your discomfort. It is perfectly fine to disagree with your supervisor.

Tales From the Field: Intern

When I began my practicum semester, I did not fully understand what having weekly supervision even meant or what the role of a supervisor was. Now looking back as I am about to finish my internship, I have been lucky enough to have had such an amazing supervisor and realize the necessity of having someone ethical and competent in your corner giving you sound advice and instruction.

Earlier this year, I began seeing a new client that instantly triggered feelings of countertransference. This was my first time experiencing this situation, and this client unfortunately reminded me of a past abusive relationship. From his physical features, to his tone of voice and mannerisms, to his age and how he spoke about women, I immediately felt my body starting to have a physical reaction during our first meeting. I brought this client up the next day in my weekly supervision, and my supervisor asked me if I thought it was a good idea for me to continue to work with him. I decided to challenge myself professionally and see if I could push past my own feelings and see this client with unconditional positive regard.

Two weeks later, this client showed up for a session on the wrong day, as he had mistakenly written down the wrong time and became very angry when he found out I was in session with another client. He began banging on the lobby door and yelling my name. He made such a ruckus that another therapist could hear him, and she came out to address him. He was furious and yelled at her, and she asked him to leave and told him that I was not available. After my shift had ended, I gave him a quick phone call to address the situation, but he did not answer my call. The following week (when he was actually on my schedule), I was filled with anxiety about seeing him and wondered if he would even show up. My supervisor spoke with me on the phone the night before, checked in on me in the morning of the session, and let me know that she had my back. She instructed me to set boundaries with this client and to let him know that I would not be disrespected.

The client did end up showing up to his scheduled session and was fired up and very angry with me. I simply addressed the situation and explained the scheduling issue, and he demanded that I do something about it in an extremely hostile tone. I felt my body start to get hot, but then I remembered what my supervisor told me: I did not have to put up with him. If he was going to be disrespectful or rude, then I could make the call to no longer see him. After the client accused me of "trying to screw [him] over," I calmly told him that perhaps he would be better off seeing another therapist and that we should end the session right now. As soon as those words came out of my mouth, his entire demeanor and attitude changed, and he apologized. We went on to have a great session, and I have had no issues with him since.

It was my supervisor that got me through that day and had encouraged me to "take my power back." I learned about setting boundaries with clients and that I am a professional and do not have to put up with being talked down to. My supervisor texted me as soon as she knew the session had ended to make sure I was safe. I was so grateful to have such a good support system in her; she really helped build my self-confidence that day.

Erin Zubia, MA in Clinical Mental Health Counseling, Colorado Christian University

Supervisee–Supervisor Alliance

During your schooling, you probably learned that one of the most important ingredients to successful therapy is a strong therapeutic alliance with your client (Bailey & Ogles, 2023). This is certainly the case and something to keep in mind during your practicum/internship. You should constantly think about how your increased connection with the client is related to positive therapeutic outcomes.

Not only should you think about your alliance with your clients, you should consider your alliance with your supervisor as well. This is important since the alliance between supervisee and supervisor is more complex than that between therapist and client (Ybrandt et al., 2016). One of the reasons for this is that your supervisor is both a teacher and an evaluator. Their evaluation of you may lead to stress and anxiety for you. Depending on how many semesters you will be in your placement, there may be one, a couple, or many times that your supervisor provides a formal assessment. This assessment is probably tied to your grade for that class. You shouldn't try to get along just to get a good grade. Rather, when you have a negative perception of your supervisor, you will likely not want to be active during these meetings, which will decrease the amount you get out of them.

Good and Bad Supervision Experiences

We would like to be able to tell you that all of your supervision experiences will be great. Even with a supervisor that you get along with, that will likely not happen. Salvador Minuchin, one of the founding fathers of family therapy, told Michael that he didn't think he was being a good supervisor if at some point the supervisee didn't hate him. What he was saying was that his job was to push the therapist out of their comfort zone. In this process, people usually became quite off-balanced and would become frustrated at him (the supervisor). Not all of your supervisors will try to do this. Some will try to get you to really like them and not try to upset you at all. Whichever approach, your supervisor's job is to help you along in the process of developing into a competent and skilled psychotherapist.

It will be important for you to ensure that you are frequently meeting with your supervisor. One of the things that has been found is that frequent and thorough meetings with your supervisor are associated with better supervisory experiences (Anderson et al., 2000). And that is one of the main things you are trying to achieve—good supervision meetings which will help you grow as a therapist so that you can be more efficient and effective with your clients.

We also want to note that bad supervision experiences can be good supervision experiences. More specifically, bad supervision experiences can be good in the end because you will absolutely still learn from these experiences, which is what supervision is really all about. Even if you learn from supervision in a way that you weren't hoping for (e.g., having a supervisor who you do not get along with), you will still learn. You will learn about what you like and don't like about supervision, how you want and don't want to be as a therapist, and how you want to be able to respond as a professional in these tough situations. Kayleigh frequently conveys this message about life to her clients as well: The undesirable experiences are still a necessary part of life because they provide more information about the situation and ourselves for us to grow.

Tips From a Supervisor

As a supervisor, I find that many of my supervisees come to our sessions and put the onus of what happens during those times on me. They look to me to tell them what we should talk about, tell them what their growth goals should be, and assess how they are doing as student therapists. While I am perfectly able to do all of these things, I don't think it is as useful as if they did these things as well.

Just like therapy is a process that necessitates the active engagement of (at least) two people, supervision seems to be isomorphic—both people need to dance together. I find that the best supervision sessions happen when the supervisee comes in with a point of view. That is, they have spent time away from our meetings thinking about areas of growth that they want to explore, issues that have come up in session or at their site, or conceptualization questions of applying a model to a case. In essence, they have developed goals for the supervision session.

My main tip for this chapter is to view supervision as a process in which both parties need to bring something to the table. Your supervisor will have their own ideas of what might be talked about during supervision sessions. That's good, as they have a way of viewing what will be important for your growth. However, you have a viewpoint as well. Make sure that you have an agenda for every supervision session. Spend part of the week leading up to the session writing down the questions that you have about your site, your clients, and your therapeutic development. Then, during supervision, ensure some time is spent focusing on at least one of your ideas/questions. I find that, for me and my supervisees, these moments are usually the most appreciated.

Summary

Your practicum/internship experience is designed for you to further learn while you are becoming a psychotherapist. Your supervisor is your guide in this process. This chapter presented you with many ideas of how you can benefit from supervision. You may have both a site supervisor and a faculty supervisor. Each of them will bring something different to the experience. While your supervisor will have a direction they want the supervision meetings to go, you also have responsibilities as a supervisee. We encourage you to be an active agent in the supervision process.

References

Anderson, S. A., Schlossberg, M., & Rigazio-DiGilio, S. (2000). Family therapy trainees' evaluations of their best and worst supervision experiences. *Journal of Marital and Family Therapy, 26*(1), 79–91. https://doi.org/10.1111/j.1752-0606.2000.tb00278.x

Bailey, R. J., & Ogles, B. M. (2023). *Common factors therapy: A principle-based treatment framework*. American Psychological Association.

Hess, S. A., Knox, S., Schultz, J. M., Hill, C. E., Sloan, L., Brandt, S., Kelley, F., & Hoffman, M. A. (2008). Predoctoral interns' nondisclosure in supervision. *Psychotherapy Research, 18*(4), 400–411. https://doi.org/10.1080/10503300701697505

Port, M. S. (2019). Effects of supervision on a trainee's clinical internship experience in central Africa. *Training and Education in Professional Psychology, 13*(3), 180–184. http://doi.org/10.1037/tep0000259

Reiter, M. D., Jung, W. F., Popham, J., Fitzgerald, C., Garcia, E., de Perez, M. G., Lockhart, T., & Villanueva, N. (2020). Training through naming: A process of psychotherapist skill development utilizing recursive frame analysis. *The Qualitative Report, 25*(8), 2085–2099. https://doi.org/10.46743/2160-3715/2020.4330

Storm, C. L., & Todd, T. C. (2014). Core premises and a framework for systemic/relational supervision. In T. C. Todd & C. L. Storm (Eds.), *The complete systemic supervisor: Context, philosophy, and pragmatics* (2nd ed., pp. 1–16). Wiley.

Ybrandt, H., Sundin, E. C., & Capone, G. (2016). Trainee therapists' views on the alliance in psychotherapy and supervision: A longitudinal study. *British Journal of Guidance & Counselling, 44*(5), 530–539. https://doi.org/10.1080/03069885.2016.1153037

Chapter 15

Psychotherapist Growth

The purpose of your practicum/internship is to prepare you to be a psychotherapist. No one has any expectation that when you started this process, you were already a fully formed psychotherapist. Actually, it was the opposite. The thought was that you were not ready and needed the training and supervision that you receive during your placement so that your skills as well as your conceptualization about cases and yourself expanded. In essence, your practicum/internship experience is really about your growth as a psychotherapist. In this chapter, we want to talk about the process of development as a psychotherapist.

Regardless of where you currently are in the process, you should know that you are not a final product. There is more cooking to do. We encourage you to pause right now and think about how far you have come already. You are definitely not the same therapist, and we believe you are not the same person, as you were when you first began your placement. What are the ways that you have changed? How have you grown in your conceptualization of cases? How have you grown in your belief in yourself? How have you grown in your use of self in the therapy room? What can you do now that you weren't able to just a few short months ago?

Myth About the Field

"I will learn everything I need to learn about therapy in my graduate program."

This is implicitly not true simply based on the requirement for licensed therapists to engage in continuing education units (CEUs), for example. Your psychotherapy graduate program is the beginning of your journey as a therapist. Laws will change, new theories will be created, different life events are going to occur, all of which will change the therapy field outside of what you learn during your graduate program. You—both as a person and as a therapist—will also change after your graduate program, so the way you conceptualize and approach therapy will likely change as a result as well.

Skill Development

Therapist development happens over time, usually through stages or phases. We can look at this in a variety of ways. We present here a six-phase model developed from Rønnestad and Skovholt (2003), which includes the lay helper, the beginning student, the advanced student, the novice professional, the experienced professional, and the senior professional (see Figure 15.1).

DOI: 10.4324/9781003433484-15

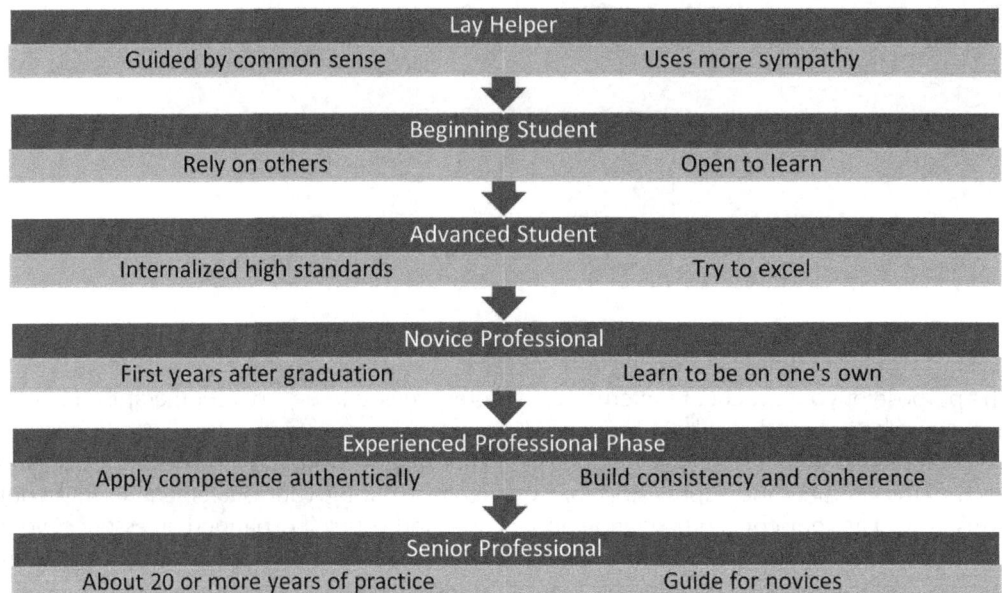

Figure 15.1 Rønnestad and Skovholt (2003) developed a six-phase model of therapist growth.

Before you entered into your therapy program, you were (without you knowing it) in the **lay helper phase** (Rønnestad & Skovholt, 2003). You were likely the person who friends and family came to when they were having difficulty. You had an open ear and were willing to listen. You wanted to help. The difficulty may have come from not having a therapeutic sense of what to do, and you were perhaps trying to solve the other person's problems in a way that would work for you rather than for them. You probably gave a lot of unheeded advice. Lay helpers tend to be guided by their common sense and will employ sympathy more than empathy.

Next, you applied, got accepted, and began a psychotherapy program. Here, you entered into the **beginning student phase** (Rønnestad & Skovholt, 2003). You began learning psychotherapy skills and theory. These were enhanced through the countless role-plays you participated in, papers you wrote, and tests you took. Beginning therapists tend to rely on external expertise to know what to do rather than internal expertise which senior practitioners use (Skovholt & Rønnestad, 1992). However, you realized that there was a lot about psychotherapy that you did not know and were open to learn.

Currently, you are probably in the **advanced student phase** (Rønnestad & Skovholt, 2003). Now, you should be able to put your knowledge into practice. For some, there is a dilemma, as they expect themselves to be perfect and not make mistakes. They may be more conservative and rigid. In this phase, many people tend to internalize high standards and try to excel. While appreciating that they have learned a lot, they also realize that they still have a lot to learn. In this process, they may seek out confirmation and feedback from senior therapists and supervisors.

Once you graduate, you move into the **novice professional phase**. This usually happens for the first few years after graduation and tend to be intense and engaging. Here, the therapist learns to be on one's own. During this process, the person tends to do a lot of shedding and adding, where they are trying on new conceptual and practical theories and skills. They tend to try to confirm what they learned in their graduate program, then maybe go through a period of disillusionment with themselves and their professional training. Lastly, they engage in a more intense exploration of self and themselves as a mental health professional.

The next phase is the **experienced professional phase**, where you have worked for several years in the field and have seen a wide variety of clientele in a variety of settings. Here, the primary developmental task is to develop an authentic way of being a professional. You have developed your conceptualizations of therapy that fit for you rather than just trying some on. This plays out by being able to be flexible and adapt skills and theories based on your own unique understandings.

Lastly is the **senior professional phase**, which happens about 20 or more years after practicing. The primary development task of this stage is becoming a guide for novices coming into the field. This phase is also filled with loss as colleagues retire and/or die, and their own advancement becomes a factor—both professionally and personally.

There is good and bad news here about growth in effectiveness. The good news is that, over the course of their training in practicum/internship, student therapists improve in the positive outcomes for their clients (Owen et al., 2016). The bad news is that this is dependent on the severity of the client's situation. Student therapists do better with clients who are less distressed. The more distressed the client, the less likely the student therapist helped them achieve a positive outcome. This is why, usually, practicum placements will use a triage system where they will give you the less involved "easier" cases at the beginning of your training. However, this is not always the case. Michael has had supervisees whose first case was a complex case involving infidelity, prostitution, substance abuse, and/or suicidality.

Overall, it is extremely unlikely that you will not grow your therapeutic skills or your personhood (what we might call self-actualization). We can just about guarantee that your growth, especially in your skills, will seriously get better. Student therapists rate themselves as increasingly improving in their basic relational skills and technical skills (Dennhag & Ybrandt, 2013). One of the side effects of improving one's psychotherapy knowledge and skills is that there is often correlated growth on the intrapersonal and interpersonal levels (Furr & Carroll, 2003).

> **Quick Tip**: Put yourself in the mindset that you are a lifelong learner. Each week, ensure that you are learning something new. Read an article or book chapter about psychotherapy. Listen to a therapy podcast or watch a therapy demonstration video. Write down what you have learned each week and then try to apply that to your next therapy session.

The Personal or the Professional

We usually talk about the notion that you should not let your personal life seep into your professional life. This is why Freudian psychoanalysts spend thousands of hours over many years going through their own analysis so that they reduce the possibility of engaging in countertransference. However, the goal of complete separation is an impossibility. Our personal life impacts our professional life and, conversely, our professional life impacts our personal life (Paris et al., 2006). This can't be helped. However, knowing this, we can better manage this interaction.

One of the things that you have probably noticed by now is that the learning and training that you've been doing in your therapy program has led to changes outside of school and the therapy room. It has to happen, and it's a good thing. You are learning how to help other people, and in the process, you are learning that you are a perpetually growing individual. Let's talk about some of the areas of your personal life that have likely been changing for you.

Wellness is a concept that we talked about in Chapter 13. Being in a program in which you are helping people to be healthy has likely led you to try to keep yourself healthy. Yes, there are times when this may become difficult, as you have a lot of demands on you. Yet maintaining sound health practices is extremely important. These components include attending to our physical, emotional, mental, spiritual, and social needs (Corey et al., 2017).

Physically, you can move toward wellness through eating and sleeping well along with exercising. Mentally and emotionally, you might provide time for yourself to relax, meditate, and detach from the pressures of the world. Spiritually, you can connect to the world through engaging with nature or religion. Our spiritual well-being involves us finding a purpose for living. Your social needs can be met by connecting with other people. Doing things with others, preferably enjoyable activities, helps keeps us grounded.

Some of the personal experiences that graduate therapy students experience that most impact their professional growth are their personal relationships, spiritual relationship, overall learning, personal therapy, and their work experiences (Paris et al., 2006). The professional experiences they have that most impact their personal growth are the practicum/internship experiences, supervision, interactions with colleagues, and their personal reactions to being in their placement.

Psychotherapy students cite incidents that occur outside of their program as being the most frequent that lead to personal growth (Furr & Carroll, 2003). These critical incidents were usually related to personal relationships that were changing based on the person being in a therapy program. This is something that you should expect. Your program is not only getting you to learn psychotherapy skills but helping you focus on self-of-the-therapist issues. You are exploring your values and beliefs. You are learning how to communicate more effectively. You are learning about really listening to someone and letting them know you are hearing their deeper meanings. In essence, you are growing and becoming more self-actualized. The issue comes in that the other person has become comfortable with you being a certain way. Now you are changing, and they may not be growing and changing alongside you. This leads to potential conflict between the two of you as you are expecting something different in the relationship while they are wanting things as they were. This disparity provides you with an opportunity to really explore yourself, your wants, your needs, and what you are willing to accept.

Tales From the Field: Intern

I worked with adults at an inpatient dual-diagnosis residential facility for practicum and with children, adolescents, and families at an intensive outpatient nonprofit agency for internship. Prior to transitioning from practicum to internship, I decided that increasing self-awareness would be a professional and personal goal. During my practicum,

I realized that a commonality between therapists and clients of all ages was the impact of trauma. The visceral experience of trauma is vicariously perpetuated from clients' life stories. As I listened to my clients, I heard how closely their life stories paralleled my own at different developmental stages. As a student intern, I was trying to manage countertransference that was bubbling up from seemingly insurmountable obstacles in my own life, including my own trauma trigger: the hospitalization of a parent.

I believe transference and countertransference are intricately woven into the fabric of the therapeutic relationship. My attempts to manage countertransference initially produced feelings of loneliness and fear, as this can be a daunting area of growth as a therapist. For me, overcoming this obstacle entailed purposefully engaging in self-awareness activities and positive social connections at my internship site. For example, listening to the concerns of my fellow student interns helped me realize how universal my feelings were. The support and structure of the internship program at my site was also pivotal in fostering growth in this area. I was paired with therapists who treated me like a partner and valued my input regarding clients, which helped increase my confidence and ability to regulate anything that came up for me during a session. After each session, the therapists welcomed any concerns, issues, or feelings that I needed to process and provided feedback on clinical notes I wrote. Receiving this feedback not only allowed me to refine therapeutic skills and administrative functions but also better understand and work through the countertransference I would feel creep up at times.

A major component of self-awareness—which I believe is integral to growth—is the balance of one's internal standards and personal values with external thoughts, emotions, and behaviors. Oftentimes, situations arose at my internship site that led to some internal conflict; however, utilizing the resources at my site allowed me to have the self-awareness to address these concerns head-on. The clinical supervisors and therapists at my site provided me with knowledge that a textbook alone could not, and I have my time at my internship to thank for this development in my therapeutic growth.

Amanda Mohammed, MS in Clinical Mental Health Counseling program, Lynn University

---

Exercise 15.1   Changing Personal Relationships

Take a moment to think about a couple of significant relationships that you have in your life. Answer the following questions for each one.

1. What was this relationship like before you started your therapy program?
2. How has the person seen you change?
3. How have these changes impacted the dynamic of the relationship?
4. In what ways would you like the other person to change along with you?
5. How do you foresee the relationship may recalibrate?

In learning the information of psychotherapy, how this learning happens is quite important. Students find cognitive learning to be useful; however, what they find as most influential are experiential learning activities (Furr & Carroll, 2003). When students can link the theory to the application, they perceive these moments as most helpful in them really understanding the material.

What does this mean for you? Probably that your field placement—which is basically a prolonged experiential learning activity—will be the biggest learning experience you will have in your whole program. As we described in Chapter 3, getting in the right mindset is extremely important. We encourage you again to view your practicum/internship in a way that you are able to suck all of the marrow out of it. This isn't about getting hours. It is about you becoming a better psychotherapist. Each day you go to your site is an opportunity for your growth. It is up to you to make sure that happens.

Tips From an Intern

During the writing process of this book, we asked some fellow colleagues and current students about what they think could be included in each chapter. One of them asked, "How much experience and growth should we expect during our two internship semesters?" (her particular program required two off-site internship semesters) in reference to this chapter. This question provided the inspiration for this tip: Pay attention to the small differences in growth.

Becoming a therapist—especially a *good* therapist—is quite a daunting task. In my experience, I was determined to go from being a novice therapist to being a master therapist pretty quickly. In an unsurprising turn of events, I learned that this is not how it works. I wanted to see huge leaps and bounds in my growth from the start. I wanted to be like the great founding therapists who seemed like magicians in the therapy room. I found that my growth, however, was most noticeable in the little things.

When you first start your practicum/internship, you will not yet have found your groove with the small, everyday aspects of therapy. For example, many student therapists struggle with their language in their progress notes (as we talked about in Chapter 4). Another example is how you are going to talk with a client when they don't show up to their session and are going to get charged a no-show fee. These are little things that can get you frustrated or get in the way of focusing on the big picture stuff if you haven't figured out how to handle them yet. At the same time, these little things wind up being the noticeable skills that you develop that really highlight your growth. At first, they are annoying nuances that seem to trip you up. As you practice them at your practicum/internship site, however, they will become aspects of the job that are second nature.

For me, these small things were noticeable areas of growth during my practicums and internships. They left me feeling more confident in my abilities as a student intern—I actually felt like a therapist who knew the ins and outs of the system/field and could trust in what I was doing. My growth in these smaller intricacies of being a therapist freed me up to more purposefully refine the course of therapy as a whole with my clients. So when you are thinking about your own psychotherapist growth during your practicum/internship, allow yourself to focus on the small areas of growth instead of getting bogged down by wanting to go from zero to a hundred really fast. I'm willing to bet that you will realize you grew more than you think you did, and this realization may allow for you to feel more confident in your capabilities.

Change

When it comes down to it, what is therapy all about? Change. We work with clients, in whatever modality that we use, because there is something happening in their life that they either don't want or they want more of. If they leave our therapy office and there is no change, then we were ineffective and didn't do our job. We can look at personal growth in the same way. If we are the same person a week, a month, or a year from now, we haven't grown. This prevents us from experiencing ourselves in new ways and can impinge on our understanding of therapy as a process of growth.

There are many different models of change. The one that has perhaps permeated the therapy field the most is the **stages of readiness for change** (DiClemente & Prochaska, 1982; Prochaska & DiClemente, 1992; Prochaska et al., 1992). These stages include precontemplation, contemplation, preparation, action, and maintenance (see Figure 15.2). The model is a circular, rather than linear, model in which people may move forward and then back over time. This is why (along with originally being developed for people dealing with addictions) there is also a relapse stage, although not everyone will go through that.

In the **precontemplation stage**, the person does not think there is an issue and thus does not think that they need to change. Depending on the behavior, they may be unaware that

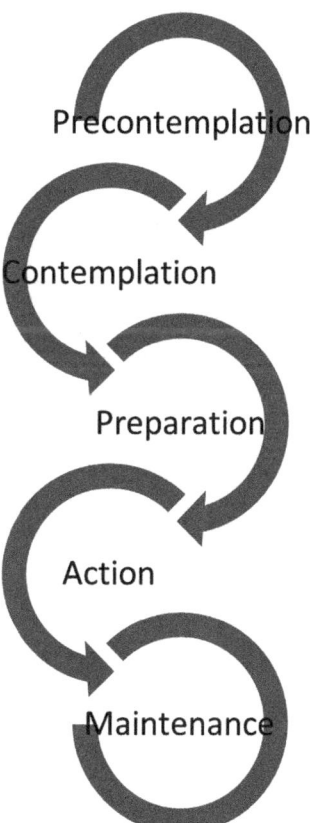

Figure 15.2 The stages of readiness for change model highlights how people go through a circular process of change.

there is a need to change or might not see that their behavior is leading to negative consequences. In substance abuse, we would say that someone in this stage is in denial.

In the **contemplation stage**, the person is aware that their behaviors are somewhat problematic and that there is a need for change. However, they don't take action yet. They are still considering things and might think that they will change but in the future.

During the **preparation stage**, the person has decided that they are going to change and starts to prepare for that process. This might include searching for therapists, telling others of their desire to change, or ordering self-help books.

In the **action stage**, the person is actively trying to change their behaviors. This is the stage that we usually expect clients to be in when they come to therapy, but that may not always be the case. For those in the action stage, we can give homework for them to do something since they believe that change will come through their own personal agency.

In the **maintenance stage**, the individual has made the desired change and are now trying to make sure that they continue the positive actions they are doing. A big aspect of this stage is relapse prevention, in which the person anticipates potential roadblocks and snares to their progress.

Some people, when thinking about the stages of readiness for change, add a sixth stage—**termination**. Here, the person has been doing the positive behaviors for so long that they don't really think about them anymore. They have become so habitual that they are a part of the person's lifestyle.

Everyone has experienced going through the stages of this model, although they didn't attribute the change in this way. Now that you know the model (or are reminded of the model if you learned about it previously), you are able to think about it for past events or for future behavior change. Exercise 15.2 allows you an opportunity to explore your past change and growth through this model.

Exercise 15.2   Your Stages of Readiness for Change

Look back on the stages of readiness for change model and think about how you have gone through this process. Choose two different behaviors in which you went through all five stages. Describe what it was like for you at each stage. Include some markers that let you know you were moving from one stage to another.

Change Process 1

Precontemplation:
Contemplation:
Preparation:
Action:
Maintenance:

Change Process 2

Precontemplation:
Contemplation:
Preparation:
Action:
Maintenance:

Tales From the Field: Supervisor

Christina was a passionate novice therapist, eagerly embarking on her first internal practicum course as part of her master's program in Marriage and Family Therapy. Her journey into the world of therapy began with a bachelor's degree in psychology. She chose her current program for its unique live supervision/observation practicum experience. This program brought together a small group of students and a licensed supervisor in an observation room with a phone for immediate supervision during therapy sessions. I was Christina's—and her other classmates'—supervisor during this practicum.

One morning, we found ourselves immersed in a particularly challenging case. The client vividly described a traumatic experience that sent shivers down Christina's spine. The raw emotions and graphic details triggered a personal reaction in her, making it difficult for her to maintain composure. Feeling overwhelmed, Christina excused herself and hastily left the observation room, desperately needing a moment to regain her emotional balance. As therapists, we know that we are going to have some heavy conversations with our clients. However, it is often a lot to handle, especially for first-time therapists hearing extremely intense information. This usually becomes a huge area of growth for student therapists—being able to hear and understand but not absorb the difficult experiences of clients.

Despite the initial distress, Christina did not let this challenging experience deter her. She knew she had to address her own reactions and emotions if she wanted to be an effective therapist. With unwavering determination, she turned to me and opened up about the emotional impact the session had on her. Christina was able to process her feelings and understand why this case had affected her so deeply through communication and transparency during supervision meetings. Over time, with continued support and guidance, Christina became more comfortable working with clients who had experienced trauma and their intricate family systems. This pivotal moment—and purposeful consultation in supervision—marked the beginning of her growth as a therapist, ultimately helping her provide more empathetic and effective care to her clients.

Lori Pantaleao, PhD, LMFT, Couple and Family Therapy program, Nova Southeastern University

Self-Actualization

As human beings, we have developmental growth, which can be seen in our physical maturation from birth, to childhood, to adolescence, to adulthood. Yet we also grow in terms of our potential. One way we can look at this is through the notion of self-actualization that was put forth by Abraham Maslow (1970). **Self-actualization** is the notion that people try to fulfill their highest potential and be the best version of themselves that they can. However, to be able to do so, lower-level needs must be satisfied first. This notion is called the **hierarchy of needs** and, starting from the lowest level, includes physical and survival needs, safety needs, love needs, ego and esteem needs, and the need for self-actualization (see Figure 15.3).

Our **physical and survival needs** include ensuring that we have food, water, air, and shelter. It is difficult for people to think about who they are and how they want to grow as an individual when they need to find something to eat and a place to sleep. **Safety needs** are about protection from physical or psychological threats. This provides us with security

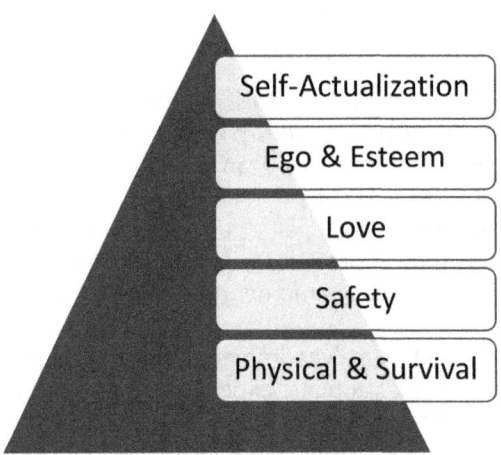

Figure 15.3 In the hierarchy of needs, people must satisfy lower-level needs first to be able to attain higher-level needs.

whether it be personal safety, financial security, or our health. **Love needs** lead us to try to make intimate connections and feel like we belong. This need is fulfilled by our relationships with family, friends, significant others, and those in our communities. **Ego and esteem needs** are related to our self-esteem as well as recognition from others. In this part of the hierarchy falls our desire for self-respect, self-confidence, competence, creativity, and achievement. Once all of these needs are met, we can focus on **self-actualization**. This is when we strive to become fully ourselves. Here, we move toward fulfilling our unique potential as we move forward on our journey of self-discovery and personal growth.

What Would You Do?: 15.1

As a student therapist, you may not be making the income right now that you one day hope to make. Further, your time is likely spent prioritizing school, completing all necessary coursework and clinical hours. You find that you do have a stable place to live and enough money to ensure you do not experience food insecurity. However, the place you live is in a bad neighborhood and you find yourself quite isolated from other people, not having a romantic partner. Your program is encouraging you to do self-of-the-therapist work, moving towards self-confidence and self-actualization; however, you find yourself frequently anxious and unable to concentrate on what the program wants you to focus on. What would you do?

How is this information useful for you? The more that you can focus on ensuring that you are meeting the needs of each lower level, the more you can move up the pyramid so that you will have energy to engage in self-actualization. Take a second and look at Figure 15.3 and try to determine how much energy you expend on each level. How might you fulfill the current level you are struggling with?

One thing to remember is that we never become fully self-actualized. It is always a process. And as the famous saying goes, "It is not the destination, it is the journey." One of the things you will likely find is that the more you are able to focus on your path toward self-actualization, the more self-aware you will become. You will be able to move beyond black-and-white thinking, understand what you desire (rather than what others are wanting of you), be more honest and caring with others and self, and have greater purpose in your life.

Developing Goals for Self

As therapists, we are usually quite aware of goals and help the people we work with move steadily toward those goals. But how much do we apply the same principles to ourselves? Have you developed your own goals, both as a person and as a clinician? If so, good. If not, how come? In this section, we want to cover goal development and ensure that you understand the components of good goals.

You have likely learned about **SMART goals** in your program:

S: **S**pecific
M: **M**easurable
A: **A**chievable
R: **R**elevant
T: **T**ime-Bound

Specific goals are clear and focus on the who, what, when, where, and how. Measurable goals allow an outside person to know when it happens. Thus, they will be behavioral. Instead of, "I will feel happier" the goal might be, "I will go to the park at least two times per week." Achievable goals are important, as we would never want to set a goal that the client is not likely to reach. They are already coming into therapy toward the end of their rope with diminished hope and motivation. The longer it will take the client to reach the goal, the less likely they will hang in there. This relates to the next goal of being relevant. The client must find the goal to be meaningful. They are more likely to work hard to achieve a goal they believe in rather than one that is forced on them. Lastly, goals should have a deadline. This allows the person to track their progress and see if they are on pace to reach it.

We also like the characteristics from de Shazer (1991) that overlap with SMART goals. These are that goals should be

1. small rather than large;
2. salient to clients;
3. described in specific, concrete behavioral terms;
4. achievable within the practical contexts of clients' lives;
5. perceived by the clients as involving their "hard work";
6. described as the "start of something" and not as the "end of something";
7. treated as involving new behavior(s) rather than the absence or cessation of existing behavior(s). (p. 112)

Two significant aspects we like about these goals as a complement to SMART goals are that they ensure the person (client) is doing something and not relying on someone else (e.g., "My partner will be nicer to me" or "My clients will be more engaged in therapy"), and they

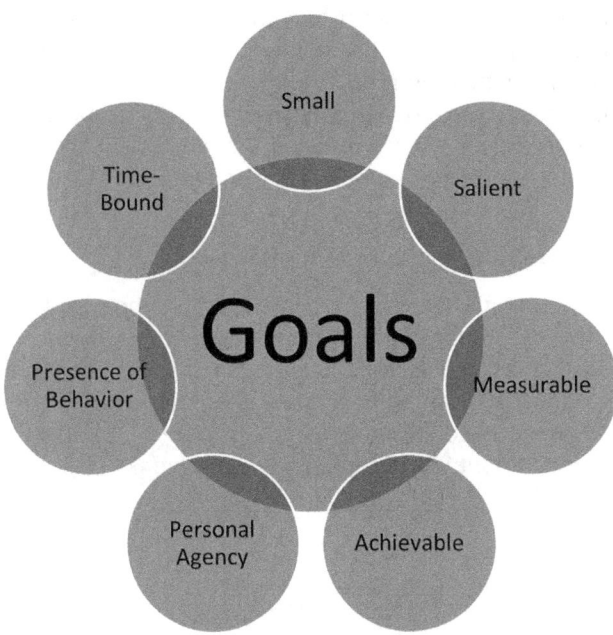

Figure 15.4 Good goals are comprised of specific factors that lead to greater likelihood of attainment.

focus on the presence rather than the absence of behavior (e.g., "I will engage in mindfulness meditation for 20 minutes" rather than "I won't be as depressed") (see Figure 15.4).

Exercise 15.3   Developing Professional Goals

For this exercise, develop three professional goals for yourself. Make sure that each goal fits the described characteristics of good goals. One goal should be able to be achieved within one week, one within one month, and one within three months. Figure out how you can keep track of your progress on each goal.

Goal 1 (achievable within 1 week):
Goal 2 (achievable within 1 month):
Goal 3 (achievable within 3 months):

Tips From a Supervisor

Exercise 15.3 asked you to develop three goals, all to be achieved in a variety of time frames. My main tip for you is to continuously develop goals and challenge yourself to maintain the mindset of growth. Many of my supervisees find themselves pretty tired toward the end of their field placement. They kind of just want it all to be over so that they can go out into the world and practice (and get paid for it while not paying for school anymore!).

At this point in your therapy career, you would be considered to be in the advanced student stage of development. There is still a lot of growth and development left for you. That growth happens passively but I think more so actively. You should be consciously thinking about what you can do in the advanced student stage to move into the novice professional stage. Then, you can set small but steady goals that will help you, one day, move into the experienced professional stage. Then, you would set more goals so that you can one day be in the senior professional stage.

This progression doesn't just happen. It is thoughtful. Some of it does happen without you planning it. However, you are likely to work closely with your clients to make small, measurable, and realistic goals for them to move forward in their lives. The same should hold for you. The main tip I have is to not view yourself as an end product but someone that is always cooking and developing flavors. Perhaps this metaphor comes from my enjoyment of watching food competition shows where I have heard many times from professional chefs that a layering of flavors happens over time. Some dishes take hours or even days to marinate or cook down. Your growth as a therapist will also take time. While some of it will be spontaneous, you do have influence over many of the other aspects. Setting and actively working on these small goals will help you get there.

Summary

This chapter has explored the notion that, based upon you (a) being a human being and (b) being in the therapy field, self-growth is an integral and inevitable process. Our hope is that you both embrace it and create it. However, this process can be discomforting and even scary as you learn more about yourself (Corey et al., 2017). We believe that the most significant change for people comes when they are challenged (either by self or others) to get out of their comfort zones. That is our challenge to you: Challenge yourself to get out of your comfort zone as you really explore who you are/who you want to be and find pathways to get there.

References

Corey, G., Corey, M. S., & Muratori, M. (2017). *I never knew I had a choice: Explorations in personal growth* (11th ed.). Cengage.

de Shazer, S. (1991). *Putting difference to work*. Norton.

Dennhag, I., & Ybrandt, H. (2013). Trainee psychotherapists' development in self-rated professional qualities in training. *Psychotherapy, 50*(2), 158–166. https://doi.org/10.1037/a0033045

DiClemente, C. C., & Prochaska, J. O. (1982). Self-change and therapy change of smoking behavior: A comparison of processes of change in cessation and maintenance. *Addictive Behaviors, 7*(2), 133–142. https://doi.org/10.1016/0306-4603(82)90038-7

Furr, S. R., & Carroll, J. J. (2003). Critical incidents in student counselor development. *Journal of Counseling & Development, 81*(4), 483–489. https://doi.org/10.1002/j.1556-6678.2003.tb00275.x

Maslow, A. H. (1970). *Motivation and personality* (2nd ed.). Harper & Row.

Owen, J., Wampold, B. E., Kopta, M., Rousmaniere, T., & Miller, S. D. (2016). As good as it gets? Therapy outcomes of trainees over time. *Journal of Counseling Psychology, 63*(1), 12–19. https://doi.org/10.1037/cou0000112

Paris, E., Linville, D., & Rosen, K. (2006). Marriage and family therapist interns' experiences of growth. *Journal of Marital and Family Therapy, 32*(1), 45–57. https://doi.org/10.1111/j.1752-0606.2006. tb01587.x

Prochaska, J. O., & DiClemente, C. C. (1992). Stages of change in the modification of problem behaviors. In M. Hersen, R. M. Eisler, & P. M. Miller (Eds.), *Progress in behavior modification* (Vol. 28, pp. 183–218). Sycamore Publishing Company.

Prochaska, J. O., DiClemente, C. C., & Norcross, J. C. (1992). In search of how people change: Applications to addictive behaviors. *American Psychologist, 47*(9), 1102–1114. https://doi.org/10.1037/10248-026

Rønnestad, M. H., & Skovholt, T. M. (2003). The journey of the counselor and therapist: Research findings and perspectives on professional development. *Journal of Career Development, 30*(1), 5–44. https://doi.org/10.1177/089484530303000102

Skovholt, T. M., & Rønnestad, M. H. (1992). Themes in therapist and counselor development. *Journal of Counseling & Development, 70*(4), 505–515. https://doi.org/10.1002/j.1556-6676.1992.tb01646.x

Chapter 16

Navigating Termination

Leaving Your Site

Congratulations! If you've gotten to this point of the book, that means that you are soon to be leaving your site. When you started your practicum/internship, it probably seemed that it would last a long time. But time tends to move quite quickly, and now you are at the end of the journey. However, just as there are processes for you to engage in when you are starting a placement, there are also processes that will help you, your clients, and the people at your site to have a beneficial parting of one another. This chapter covers some of the major topics for you to think about when you are about to finish your practicum/internship.

Myth About the Field

"Termination happens because therapy was a failure."

Therapy is not a typical business endeavor because our job is to get our clients to fire us as soon as possible. Now, we don't want them to curse us out, flip over a table, and storm out of the office. We want them to fire us because they have gotten what they need from therapy and can continue to uphold these changes in their life on their own. In the therapy world, this is considered to be termination, and this is the ultimate goal for every client in therapy.

Why Does Termination Happen?

Psychotherapy is set up from the very first moments that it will not last forever. Even old-school psychoanalysis, where analysand and analyst met three to five times per week for an extended amount of time, had a view that the analysis would end in 3–5 years. While some ethical codes hold that a client is a client in perpetuity (forever), this doesn't mean that we are actually continuing the therapeutic relationship with them. All therapy will eventually end, as it is a natural part of the therapeutic process (Reiter, 2022). We call this process **termination**. There are four different ways that termination can happen: client initiated, therapist initiated, mutually initiated, and forced termination (see Figure 16.1).

Client-initiated termination occurs when the client, on their own, decides that they will not come back for any more sessions. This may be because they have gotten what they wanted out of therapy, they didn't get what they wanted, or they can't come anymore because of financial or logistical reasons, such as they are moving away from the area. Therapists tend to be a bit blindsided by client-initiated termination, as they were unaware or partially unaware of the client's dissatisfaction with therapy or the client's perceived self-improvements (Westmacott et al., 2010).

DOI: 10.4324/9781003433484-16

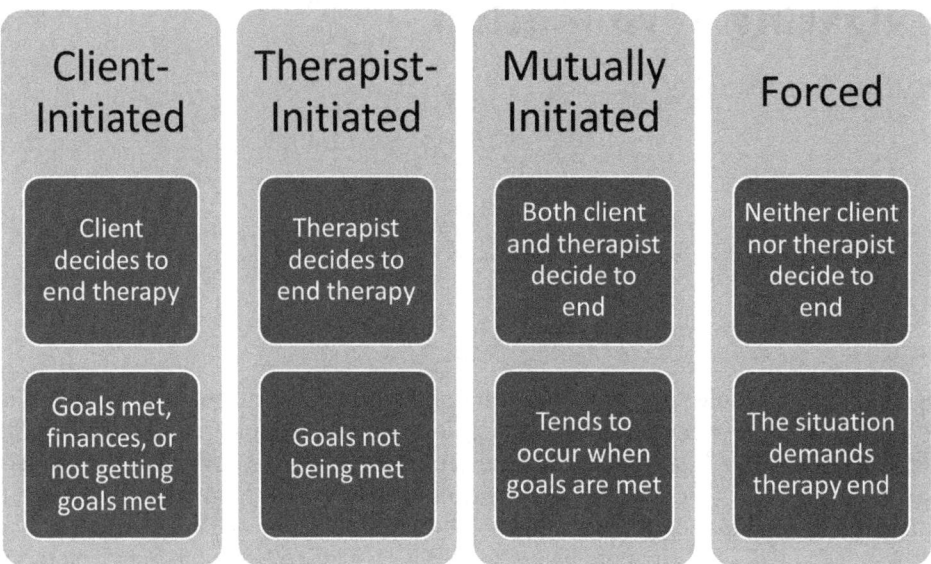

Figure 16.1 There are a variety of ways that termination happens in therapy.

Therapist-initiated termination happens when the therapist decides that termination is the best move. Here, the therapist may end therapy because they do not believe the client is progressing and that they need to ethically end therapy or because the therapist is leaving the site (because it's the end of their placement or they are moving out of the locale). For those therapists who do not believe their client is benefiting from therapy, ethically they need to address this. Just about every ethical code holds that therapists discontinue therapy when they see that it is no longer beneficial for the client. However, this is where the gray area is of psychotherapy. We also have an ethical mandate not to abandon our clients. How many sessions of non-improvement are needed for us to say that we shouldn't continue working with that client? Two? Ten? Twenty? This is where frequent conversations with your supervisor will come into play. When you find that what you are doing with your client is not working, you will need to change what you are doing. How can you take a different approach with them to see if maybe that will work? How might you have an open conversation with the client to gain their thoughts on what has and has not been helpful?

The third way that termination can happen is through **mutually initiated termination** in which the client and therapist both agree that ending the therapeutic relationship is the best move at that time. This is the preferred modality of termination. Most things in therapy (and in life) are better when both people agree on it. While this is the preferred way of initiating therapy, it is one you cannot control. But you can be on the lookout for the possibility.

The last way termination might occur is through **forced termination** when, for reasons outside of the therapist's and client's wants, the therapeutic relationship might need to end. Usually, forced termination happens when one person is leaving, either geographically or professionally. This will happen for you at the end of your internship/practicum experience when you must leave the site. You might be in the middle of the therapeutic process with a client making good progress, but your last day at the site comes before you finish therapy.

Clients have their reasons for stopping therapy. And therapists have their perceptions of why clients end therapy. In one study, therapists reported that clients terminated primarily because they had made progress or had met their goal (Bischoff et al., 2020). This is good news for us, as this is the intent of therapy. The next three most common reasons for termination included no-show/no response, no reasons provided, and school break. These reasons can bring a lot more stress for you since there is a high level of ambiguity involved. You don't know why the clients are ending the relationship, which can sow a seed of self-doubt in you. Did they end therapy because they didn't like you or find you helpful?

Fortunately, various researchers have asked clients about why they terminated, so we can understand this process from their perspective. Some of the reasons for client-initiated termination includes feeling better (based on a strong therapeutic alliance and benefits from the therapeutic tools); issues with the group setting (for those who were in group therapy); a breakdown in the therapeutic alliance; miscommunication (forgotten appointments); and impracticalities, such as work, childcare, and physical issues (Ghaemian et al., 2020). Clients also terminate because of financial and logistical reasons, or when there is a rupture in the therapeutic relationship and the client has a severe negative experience and will likely engage in an abrupt termination (Knox et al., 2011). You will have clients who terminate for all of these reasons as well as others.

Terminating With Your Clients

As mentioned, we have a very odd job as therapists. It is one that goes against every sound business principle: To get our clients to fire us as quickly as possible. It would be best if they fired us after the first session. Now, we are being just a little facetious. The word "fired" has negative connotations, as if we did something wrong. We can substitute "no longer need us" instead (but it doesn't have the same ring to it). Regardless, from the first moments we meet with a client, we should be having the ending of the relationship in mind.

One way to ease the discomfort of termination is to engage in **foreshadowing** (Reiter, 2022). Here, you can let the client know about the ending of the relationship with as much ample time as possible (you should know when your last week at your site will be). If you know that you only have a certain number of sessions, you can periodically inform the client. This is similar to letting a child know that they have 15 minutes before you are going to leave, then 10 minutes, and then 5 minutes.

Another way of easing the transition of termination is to begin to space out your sessions. Depending on your placement, you probably are meeting with your client once a week. As the client starts to progress, you can shift the frequency of sessions from once a week to once every other week. With continued progress, this can be moved to once a month. This gradual weaning of frequency allows the client more autonomy and deflects away from potential dependency that clients sometimes feel on their therapists.

When you do get to your last session, we encourage you to highlight all of the client's positive changes. They will likely try to put a lot of the responsibility for this change on you, saying things such as, "I couldn't have done this without you" or "You really changed my life." It is very important here to acknowledge the client's statement yet figure out a way to enhance their personal agency. You might say, "Thank you. It was nice being on this journey with you. And I am very impressed by what *you* did during therapy. You really used this opportunity well to make the changes in your life that you wanted to."

Tales From the Field: Intern

Leaving a practicum site can be difficult. Not only are you leaving the site, but you are experiencing loss on some level. I had been at my practicum site as a doctoral student for a year and had made connections with other therapists and staff. I knew it would be sad to not see them every day. But I also knew my time as a student would be brief; the reality is that people leave jobs all the time. I knew I wanted to have professional connections with these individuals after my time at the agency ended. I am happy to report that I still connect with a few of these people, and they are great referral sources.

The other challenging part about leaving a practicum site is ending professional relationships with clients. This too presents challenges because you have established rapport and therapeutic relationships with people. Clients build trust and a connection with their therapist as they divulge personal and private information about their lives. Ending these relationships must be done professionally and respectfully. I began informing clients whom I worked with about my time frame at my site almost three months prior to my end date so that it wasn't a surprise. The focus of therapy shifted to maintenance after the therapeutic relationship ends and discussion of transferring their care to other therapists at the agency, if the clients were open to this. The challenging part is when clients inquired about where I would be practicing after I left and requested to follow me to continue therapy. I attempted to delicately, yet professionally, explain that I could not divulge that information due to contractual agreements with the practicum agency. I certainly did not want to "poach" clients, but I also did not want these individuals to feel abandoned either.

What put my mind at ease regarding what felt like abandoning clients is that I was able to speak to the therapists to whom my clients would be transferring. I was able to discuss the cases in depth, including what their presenting issue was at the beginning of treatment, how goals were identified, and the progress each individual had made. This helped each therapist have a solid understanding of each case. I was able to inform each client of these conversations, and I believe this put their minds at ease as well. Many thanked me for this "warm" transfer of their care because they did not want to have to repeat their story and start over with someone new. The collaborative approach I took for each individual helped maintain the relationship clients had with the agency. Not only did the clients thank me for this, but the receiving therapist also did as well, as it eliminated the need to review all case notes for each client and provided a seamless transition.

As a practicum student and professional counselor, I realize it may not always be possible to transition clients with such a hands-on approach. But in this instance, I felt I took a client-centered approach that would allow each client to continue to make progress toward living happier, healthier lives. In the grand scheme of things, isn't that the goal?

Shauna Putzy, PhD in Clinical Psychology program, Capella University

---

What Would You Do?: 16.1

For this scenario, we will give you a common one that has happened to both of us and to many of Michael's supervisees (and Shauna's in the previous tale). You have a client that you have worked with for a while and are making good progress; however, you and they know that they still have a way to go in therapy. You let them know that you will be leaving the site. They tell you they do not want to be transferred to another therapist as they don't want to start over. They like working with you and want to continue. They ask whether they can go to your new placement or location. You quickly ponder whether your site will like this, as the client is not your client but the site's client. Saying "yes" to this client might come across as poaching. What do you do?

Relapse Prevention

Depending on the client's presenting symptoms, you might consider a focus on **relapse prevention** toward the end of the treatment with a client. Why would you consider doing so? Think back to Chapter 15 when we talked about the stages of readiness for change model. We presented it as a five-stage model (precontemplation, contemplation, preparation, action, and maintenance). We had mentioned that some people consider another stage in there, termination. However, given that this model was originally developed in the substance abuse field, there is sometimes a stage called relapse.

People don't always make a linear progress around the issue(s) they are dealing with. This is why it will be important for you to normalize the possibility of a relapse. But not every time the client experiences that issue again should be considered a relapse. Let's briefly talk about the differences between slips and relapses. In substance abuse parlance, a **slip** is when the person, after some period of abstinence, uses the substance, while a **relapse** is a repetitive use that leads to problematic consequences (Reiter, 2019). As an example, your client has been seriously drinking for three years. They then stop for four months. If they go out one night and drink, then don't drink again, this would be a slip. If they go back to binge drinking and their relationships start to suffer, we would consider it a relapse.

A focus on relapse prevention is extremely important since it is the most common outcome for clients dealing with substance abuse or serious mental disorders (Prochaska & Norcross, 2007). However, it is important to think about for any client dealing with any issue since clients tend to get into habits of being. Sometimes, getting out of these patterns is hard to change. If a client leaves therapy and three weeks later engages once in the problem behavior, they may say to themselves, "This just shows that therapy wasn't effective." We don't want that to happen. Rather, if you talked with them toward the end of therapy that relapse was a normal possibility, when they do engage in the problem (e.g., fighting with a spouse, watching porn, or drinking), they may then say to themselves instead, "Oh, this is one of those times my therapist told me about. This is now a sign that I need to be a bit more vigilant about focusing on maintaining my gains."

The solution-focused therapists have a unique way of viewing relapse as it doesn't mean that the client is back to square one. Instead, they view it twofold. First, it is a sign that an expectable but not inevitable situation happened because the solutions the client has been employing that were working to some degree haven't fully taken hold yet (McCollum & Trepper, 2001). Second, the fact that there was a time the client wasn't engaging in the problem demonstrates that there was an exception, which can then be focused on (Berg, 1994). So if a client comes in and says they are back to square one, you can let them know that's not quite accurate. They have had the experience of being in a certain way for some time period that the problem was not present (or not as severe). You might then focus on how they can do more of what previously worked for them before the slip or relapse.

Transition Sessions

When you are about to leave your site, you will probably have clients who still want therapeutic services. Their therapy journey isn't over just because you are finished with your practicum/internship. Almost all sites will have licensed therapists on staff who can work with the clients, or perhaps there will be new interns starting.

One of the things that you can do to facilitate the client ending therapy with you and starting with someone else is to have a **transition session**. Here, you and the new therapist both meet with the client. This session is for you to help ease the client from the ending of their connection with you to assist in the development of a new therapeutic relationship with someone else. Perhaps you were the new therapist in a transition session when you first started at the site.

In this session, you will probably summarize the therapeutic goals and assess where the client is with each of them. This is also a good time for the client and the new therapist to perhaps develop new goals, depending on the attainment of the previous goals.

Leaving Your Clients With Something

Depending on your therapeutic orientation and what you think is useful for clients, you might leave them with something more than the positive change that they have made. This wouldn't be something big but a small token, note, or letter. For instance, Michael supervised a student therapist who worked with a client who was dealing with interpersonal difficulties. People seemed to not like her that much. She didn't like herself that much. Throughout the course of therapy, the client had talked about herself in quite negative terms, viewing herself as a hardened individual. During therapy, the student therapist likened the client to a cactus, where she was rough and prickly on the outside yet soft on the inside. This had made sense to the client and led her to appreciate that while she seemed hardened, there was a soft side to her that she wasn't fully allowing to come out. At the last session, the therapist gave the client a small cactus. The client laughed and expressed her appreciation for the gift and the therapy. This cactus, which cost only a few dollars, went a long way in ending therapy on a very positive note and serving as a reminder to the client, when she would look at it in the future, of her growth and change in perspective.

What might you leave your clients? One thing we like to do is to end therapy with a **therapeutic letter**. While you might give a therapy letter anywhere along the course of therapy, even in the first session, they work extremely well as a closing letter, summarizing the positive gains the client has made. We are particularly fond of the use of **temporal therapeutic letters** (Reiter & Brown, 2020) in which you organize the letter into three paragraphs. The first paragraph focuses on the past and the various concerns the client brought with them to

Table 16.1 Sample temporal therapeutic letter.

Dear Yumi,

I wanted to take a moment to summarize our time together. You initially came to therapy expressing your upset about the breakup of an important relationship. You were quite sad and were wondering whether there was something wrong with you. This led you to really doubt yourself.

However, in therapy, we heard a different story. This story was of a woman who had a view of what she wanted in life. It was a story of a person who said to herself, "I deserve to be treated well and loved." You began to see not only what you could bring to relationships but really appreciated yourself as a human being.

What will it be like for you as you continue to treat yourself with kindness and respect? How will your relationships change when you keep demanding respect from people and from yourself? What other aspects of yourself will you acknowledge and prize? With this way of viewing yourself, what will you do that you didn't do when you first came in?

Sincerely,
Your therapist

---

therapy. The second paragraph focuses on the present, discussing the changes the client has made in therapy. The third paragraph is about the future and asks clients questions about what their life will be like when they maintain or increase the changes they've made. We usually read the letter to the client in the session and then give them a copy of it to take home so that they can read it whenever they want (we then put a copy of the letter in the client's chart). Figure 16.1 presents a sample temporal therapeutic letter.

Exercise 16.1   Constructing a Temporal Therapeutic Letter

Choose one of your clients, perhaps one that you are terminating with, and construct a temporal therapeutic letter. Before you give it to your client, go over it with your supervisor. The letter should have the following three sections:

Paragraph 1: The Past
Paragraph 2: The Present
Paragraph 3: The Future

This is only one letter format you can write to your client. There are many others, where you might consider general guidelines and structuring (see Reiter, 2023). What is important is that you are maintaining and/or bolstering the positive therapeutic experience the client has had. You want them to leave so that they would (a) come back in the future if they thought it might be useful and (b) tell other people that they should go because of their positive experience.

Your Clients Leaving You With Something

We talked about how you might give your clients a small token that signifies the positive changes they've made in therapy or just a small note that puts a closure to the therapeutic relationship. Clients may do the same for you. If they do, we—in general—recommend that you humbly accept this token, as your refusal of it might leave a negative experience for the client right at the end of therapy. When clients have given us a token at the end of therapy, it is usually something quite small. For instance, in our team therapy, Kayleigh was working with a client in which one of the themes was about a tree. The therapeutic conversation centered around an analogy of how the client was like a tree with roots, branches, leaves, etc. Trees came into play in many of the sessions. At the termination session, the client brought in a very small book about trees of Florida (where we were located). This was the client's way of giving Kayleigh (the therapist) and the team a token of appreciation.

Is it ethical to receive gifts from your clients? Yes. For instance, American Counseling Association (2014, Section A.10.f.) Receiving Gifts states:

> Counselors understand the challenges of accepting gifts from clients and recognize that in some cultures, small gifts are a token of respect and gratitude. When determining whether to accept a gift from clients, counselors take into account the therapeutic relationship, the monetary value of the gift, the client's motivation for giving the gift, and the counselor's motivation for wanting to accept or decline the gift.

Now, you won't accept every gift. We accepted a book that cost only a few dollars. But what if the client brought you a gift certificate for a cruise? This would probably be too large of a gift. As with most ethical standards, there is a gray area. How much value is too much? You can't quite put a price tag on it. Not all gifts will be bought. What if the client made you a gift, such as a painting or a sculpture? These are all important questions to ask yourself.

What Would You Do?: 16.2

You are working with a 30-year-old client who is an artist. They regularly sell their art at fairs and festivals for an average of $500. At the end of therapy, when you are having the termination session, they bring you a gift of one of their art pieces. Based on conversations you had in therapy, you know that this type of piece tends to sell for $500–$600. What do you do? Do you keep it, even though it is worth a lot of money? Do you refuse the gift? If so, what would you say to the client? How would you keep in mind the positive changes the client has made and their appreciation of the work that you did together, regardless of the decision that you make to accept or not accept the gift?

Dealing With Ambiguity

One of the hardest things for new therapists is realizing that you will no longer be a part of your clients' lives. The therapeutic relationship is a unique one in which you know intimate details of your clients' lives and are close with them but for a professional reason. Some of your clients are likely to see you and tell you intimate details of their life more often than they see and talk with some of their own family members while they are in therapy. Unlike most relationships, however, the therapeutic relationship ends once the client has hopefully met their goals (or needs to be discharged for other relevant reasons).

When you have developed a good therapeutic relationship with your clients, this can be a hard bond to break once therapy is over. Although a different type of relationship, the therapeutic relationship is still a relationship. It can feel odd for therapists to have someone whom they knew well and saw frequently suddenly not be there anymore. It is also tough because we are in a helping field—you probably genuinely care about your clients, so this makes the parting process a bit more difficult as well. Part of being a therapist is trusting that your work with clients has helped them on positive paths. Trust that they will continue without you on their journeys.

Quick Tip: Have a session with your clients where you are primarily focusing on where they are at with each of their goals. This will help the client to reconsider whether they think they need to continue therapy with another therapist. Perhaps they haven't reached all of their goals yet, but they can see that they are on the path and can continue on their own. Make sure you know the site's practices for transferring a client to a new therapist and offer that as a possibility to the client.

Tips From an Intern

I am usually not a metaphor person, but the experience of leaving a practicum/internship feels, for me, exactly like ending one book and then beginning the next one in a really good series. There is that twinge of bittersweetness because you have really loved reading the former book. Maybe you learned so much from it and it was quite an adventure; perhaps it was exactly what you expected it to be and was quite satisfying. At the same time, there is the excitement and anticipation that starts to bubble up as you realize that you have a whole other book to read that continues the story. The end of your practicum/internship may very well be the end of your academic program as well. This means that the next "book" is going to be about what you do with this degree in the real world. It is both the continuation of your therapeutic journey and the start of that therapeutic journey in a completely different context.

As you leave your site, soak in everything that made it a great experience and learn from the moments that weren't so great. Be able to close the book with satisfaction, put it back on the shelf, and then grab the one that follows.

Getting Everything Signed

Throughout your placement, you've learned about the importance of paperwork. You've had to document the introduction of clients to the site (usually through intake and biopsychosocial forms), their therapy (through treatment plans and progress notes), and their exit from the site (through closing letters or discharge paperwork). These are documents that you wrote for the benefit of the client (or at least about the client).

Before leaving the site, make sure that you've taken care of the paperwork that is your responsibility. The primary forms are likely the signing off of your clinical hours. We recommend that you don't wait until the end of the term like many of the interns that we've known. The longer you wait to document hours, the greater the likelihood there is that you will forget an hour or two or three or ten. Further, it also puts pressure on your supervisor to sign everything at once. However, some supervisors would prefer doing them all at once rather than each week. But from all the supervisors we know, most are okay signing off at the end of the supervision session or soon after. We just don't want you to be in the situation of someone we knew who waited until the end of the placement to get their clinical hours signed off. When they tried, the supervisor had moved without leaving a forwarding address, and they were not able to get in touch with them. There was quite a bit of chaos as they tried to figure out how to get documentation that they conducted sessions and was supervised for the hours that they worked with clients.

Supervision Notes

Remember, you are learning not just from your active time at your site but also from the supervision meetings in which you will engage to discuss what you have been doing at your site. We mentioned in Chapter 14 that we recommend you take notes during each supervision meeting. These notes are there for you to utilize and build upon throughout the semester at your practicum/internship. You will go back to certain cases you spoke to your supervisor about earlier in the semester and then conceptualize them further as therapy continues.

The beauty about these notes is that they do not cease being helpful once you finish your time at your site. Your supervision notes are likely going to be beneficial in a variety of other contexts outside of your practicum/internship, so these notes are something else we recommend that you hold onto once you leave your site.

One thing that your supervision notes will continue to be helpful with is supervision (we bet you didn't see that one coming). In our experience, past supervision can be just as helpful as present supervision. Let's say you come across a similar case in another context once you leave your site (e.g., perhaps at a job you begin working at after graduation). You may think to yourself, "Wow, this case is really similar to when I worked with that other client. I remember we talked about a certain technique in supervision that wound up being really helpful for this person; maybe I can try this with my current client."

If you can remember exactly what you did on your own, then that is great. Sometimes, though, when we see a lot of clients, the specifics of the techniques (and even the rationales behind them) can get muddled in our memories, especially as new therapists who are navigating the field. This is where your good ol' supervision notes can come in handy. If you took detailed notes, you likely wrote down the why and the how behind using this technique with the previous case. A quick glance through your notes provides a nice refresher that can lend more confidence when using a technique from a previous case.

If your degree does not end once you complete your practicum/internship or if you decide to continue your therapy education (e.g., go into a doctoral program), then your previous supervision notes can even be helpful for school assignments. Most psychotherapy graduate programs have some assignments that require students to confidentially reflect on cases that they have worked to further their therapeutic development (e.g., writing a case study about a client you had and a psychotherapy theory you utilized with that client). Once again, it can sometimes be hard to remember everything that you did with a previous client (especially if you don't have access to the progress notes anymore). Your supervision notes can help jog your memory and remind you of your case conceptualization and interventions to more easily and accurately write any academic papers.

Ending Relationships at Your Site

During your time at your site, whether it is for one semester, half a year, or a whole year, you have made genuine connections with the people there. We have already talked about ending your relationships with the primary individuals you work with—your clients. Now, we'd like to take a few minutes and honor the relationships you have made with the support staff, other therapists, and supervisor at your site. These individuals have played a key role in your development as a therapist.

The bad news is that there will be some of these individuals that you will be saying goodbye to. Leaving them will lead to some feelings of loss, and that is perfectly okay and expected. Endings are hard for many people. You have perhaps come to rely on these individuals for connection, support, information, and guidance. They likely played a key role in your learning experience during the practicum. So the ending of the relationship will be a dual experience: happiness because you are moving on and sadness because things are changing.

The good news is that there may be some of these individuals with whom you will stay connected. Besides your clients, it is perfectly fine to maintain a relationship with various people at the site, such as the administrative staff or other therapists. Staying in contact with everyone from your site after you leave is probably not likely. However, there will be certain people whom you resonate/connect with and want to keep in contact with after finishing up at your site. We see students who meet other colleagues in similar psychotherapy programs at their sites and then remain friends with them after leaving. Your practicum/internship experience is a great way to meet other people who are going through the same process as you and expand your network of support.

Tales From the Field: Supervisor

I consider myself incredibly lucky to have had the honor and privilege to guide interns through their first real experiences in the field. At the time, I was the clinical director of a nonprofit facility. Part of my job included supervising the student interns for our internship program. There's something very fulfilling in watching an intern blossom into who they are as a therapist. I believe our role as supervisors is not to mold interns into what we need nor train them to play the part we want them to play. Rather, our role is to guide them in finding themselves as therapists, connecting all of the important parts of therapy to create who they are as an authentic therapist when working with clients. I like to think that the way I held space for them to grow made them feel seen, heard, and appreciated for not only what they brought to the program but also for who they were as individuals. This partly led to many interns applying for paid positions at my workplace as they graduated and became registered interns.

This hiring of interns as they graduated and completed their externship hours was probably one of my favorite things to do during my time as clinical director. To be transparent, I selfishly wanted to continue to get to see their growth and be a part of their continued therapeutic development. At a larger scale, however, doing so also greatly benefited the program. It was far easier to continue to train someone who was familiar with our policies and procedures then it was to bring in someone brand-new. I like to think that it benefited the interns as well to step in to their first paid experience in the field within a dynamic they already were familiar with. Perhaps it made the next step in their professional careers feel safer and a little less daunting. There were common characteristics of the interns that we hired postgraduation. The majority of the interns we hired had shown that they were organized, efficient with documentation, and dedicated and committed to their clients. The interns we chose to hire were also incredibly proactive and sought out additional supervision whenever they were unsure or had questions. When you are the clinical director of an incredibly busy program, interns who proactively come to you with questions are priceless. Those that didn't tended to have difficulties in their caseload and therapy sessions. But what had always been most important for me was how authentically the interns approached what it means to step into client's lives in the way we do as therapists.

When I think about where the first two wonderful interns we hired after their externship experience are now, I am filled with contentment and pride. They have continued to grow and flourish. Both are now a part of successful private practices and are making a name for themselves in the therapy field. Amongst all this growth, I still see in them the same values I saw in them the day they walked into my office for their initial student intern interviews: They are dedicated and committed to their clients, they understand the immense honor it is to do the work we do, and perhaps most importantly, they are genuinely themselves.

Katherine Lewis, MS, LMFT, private practice

In addition to keeping in touch with newly made friends from your site, it would also be prudent to ask for the contact information of any supervisor and/or therapist in the field whom you would like to work with again or want to learn more from. For example, let's say there is another therapist who works at your site who used to work with military families, and this is the specialization you want to go into after graduation. This would be a good person to stay in contact with after you leave your site so you can reach out to them with any relevant questions in the future. This is the networking aspect of your practicum/internship experience that you should think about as you prepare to leave your site.

Tips From a Supervisor

Termination is a tough thing for many of my supervisees, especially when they are leaving their practicum/internship site, as it is a marker of their movement from one stage of their career to the next. The end of your field placement is usually associated with your graduation from your program. This is an event that you have dreamed and fantasized about for many upon many years. It has significant meaning for you.

The tip here is to not see it as an end goal but a stepping stone. Practicum and internship experiences were developed to assist you in the *process* of learning how to become a psychotherapist. I think it is useful to view it as such: a process. It is not the end of something but a part of something larger. This way, you can look at it from a wider perspective, from what happened before, during, and then after—what is to come next in your continued development of being a therapist?

Just like you might have a final session with a client during which you review many of their gains in therapy, you can do this for yourself as well. Perhaps you will do this with your supervisor. How have you grown as a therapist? What skills did you develop? What have you been good at doing? What areas could you still improve upon? Where would you like to continue to grow as a therapist? Your leaving your practicum/internship site can be used as a check-in point with yourself—and possibly your supervisor—to assess whether the goals that you had for yourself at the start of this process were met and what new goals you have developed for yourself.

Summary

At some point, you will be exiting your site. As this time approaches, you will need to consider how to end your relationships with your clients and the professionals at the site. Termination is often an anxiety-producing event. Rather than just let it happen, there are many things that you can do to prepare for termination to make it a successful and useful endeavor. While you are figuring out how to make termination significant for your clients, ending your time at your site is important for you to leave in a positive way. As with many of the other situations that have occurred during your practicum/internship, you are not going through this process alone. Make sure you work closely with your site supervisor and program administrator to ensure that all of the requirements for you are being met.

References

American Counseling Association. (2014). *2014 ACA code of ethics*. www.counseling.org/resources/aca-code-of-ethics.pdf

Berg, I. K. (1994). *Family based services: A solution-focused approach*. Norton.

Bischoff, T., Krenicki, L., & Tambling, R. (2020). Therapist reported reasons for client termination: A content analysis of termination reports. *The American Journal of Family Therapy, 48*(1), 36–52. https://doi.org/10.1080/01926187.2019.1684216

Ghaemian, A., Ghomi, M., Wrightman, M., & Ellis-Nee, C. (2020). Therapy discontinuation in a primary care psychological service: Why patients drop out. *The Cognitive Behaviour Therapist, 13*, e25. https://doi.org/10.1017/S1754470X20000240

Knox, S., Adrians, N., Everson, E., Hess, S., Hill, C., & Crook-Lyon, R. (2011). Clients' perspectives on therapy termination. *Psychotherapy Research, 21*(2), 154–167. https://doi.org/10.1080/10503307.2010.534509

McCollum, E. E., & Trepper, T. S. (2001). *Family solutions for substance abuse: Clinical and counseling approaches*. Haworth Clinical Practice Press.

Prochaska, J. O., & Norcross, J. C. (2007). *Systems of psychotherapy: A transtheoretical analysis* (6th ed.). Brooks/Cole.

Reiter, M. D. (2019). *Substance abuse and the family* (2nd ed.). Routledge.

Reiter, M. D. (2022). *Therapeutic interviewing: Essential skills and contexts of counseling* (2nd ed.). Routledge.

Reiter, M. D. (2023). *A therapist's guide to writing in psychotherapy*. Routledge.

Reiter, M. D., & Brown, A. (2020). Temporal therapeutic letters: Utilizing time as a structural guide. *Journal of Systemic Therapies*, *39*(2), 1–16. https://doi.org/10.1521/jsyt.2020.39.2.1

Westmacott, R., Hunsley, J., Best, M., Rumstein-McKean, O., & Schindler, D. (2010). Client and therapist views of contextual factors related to termination from psychotherapy: A comparison between unilateral and mutual terminators. *Psychotherapy Research*, *20*(4), 423–435. https://doi.org/10.1080/10503301003645796

Chapter 17

What's Next?

Licensure and Job Acquisition

Your practicum/internship should be a primary ingredient in your initial career development. It allows you to network with professionals, implement competencies you learned in class, gain exposure to a variety of clientele and settings, and learn along with peers (Hernandez et al., 2014). Usually, your practicums/internships are during the latter half of your academic program. This means that you will likely graduate after you finish your last semester of practicum/internship. This makes sense, as practicums and internships are the culmination and implementation of everything that you have learned in your program thus far and provide that exposure to real-world therapy workplaces. After you wrap up your practicum/internship experience and graduate, there are two main steps to move forward in your psychotherapy career: (a) get a job and (b) get licensed.

Myth From the Field

"My site will automatically hire me if I do a good job during my practicum/internship."

Many students choose their site because they thought that, when finished, they would get hired at that location and that this would be a place they would want to work at. While we have seen it happen, and even happened for Kayleigh, this is not the rule. There are sites that do utilize the practicum/internship as a long-term job interview, but many sites do not since having students come through provides them a way of having therapists that they do not have to pay. Our recommendation is to think about doing such a good job not only with your clients but with the site that if they do have a paid opening, they would want to hire you. This requires you being professional, coming on time, being dressed appropriately, being collegial, and doing good clinical work.

Tips From an Intern

Luckily, therapy jobs seem to be in high demand. Between the COVID-19 pandemic and the subsequent expansion of teletherapy, more people appear to be seeking out therapeutic services which can be conducted via multiple mediums (i.e., in person, phone call, video chat, online chat). You will thus hopefully have several options as you begin your job hunt.

DOI: 10.4324/9781003433484-17

However, we usually want to work smarter, not harder. If you like your site and would be interested in working there, start there first. If you are not already aware, ask questions about the types of job they offer (e.g., full-time, per diem), the pay, and the responsibilities. Come from the perspective of a curious intern learning about the inner workings of the therapy world. If you come to the conclusion that you are happy with the logistics of your site, make it known to your supervisor at that site that you would like to work there after graduation—regardless of if they are officially hiring or not. The nonprofit site that I interned at was not advertising a new therapy position; however, I told the clinical director that I would be interested in working there after graduating, and then they offered me a position.

If you make a good impression on your site supervisor and are proactive and vocal about your desire to work there, it is possible for you to get a position even if they are not actively looking for a new therapist. I didn't have to worry about looking for a job after graduation because I considered and obtained a job at my internship site first.

Now, not everyone winds up loving their practicum/internship site. That is just the way things work sometimes. If this winds up being the case for you, then obviously this tip may not apply. However, if you did enjoy your experience at your site, look there first if you are hoping to acquire a job after graduation. It might help make the process shorter and easier.

Registering With Your State

A necessary first step in becoming licensed is to register with the state you are in after graduation. Now, what you will register as will be different depending on the state. For example, for marriage and family therapy in Florida, you will be a Registered Marriage and Family Therapy Intern, while in Georgia you would be considered an Associate Marriage and Family Therapist. This is just basically the official title/designation that you would go by in between graduating and becoming fully licensed. In Ohio, you would need to register as a Marriage and Family Therapy Trainee before you saw any clients in your practicum/internship, then become a Licensed Marriage and Family Therapist while accruing your supervised hours until you become an Independent Marriage and Family Therapist. This is why we encourage you to spend a lot of time on your state's (or country's) licensing website, even before you begin your internship (sorry to say this at the end of the book), so that you are clear of what you need to do and when. For instance, Michael had a marriage and family therapy supervisee in Ohio who couldn't see clients because the paperwork for her to register as a Marriage and Family Therapy Trainee was taking quite a long time. Most students in other states do not need to register with their state until they finish seeing clients through their graduate program and will be practicing outside of the school arena.

Usually, once you have registered with the state, you can see clients, count your supervised therapy hours, and register for the licensure exam. This means that you want that registration status as soon as possible. Again, the minutiae of how you go about this registration process of course differs for each state. Most states require things such as your degree and a letter from your approved supervisor agreeing to provide supervision for you. Even these requirements have nuances in them—your degree can only be submitted to the state once it has been officially conferred by your university, and the state has to approve your supervisor first before you can start counting hours (i.e., you can't just count your hours as soon as you submit your letter).

We won't lie to you and say that all of this is an easy process—it's not. It consists of a lot of moving parts which you need to be on top of if you want your registration status as soon as possible (which we recommend so you can be licensed as soon as possible as well). We wish we could provide you with the exact steps you need to take in order to register with your state, but that is beyond the scope of this book. Our goal instead is to make you aware of these little things so that they won't hit you like a freight train once you graduate. We have seen so many students get bogged down and overwhelmed by everything they need to do, so make sure you know exactly what you need to submit and when beforehand. You can usually get this information from a professor/supervisor or your state's website, but we recommend that you call your state to verify with a representative everything that you need and the best way to submit all the required documents. Your state will have some sort of board office number for your field that you can call if you look it up online.

Even if you are on your game and get everything submitted as soon as you can, states are usually slower rather than faster at processing these sorts of things because of the high influx of documents that they need to sort through. Processing times can range from a few weeks to even a month or two. Our suggestion is that you see how long the state says it will take to process a document submission (it usually says this in a confirmation email they send you after you submit something). Then, if that amount of time passes and you still haven't heard anything about the status of your submission, call them. Kayleigh's supervisor letter got lost in the paperwork shuffle once, and it sat for two months; she only found out that it hadn't been reviewed or processed yet because she called the state to check on its status. It got processed within the next few days, so being vigilant paid off (and it probably could have been processed earlier if she had called sooner!).

Preparing for Licensure

Okay, you have your registration status with your state! Now we can go over the other aspects of preparing for licensure. We listed getting a job as the first step because you have to have a job to become licensed. You will need to log a certain amount of therapy hours postgraduation in order to qualify for licensure (much like counting hours at your practicum/internship to qualify for your degree), and the easiest way to attain these hours is to obviously get a job in the field. However, we want to talk about preparing for licensure first because you should start this process during or perhaps even before getting a job. If you wait to work on this step only after you have acquired a job and attained your therapy hours, you will probably be behind in the licensure process.

It shouldn't be a surprise at this point, but we want to repeat that the specifics of licensure requirements are going to differ for each state (and country). These requirements can be found with a quick search on the internet or a phone call to the state, so we recommend that you look into the parameters of the licensure process for your state. This information is going to be integral for you to complete these requirements and get licensed as soon as possible. While these specifics may differ, there are three general requirements for licensure that we want to go over: therapy and supervision hours, the licensure exam, and continuing education units (CEUs).

Therapy and Supervision Hours

We already mentioned the therapy hours—these are just the amount of direct therapy hours (that you will obviously give, not receive) that you need after you graduate and become registered with your state. The number of hours required for licensure will vary a bit between some states; so once again, just make sure you know how many you need. Map it out like we recommended you do with your practicum/internship hours: Calculate how many therapy hours you will need on average per week based on the time you register with the state and the time you are eligible for licensure postgraduation. This will give you an idea of how many sessions per week you will need in order to get licensed as soon as possible. If you aren't able to work that many hours every week (e.g., perhaps you continue your education in pursuit of a doctoral degree after graduating with your master's, you have a family, or you have a non-therapy-related job), then that is perfectly fine, too. It will just give you a sense of how long it would take you to become licensed based on how many hours you work per week.

Just like for your practicum/internship, you will also need to accumulate supervision hours for licensure. This is basically the same type of supervision you received during your practicum/internship. A certain amount of licensure supervision hours can also be done in groups of up to a certain number of people (again, depending on the state). You may have encountered group supervision already during your practicum/internship.

Now, your supervision during your practicum/internship was free (we know you pay for the practicum/internship credits, so it is not really free if we are getting technical). However, you may have to directly pay for supervision for licensure. To provide supervision for licensure, your supervisor has to be a qualified/registered/approved supervisor in your state. Some jobs provide supervision for free; others don't. This is something you can consider when looking for a job after graduation. Oftentimes, there will be professors at your university who are qualified supervisors and provide a discounted supervision rate for students. So if your job does not provide free supervision, try your professors next. If that doesn't work out, each state has a list of qualified supervisors that you can comb through and research further. Remember, part of the registration application with the state includes confirmation of a qualified supervisor. You usually can't be registered to practice therapy without a supervisor on file, so you should look into this sooner rather than later.

If you followed our advice in Chapter 3, then you have some sort of efficient process in which you have kept track of your therapy and supervision hours for your graduate program (e.g., an Excel spreadsheet or paper forms). You can use this exact same process to keep track of your licensure therapy and supervision hours. Perhaps the details of the hours differ (e.g., maybe you needed relational hours for your program but don't need to make that distinction for licensure hours). This is fine because you can easily adapt this log in any way that you need.

We've talked about the supervision hours necessary for licensure, now let's talk about the supervisors themselves. In addition to making the aforementioned considerations about the cost of supervision, it is also important that you consider the qualities of your potential supervisor. We mentioned this in Chapter 14. For your practicums/internships in your program, you may have less flexibility with you being able to choose your supervisor. This is true in some cases with licensure supervision; for example, you are probably going to stick with your free licensure supervisor if it comes with your job because it can save you a lot of money. However, in the end, you are able to choose your licensure supervisor. Aten et al. (2008) discussed the importance of self-reflection when it comes to determining what supervisory characteristics resonate and do not resonate with you as a supervisee. This is something that you should give quite a bit of thought into, and you should even interview and chat with potential supervisors to find the best fit for you.

The Licensure Exam

The next big thing you will need to tackle is the licensure exam. The licensure exam is a comprehensive, standardized exam that tests you on information relevant to your specific therapy field. The exact setup of the licensure exam varies between fields. For example, the mental health counseling exam (as it stands at the time of us writing this book) consists of multiple choice questions based on case studies, whereas the marriage and family therapy exam consists of multiple choice questions based on various categories (e.g., diagnoses, theories, laws and ethics).

Generally, you can technically take the licensure exam at any point between you registering with your state after graduation and you being eligible to become licensed (i.e., the two-year mark after registering with the state), but we recommend you take this exam as soon as possible. This is for two reasons: (a) The information from your graduate program will be fresh in your head, and (b) if you don't pass the exam the first time, you'll want to have wiggle room so you have more time to take it again.

Once you decide when to take the exam, you will register for it based on how the registration process works in your state. The next step is to actually study for the exam. Did you think that you are ready to take it because you have all your knowledge from your graduate program? Oh, if only things were that easy. Yes, your psychotherapy graduate program will have prepared you greatly for this exam, as you will have learned the bulk of what you will be tested on. At the same time, the licensure exam is a standardized test that asks questions in a standardized way and thus has standardized answers. In therapy, we know that context is important, and things are not always black-and-white. However, the licensure exam—being a multiple choice test—requires black-and-white answers. That means that the exam usually looks for a consistent answer for a scenario, for instance, even if we would treat that situation differently in real life depending on the context.

If you have ever studied for another standardized test in school through a study program, you may remember that the study program likely not only focused on the content of the test but also *how* to take the test (i.e., looking for patterns in similar questions so you know how to answer it or how to solve for the answer). The licensure exam is set up in this way as well. Consequently, we recommend that you don't just rely on your own studying for this test. You can go over the content all you want, but if you don't also learn how to take the exam, you will likely get more questions wrong that you could have gotten right.

Utilizing a study program for the licensure exam is most likely going to be most helpful in passing the exam. Usually, study programs can be around one or two months long if you follow their study schedule. Make sure you register for an exam date that allots for this study time. If you know you will take a bit longer to complete the study program, make sure your exam date reflects the appropriate amount of time you need to study.

Choosing the right study program is also an important consideration. Unfortunately, there are study programs out there for the licensure exam for each therapy field that just don't quite do it. Talk to professors and colleagues who have taken the exam already to see what study programs they would recommend. Do some further digging yourself on each program's website to see what they offer and for how much. We want to inform you that some study programs cost just as much as the licensure exam itself. While this may seem like a steep price, it is often worth the investment if it is a good program and you put the necessary effort into completing the program.

Last but not least, don't be hard on yourself if you don't pass the exam the first time. It is not rare for individuals to need another try or two before they pass. This does not mean that you are not a competent therapist or you are an unintelligent person. Oftentimes, we have seen that it is people's nerves that get the best of them when taking this exam. Even when completing a great study program, the anxiety when you sit down at the testing center can set in, and a lot of what you learn from the study program can fly out the window. For example, we know of one student who completely forgot to take a break at the halfway mark of the exam (which helps you refuel with a snack and gives your head a break) despite the study program talking about the necessity of this break. This is why finding strategies to stay calm throughout the entire exam is going to be instrumental in passing.

Quick Tip: Don't put off tomorrow what you can do today. The more that you do to prepare for licensure when you are in school and still in student mode, the better. The longer that you put it off, the more you forget what you have learned, and the more likely you will continue to put off your registration and licensure testing. Think about forming a study group with your colleagues and purchasing a licensure preparation program.

What Would You Do?: 17.1

You have completed all of the necessary coursework for your specific license. Now, you need to pass the licensure exam. In your program, you were able to take a couple of practice exams and scored just under the minimum passing mark. You have a few friends who have paid for study programs, and they have all passed. You have a few other friends who didn't use a program and half passed the exam, while the other half did not. You want to take the exam within the next few months. You can pay around $300–$400 for a study program or try to do it on your own. What would you do?

Developing a CV

Now that you are finishing your practicum/internship, you are likely getting close to graduating from your program. It is time for you to get a job so that you can put what you've learned at your placement into practice; plus, it will probably be nice for you to actually get paid for all of the hard work that you've put into this profession. Perhaps one of the first steps in this process is for you to develop a CV—a curriculum vitae—which provides people with a brief overview of your education, work experience, and other qualifications. If you recall in Chapter 2, we went over developing a CV to submit to potential internship sites. Now you will be adding to it to submit to potential employers. However, you will have a lot more skills and experiences to put on it, specifically related to your therapeutic work.

You might be asking, "Isn't that just a resume?" Yes and no. A resume and CV both provide an overview of you as a potential employee. Perhaps the biggest difference is that the CV is more detailed. Usually, a resume is a one-page summary of you as a professional. The CV can be several pages long. Currently, Michael's CV is nine pages long, as it highlights five earned degrees, five different universities and departments he's worked for, over 30 publications, 25 workshops and presentations, awarded grants, clinical experience, professional memberships, and professional and administrative functions. Your CV will not look like this, as you do not have 30 years in our field. Kayleigh's CV isn't like this. Hers is about four pages. Her CV, however, includes more descriptions (like a resume) of each category, like the courses she has guest-lectured in, for example, since she does have less experience. There are two different types of CVs—ones that are longer based on experience but less detailed (like Michael's) and ones that are shorter but more detailed to compensate for having less experience (like Kayleigh's).

CVs are sometimes mainly used for academia, but you can sort of think of a CV as a master resume even if you aren't going into academia. Some jobs will ask for a CV, some will just ask for a resume. If the jobs you are applying for require resumes, tailor each resume to each job. Basically, take relevant information from your CV and create a resume with the most pertinent information based on the job you are applying for (and adjust the level of detail as necessary).

Most CVs have the following components to them: demographic information, education, professional experience, publications, presentations, awards/scholarships, professional training, and professional affiliations. Depending on where you are at in your program, you may or may not have any publications or presentations. If you do not, leave these sections off of the CV. They are usually more important if you are trying to get into a doctoral program, a post-doctoral program, or a job in academia. One thing you might substitute is a section on graduate coursework. An optional section is a personal statement. However, this usually is more present on a resume than a CV.

Exercise 17.1   Developing Your CV

Your CV will be one of the first ways that a potential employer will come in contact with you. It is important to have a CV that is representative of who you are, helps you stand out from other applicants, and gets the potential employer interested to talk with you in person. For this exercise, develop your own CV. Perhaps use a template that is easily found online. Once you have created your CV, ask someone at your university to review it. This might be a faculty mentor or a career services office at your school that works with students to help with resumes and CVs. By the end of this exercise, you should have a CV that you feel comfortable sending to prospective employers.

Job Searching

Why did you decide to enter your graduate program? A safe assumption is that you did so to become a psychotherapist so that you could help people. Plus, you probably want to make money to pay off your student loans but more importantly to live a lifestyle that you would like. Thus, you will be wanting to gain employment. In this section, we will talk about some ideas for you to think about in your pursuit of a job.

Private Practice, Agency, or Residential Treatment Centers

Three of the main types of psychotherapy workplaces are private practices, agencies, and residential treatment centers. These varying contexts all have different clientele, responsibilities, pay, and general dynamics that are important to consider when looking for a job. While the specifics of each particular facility will of course be different, we thought it would be helpful to go over the general experiences/differences of these therapeutic workplaces.

Private practices typically provide outpatient therapy only—that is, you come in once a week or every other week for a session with your therapist. The particular frequency of sessions each week varies per client, but the gist is that clients are generally not receiving intensive therapy (which we will talk more about when discussing agencies and residential treatment centers). Private practices are oftentimes owned by one or more therapists (rather than a larger entity) and can be a solo or group practice. In group practices, therapists can typically either rent out office space for their sessions or just get a percentage of each session. Private practices can also either take both insurance and private pay or just accept private pay. This can affect whether you are required to diagnose or do specific paperwork with your client. A lot of therapists will only accept private pay so they do not have to do things such as biopsychosocials and monthly documentation (as talked about in Chapter 4). Others, however, will accept insurance because it allows for more referrals. For lack of a better word, private practices are generally more low-key than agency or residential treatment centers. From our experience, you can make the most money in private practice (especially if you take private payment only) because you are getting a larger chunk of the profit.

Agencies can oftentimes be a mix between private practices and residential treatment centers. Agencies often have more therapists working there than a group private practice because they are larger entities usually run by individuals who may not be therapists. You can often be a full-time therapist or an independent contractor and make your own hours. Agencies usually pay less than a private practice because they are taking a larger cut of the session fee. Some agencies have only outpatient therapy services (described earlier when talking about private practice) in which the clients come in just for therapy services and then go home after. Agencies can both take insurance and accept private pay. Agencies can sometimes offer intensive outpatient therapy (IOP) in which clients come in for either their individual sessions and/or group sessions multiple times a week. These are for people who need more than your average once-a-week therapy but aren't quite needing residential treatment.

Residential treatment is as it sounds—clients stay at these facilities for a certain period of time. These facilities are usually for more intense situations, such as substance use, eating disorders, or self-harm. Therapists whom we know have reported that while working at a residential facility can be a lot because of the intense nature of the presenting problems, they have also shared that this work is incredibly rewarding.

Tales From the Field: Intern

At the time I'm writing this, I'm a third-year doctoral student in a family therapy program and a registered marriage and family therapy intern in Florida. As soon as I got my intern number, I started working for an agency, but I knew I wanted to also work for a private practice at some point. I got my first private practice job after being a registered intern for about a year.

After working for the private practice for five months, my bosses asked if I wanted to take on a high-conflict case as a co-therapist and replace another co-therapist, as she wanted to lighten her caseload. My bosses explained that we would be seeing this client twice a week and I would join in on these sessions as the other co-therapist transitioned out. The other co-therapist transitioned out and then decided to just come back and join the sessions on Thursdays. My bosses then explained to me that I would be "shadowing" on Thursdays because of "being an intern." My bosses said, "Shadowing is a part of being an intern and almost every private practice does this."

Being a student intern for school and working at a practicum/internship to get a master's degree is different from being a registered intern with the state preparing for licensure. You should be getting paid for every service you do with your master's degree, even in those two years of being a registered intern (based on Florida's requirements, at least). We did not go through two years of coursework and internships as a student to not get paid for our services postgraduation.

I thought about the logistics of the dilemma, and I asked my supervisors and my colleagues for advice on how I should go about this. Based on what was right and what wasn't right, I decided that I wouldn't shadow anymore because it was not fair to me based on my credentials. I was a registered intern at that point, not a student intern. I should have been getting paid for all my sessions. I set up a meeting with my bosses and told them that I would not be shadowing anymore. From then on, I made sure I got paid for my work.

Bailey Rich, PhD candidate in Couple and Family Therapy program, Nova Southeastern University

---

Quick Tip: There are many different ways to search for a job. Don't put all of your eggs in one basket. Use all of them. Engage in networking. Ask your colleagues, as they may know of a job that they didn't want but would be good for you, or there might be something open at their job. Look on job search engines like Indeed, ZipRecruiter, or Monster. Also, begin cold-calling (or emailing) the various sites and agencies in your area (or an area that you would like to move to). The more connections you make, the greater likelihood that something will come of it.

Post-Internship Supervision

We have mentioned this a few times, but once you finish your practicum/internship experience, you will likely be close to graduation. However, depending on where you are with clinical hours, you are probably not close to licensure. You will need to still be supervised while seeing clients postgraduation. However, your supervisor will likely not have as much direct in-session oversight as your school-based supervisor might have in your graduate program. Rather, you would meet periodically (if you are working full-time, then it will probably be once per week for one hour) and you go over your cases. For many fields, this will last for two years to get you to the point where you are fully licensed and do not need to be supervised any longer.

However, that doesn't mean that you can't ever be supervised. Michael supervises a couple of licensed therapists who are working in private practice. They have completed school and in many ways are feeling somewhat isolated. They want to continue to grow, ensure they are engaging in ethical and effective therapy, and be challenged to evaluate their skills, conceptualizations, and therapy. They are not required from any body or organization to have supervision but do so voluntarily for continued growth and learning.

Lifelong Learning

In the not too far future, you will be graduating. If you'll be getting a doctorate, this might be the last academic course you ever take. The same for your master's if you don't want to go for a doctoral degree. Either way, you are probably thinking about not having to read books, take exams, write papers, and going to class anymore. This is partially true, as we have good news and bad news. The good news is that, if you are not going for another degree, you do not have to go to class and do assignments anymore! The bad news is that you are not through with learning (but we hope that you can see this is also good news).

Psychotherapy is a field that believes in lifelong learning. We understand that our current knowledge is not all-encompassing. We are continually trying to understand clients, the therapy process, and ourselves better so that therapy can be more efficient and effective. This belief in lifelong learning is inherent in many of our ethical codes. For instance, the American Association for Marriage and Family Therapy (2015) code of ethics holds:

3.1 Maintenance of Competency.

Marriage and family therapists pursue knowledge of new developments and maintain their competence in marriage and family therapy through education, training, and/or supervised experience.

We already mentioned that you will need to complete CEUs to become licensed. Once you are licensed, you will need to renew your license every two years. Besides paying for this renewal, the biggest thing you will need are more CEUs.

Where do you get these CEUs from? Mainly from conferences and workshops. Going to conferences is a primary means of gaining new knowledge not only for psychotherapists but for many professionals such as doctors, dentists, nurses, and others whose new knowledge will help them stay up-to-date in their field. When you go to a conference, you also have an opportunity to network with other professionals in your field.

Perhaps the biggest tip here is to take CEUs seriously. We know many people who, when they have to complete their CEUs for licensure, look for the quickest and easiest way to do so. This usually comes in doing online courses where the only thing you have to do is take a quiz at the end to earn the CEUs. Many of our colleagues have started the course with the quiz and looked through the presented materials just for the answers. When you do this, you pretty much learn no new information. You get your CEUs, but you cheat yourself and your clients of knowledge that may be useful for your and their growth. If you do access online CEUs—which is fine—just go into it thinking, "What can I take away from this that will be beneficial for me and/or my client?" rather than "How can I get my CEUs done the quickest and cheapest way possible?"

Tips From a Supervisor

Many of the students that I work with, whether they be master's or doctoral students, think that they should have the course of their career figured out by the time they graduate. This includes working with a specific population with a specific therapeutic model. In some ways, this goes against most therapy ethical codes that promote the notion that therapists work with a diversity of clientele and continually develop new skills. My tip for you here is to relax. Don't think that you have to have your future pathway fully planned.

As human beings, we learn and we grow. As you get older, more experienced, and your life changes, your views of therapy and yourself as a psychotherapist will change as well. My suggestion is to embrace this rather than fight it. There will likely be an imperative that you impose on yourself to be a certain type of therapist who works with a certain type of clientele. My challenge to you is that if you do start to get this mindset, think about why you would limit yourself. Our field is continuously developing new ideas. Seek them out. Try them on. See how they fit. View yourself as someone in perpetual growth.

I believe that having this mindset and acting on it will help to alleviate some of the potential burnout that can occur in our field. Our job is to help clients grow and move forward in their lives. We better do this when we do so as well. Novelty is useful. Figure out how to incorporate new ideas, skills, and practices into your work. You will probably have a primary therapeutic model. I am not saying that is bad. However, be open to other ideas that may help you to learn how to be more integrative or even change what your primary model is. Or work with clients that you might not normally think you would have. In other words, keep it fresh. You can start now and not think that where you are now is where you will always be.

What's Next?

Congratulations! You have made it through this book, which probably means that you made it through your practicum/internship. We hope that this book was a trusted companion for you during your journey. We know that whatever site you were at and whatever program you are in, you learned a lot during your field placement on what it means to be a therapist. There is more for you to learn. There is more for you to experience. The ideas, tools, and tips provided in this book can be used when you are gaining your licensure hours as well as afterward, when you are licensed and practicing in whatever setting you find yourself. You'll work with a wide variety of clientele and will experience new situations that you've never encountered. You'll need to figure out how to navigate these so that you succeed as a therapist. Doing so will provide you with many different tales that will be useful for other therapists and therapists-in-training. Please share those tales with us or with others. Our field is a very collaborative one in which we learn from and with one another. Add your voice and help move our field forward.

References

American Association for Marriage and Family Therapy. (2015). *Code of ethics*. www.aamft.org/Legal_Ethics/Code_of_Ethics.aspx

Aten, J. D., Madson, M. B., & Kruse, S. J. (2008). The supervision genogram: A tool for preparing supervisors-in-training. *Psychotherapy: Theory, Research, Practice, Training, 45*(1), 111–116. https://doi.org/10.1037/0033-3204.45.1.111

Hernandez, K. E., Bejarano, S., Reyes, F. J., Chaves, M., & Mata, H. (2014). Experience preferred: Insights from our newest public health professionals on how internships/practicums promote career development. *Health Promotion Practice, 15*(1), 95–99. https://doi.org/10.1177/1524839913507578

Index

9781032559902